WRITING CLINICAL RESEARCH PROTOCOLS: ETHICAL CONSIDERATIONS

Evan G. DeRenzo, Ph.D.,
and Joel Moss, M.D., Ph.D.

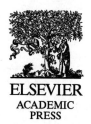

ELSEVIER
ACADEMIC
PRESS

AMSTEDAM • BOSTON • HEIDELBERG • LONDON
NEW YORK • OXFORD • PARIS • SAN DIEGO
SAN FRANCISCO • SINGAPORE • SYDNEY • TOKYO

The opinions expressed in this book are those of the authors only and do not represent any policy or position of the National Institutes of Health, Washington Hospital Center, or any other organization with which the authors are affiliated.

Elsevier Academic Press
30 Corporate Drive, Suite 400, Burlington, MA 01803, USA
525 B Street, Suite 1900, San Diego, California 92101-4495, USA
84 Theobald's Road, London WC1X 8RR, UK

This book is printed on acid-free paper. ∞

Library of Congress Cataloging-in-Publication Data
Application submitted.

British Library Cataloguing in Publication Data
A catalogue record for this book is available from the British Library

ISBN-13: 978-0-12-210751-1
ISBN-10: 0-12-210751-9

For all information on all Elsevier Academic Press publications
visit our Web site at www.books.elsevier.com

Transferred to Digital Printing in 2007

Printed in the United States of America
06 07 08 09 10 11   9 8 7 6 5 4 3 2 1

Dedication

This book is dedicated by EGD to her husband and by JM to his parents.

TABLE OF CONTENTS

PREFACE   **xvii**

SECTION I. THE BASICS: WHAT YOU NEED TO KNOW BEFORE STARTING HUMAN SUBJECTS RESEARCH   **1**

1. INTRODUCTION TO THE ART AND SCIENCE OF CLINICAL RESEARCH   **3**

I. Clinical Research Defined   3
II. Clinical Research Ethics Defined   3
III. Oversight: Origins, Relevance, and Future Role   4
IV. How to Use This Book   5

2. WHAT YOU NEED TO KNOW ABOUT CLINICAL RESEARCH ETHICS   **11**

I. Intersections of Scientific Goals and Ethical Concerns: How Study Design Influences Evaluation of Ethical Aspects   11

A. Distinctions Between Physician and
   Investigator Roles   12

B. Conflicts with Recruiting One's Own Patients   13

C. Conflicts of Interest in General   14

II. Landmark Documents in the Codification of Clinical
    Research Ethics: National and International   14

A. What Are Landmark Documents and How Are
   They Applied?   14

B. Controversies Surrounding Each Document   15

III. The Basic Principles and Theories of Clinical Research
     Ethics: Learning How to Justify Study Design   18

A. Consequentialist Ethical Theory   20

B. Deontology, or Duty-Based Ethics   22

C. Virtue Ethics   23

IV. Balancing Scientific Efficiency Against Subject
    Protection: Ensuring That the Balance Is Always
    Weighted in the Right Direction   24

3. **WHAT YOU NEED TO KNOW ABOUT THE REGULATION
   OF CLINICAL RESEARCH**   **27**

I. U.S. and International Regulatory Oversight Bodies   27

A. U.S. Department of Health and Human Services
   and the Food and Drug Administration   27

II. Radiation Safety Committees   30

III. Institutional Review Boards and Other Ethics
     Research Review Bodies and Committees   31

A. The Roles of Review Bodies and Their Purpose   31

B. The Responsibilities of IRBs and Ethical
   Requirements   32

C. Helping IRBs Do What They Do Better   34

IV. Variability Across IRBs and Other Reviewing Bodies:
    Those That Exist and Those of the Future   34

V. Project Assurances   35

VI. Initial Approval and Continuing Reviews   36

VII. Data and Safety Monitoring Boards   37

VIII. Disclosure and Minimization of Conflicts of Interest: Personal and Institutional 38

Section II. Preparing the Protocol 41

4. Designing a Clinical Research Study 43

I. Shaping the Study Question or Hypothesis 43

II. Selecting the Study Design 45

A. Distinctions Between Hypothesis-Testing and Hypothesis-Generating Clinical Research 45

B. Basic Versus Applied Research 46

III. General Design Characteristics 50

A. Expected-Direct-Benefit Research Versus No-Direct-Benefit Research 50

B. Randomization and Blinding 52

C. Placebo Controls Versus Comparator Arms 54

D. Phases of a Clinical Trial 56

IV. Beginning to Write the Protocol 59

A. Précis 59

B. Introduction: Purpose and Justification for the Proposed Study 59

C. Literature Review 60

D. Objectives, Questions, or Hypotheses 61

5. Selecting Subjects for Clinical Studies 63

I. Study Volunteers: Healthy Subjects or Patient Subjects? 64

II. Vulnerable Subject Populations: Who Is Classified as Vulnerable and How This Decision Is Made 65

A. What Makes a Subject Vulnerable? 66

B. Distinguishing Between Potentially Vulnerable and Vulnerable 67

III. Special Populations and Additional Protections   67
    A. Healthy Adult Volunteers   68
    B. Adult Patient Volunteers   71
    C. Minors   77
    D. Fetal Research   80
    E. Special Communities   81
    F. Special Protections for Special Populations   83
IV. Writing the Protocol Section on Subject Selection   95
    A. Characterization and Justification for the Proposed
      Population   95
    B. Inclusion Criteria   96
    C. Exclusion Criteria   96

6. RISKS AND BENEFITS IN CLINICAL RESEARCH   97

I. Weighing Risk of Harm Against Potential for Benefits   99
    A. Benefits to Society   99
    B. Benefits to Participating Subjects   102
II. Regulatory Requirements for Minimization of Risk   105
III. Study Procedures for Minimization of Risk   106
    A. Inclusion and Exclusion Criteria   106
    B. Rescue End Points   106
    C. Premature Withdrawal of Study Subjects   107
    D. Premature Study Closure   110
IV. Completion of a Study   111
    A. Follow-Up   111
    B. Sponsor Obligations After Study Termination   111
V. Research-Related Injuries   113
VI. Maximizing Benefits   113
    A. What Constitutes a Benefit?   113
    B. Compensation Versus Payment   115
VII. Writing the Protocol Section on Risk, Burden, and
     Discomfort   116
VIII. Writing the Protocol Section on Benefits   117

7. RECRUITING SUBJECTS 119

    I. Who Is Responsible for Recruiting Subjects? 120
    II. When Does the Recruitment Process Begin and End? 122
    III. Recruiting Subjects for Multiple Studies 123
    IV. The Professional Research Subject 125
    V. Writing the Protocol Section on Recruitment 125

8. INFORMED CONSENT 127

    I. Traditions and Purpose of Informed Consent 127
    II. When Does the Informed Consent Process Begin? 129
        A. The First Phase of the Informed Consent Process 129
        B. The Second Phase of the Informed Consent Process 130
        C. The Third Phase of the Informed Consent Process 130
        D. The Fourth Phase of the Informed Consent Process: When Does it End? 130
    III. The Difference Between Process and Product 131
    IV. Required Elements 133
        A. What Elements Are Required by Law 133
        B. What Additional Elements Are Required by Good Practice? 134
    V. Obtaining Valid Informed Consent 141
        A. Assessing Capacity to Provide Valid Informed Consent for Research 141
        B. Assent for Adults and Minors Who Are Unable to Make Decisions 143
    VI. Writing the Protocol Section on Consent, Assent, and Surrogacy Permissions 146
        A. Prospective and On-Study Subjects 146
        B. Family Members of Index Subjects 147
        C. Addressing Assent in the Protocol 148
        D. Surrogate Permission 148
        E. Consent Alterations or Waivers 150
        F. Community Consent 150

VII. Writing Consent, Assent, and Surrogacy Permission
Documents   152

   A. The Basics   152

   B. Debriefing for Altered or Waived Consent Processes   155

   C. Written Informed Consent in Health Services
Research and Quality Improvement Projects   156

   D. Short Form Documents   157

   E. Translations   158

   F. Timing   158

9. PRIVACY AND CONFIDENTIALITY   **159**

   I. Traditions and Expectations   159

   II. Management of Subject Privacy and Protection of
Confidential Information   160

   III. Provision to the Subject of Clinically Relevant
Private Research Information   163

   A. Provision of Information During Study Participation   163

   B. Provision of Information at Study Conclusion   164

   C. Provision of Information Long After Study Completion   165

   D. Counseling Subjects   167

   IV. Withholding Personal Information from a Study
Subject   168

   A. Withholding Meaningfully Uninterpretable Clinical
Research Information   168

   B. Withholding Highly Volatile and Possibly
Destructive Information   170

   V. Provision of Information at Study Conclusion   171

   VI. Release of Research Information to Others   172

   VII. Certificate of Confidentiality   173

   VIII. Writing the Protocol Section on Privacy and
Confidentiality   173

   IX. Writing Privacy and Confidentiality Statements in
Consent Forms   174

10. THE "ETHICS" SECTION 175

I. The Difference Between an Ethics Section and
a Compliance with Ethics Regulations Section 175

II. An Existing Model of a Substantive Ethics Section 177

III. Writing a Substantive Ethics Section 178

SECTION III. PROCEDURES, METHODS, STATISTICS, DATA MANAGEMENT, AND RECORD KEEPING 183

11. PROCEDURES AND METHODS 185

I. Randomization 186

II. Blinding 186

III. Drug Testing 187

    A. Drug Information 187

    B. Dosing and Administration 188

    C. Compliance 191

    D. Concomitant Therapies 192

    E. Open-Label Extensions 192

IV. Surgical Trials 193

V. Device testing 196

VI. Assessments 197

    A. The Subject's Standard Physical and Patient History 197

    B. Sexual Maturity in Minors 199

    C. Capacity to Provide Ethically and Legally
Valid Consent 199

VII. Laboratory Studies 199

VIII. Observational Methodologies 200

IX. Video and/or Audio Taping 201

X. Quality-of-Life Measurements 201

XI. Follow-up Procedures 202

XII. Adverse Reactions and Adverse Events 203

    A. Definitions, Classifications, and Attribution 204

    B. Reporting 204

12. **STATISTICS, DATA COLLECTION AND MANAGEMENT, AND RECORD KEEPING**   **207**

    I. Statistics   207
        A. Qualitative and/or Quantitative Data   208
        B. Sample Size and Power Calculations   209
        C. Variables and End Points   210
        D. Pharmacokinetics and Pharmacodynamics   211
        E. Placebos   212
        F. Modeling   214
    II. Data Collection and Management   215
        A. Instructions for Subjects, Investigators, and Other Study Personnel   215
        B. Data Entry   216
        C. Clinical Research Coordinators and Contract Research Organizations   217
        D. Academic and Pharmaceutical Industry Collaborations   218
    III. Record Keeping   219

SECTION IV. SPECIAL ISSUES   **221**

13. **USE OF HUMAN BIOLOGICAL MATERIALS**   **223**

    I. Anonymous, Anonymized, Coded, and Identifiable Specimens   223
    II. Anticipated Present and Future Use(s) of Tissue   225
        A. What Is Known and What Is or Can Be Anticipated   225
        B. Storage Procedures   227
        C. Sharing Samples with Other Investigators   229
    III. Tissue Samples from Those Who Are Deceased   230
    IV. Writing the Protocol Sections on the Use and Storage of Human Biological Materials   232
        A. Storing the Samples   233

14. SPECIAL ISSUES RAISED BY EVOLVING AREAS OF CLINICAL RESEARCH   **237**

   I. Genetics Research   237
     A. Risks to Subjects   238
     B. Subject and Family Member Conflicts   240
     C. Risks to Communities   240
     D. Genetics Studies or Genetics Study Add-ons?   241
     E. Use and Storage of Genetic Samples   243
     F. Minors: Participation in Genetics Research   244
     G. Variability in Ethical Standards, Vocabulary, and Regulations   244
   II. Psychiatric Research   245
     A. Capacity to Give Consent   246
     B. Risk of Placebo Arms   247
     C. Minors: Participation in Psychiatric Research   248
   III. Recruitment and Retention of Women and Minority Populations   249
   IV. Involvement of Pregnant Women or Fetuses   250
   V. Emergency Medicine Research   251
   VI. Community-Based Research   252
   VII. Quality Improvement and Quality Assurance Research   253
   VIII. Translational Research   254
   IX. Epidemiological Research   255
   X. Surgical Research   256
   XI. Biologics   257
   XII. Prisoners   257
   XIII. Clinical Research and Bioterrorism   258

15. CASE HISTORIES: LEARNING FROM EXPERIENCE   **261**

   I. Classical Cases in Clinical Research Ethics   262
     A. The Tuskegee Syphilis Study   262
     B. The Wichita Jury Study   263
     C. The Milgram Obedience Studies   264

II. Contemporary Cases in Clinical Research Ethics   265
  A. The Jesse Gelsinger Case   265
  B. The FIAU Case   266
  C. The Case of Brain Tissue Transplantation in
     Parkinson's Disease Studies   267

APPENDIX: WEB RESOURCES   **269**

REFERENCES   **273**

GLOSSARY   **281**

INDEX   **291**

PREFACE

We have written this book for physician-investigators, clinical research fellows, research coordinators, physicians, residents, interns, nurses, medical students, clinical research reviewers, and all other clinical research professionals. Although we presuppose that many in this audience will have experience and knowledge in clinical research, we accept that some may not. We hope we have written this book in such a way that it will provide insight, clarification, and a challenge for experienced clinical researchers and that its plain language wording will provide a baseline of understanding upon which to build future skills and insights for the inexperienced.

Both authors have had many years of experience in clinical research and clinical research ethics. Each of us is trained in different disciplines—DeRenzo in gerontology and research ethics; Moss in pulmonology, clinical investigation, and basic science. We have served as members and/or chaired Institutional Review Boards and Data and Safety Monitoring Boards. We have provided many hours of research ethics consultation about issues that arise in the conduct of clinical research across the full spectrum of study designs and diseases. And we have spent untold hours assisting both young and experienced investigators in designing and conducting clinical trials.

The conduct of clinical research is a complicated business. Protection of the safety, rights, and welfare of human subjects requires compromises in study design and execution that demand a refined balance of risks of harm to identifiable human research participants against the good of acquiring new knowledge to help the treatment and cures of diseases in future patients. This balance calls for substantial understanding of the ethical requirements for the design and conduct of clinical research and a developed sense of ethical judgment. Both are learned skills.

To assist those in the research field in learning and honing these skills, we have tried to be thorough. Although we have covered a substantial number of the ethical considerations that arise in the course of designing a research study, it is impossible to include the complete universe of issues. This is not only because we are certain to have forgotten some that we ought to have remembered, but also because, as science evolves, scientific advance generates new ethical considerations. We ask our readers to write to us about ethical issues we have omitted. Nonetheless, we have attempted to include a majority of the ethical issues encountered in the course of designing a clinical research study, and we recognize that some readers may find the number exhausting. We understand that some clinical research professionals may not appreciate how fully ethics is woven into the various components of a clinical study. We hope that using this book will assist our readers in learning how to more naturally and quickly identify the ethical aspects inherent in each step of the research process. We recognize, also, that some readers may be frustrated by the frequency with which we note that resolution of an ethical issue is not clear cut. This is because this book is about making ethical judgments. The ethical conduct of clinical research requires refined ethical judgments, some of which evolve as ethical thinking within society evolves. That is why those familiar with the regulation of clinical research will find that the recommendations in this book go beyond regulatory language. Where we have taken positions in this book about how to address certain ethical issues, we have done so based on what our experience has taught us to be optimal practice. In these cases we have proposed our own ways of resolving various ethical issues. In other cases there is simply too much disagreement within the clinical research and clinical research ethics fields, and we have noted that resolution is still under discussion. In so doing, we hope that we offer a book that provides useful guidance—a book in which such guidance has some basis and highlights areas where ethical judgments are in transition. Under both conditions, we hope we have written a book that advances the practice of clinical research and increases protection of the rights and welfare of human research participants.

For now, we are grateful to those who read earlier versions of this book. We also thank those who have contributed to it preparation. Most prominently they are Alan Sandler, D.D.S., recently retired Head of the Office of Human Subjects Research of the National Institutes of Health—for his thoughtful comments and his mentorship and guidance of JM as Chair of the National Heart, Lung, and Blood Institute's Institutional Review Board (NHLBI IRB); Jonathan Moreno, Ph.D., Director of the Center for Biomedical Ethics at the University of Virginia—for his insightful manuscript review and helpful comments; Martha Vaughan, M.D., Deputy Chief of the Pulmonary-Critical Care Medicine Branch of the National Heart, Lung, and Blood Institute—for her helpful discussions and critical review of the manuscript; and Elizabeth Griffin of Falmouth, Massachusetts—for her editorial assistance. We also thank Maria Stagnitto, Melissa Bryant, and Patricia Magno—members of the Office of Clinical Affairs of the NHLBI—for their outstanding efforts in coordinating the activities of the NHLBI IRB. We thank Dorothy Honemond, who provided expert assistance in the preparation of multiple iterations of this manuscript.

Evan G. DeRenzo, Ph.D. and Joel Moss, M.D., Ph.D.

THE BASICS: WHAT YOU NEED TO KNOW BEFORE STARTING HUMAN SUBJECTS RESEARCH

∙∙∙∙∙∙∙∙∙∙∙∙∙∙∙∙∙∙∙

chapter

1

··········

INTRODUCTION TO THE ART AND SCIENCE OF CLINICAL RESEARCH

················

I. CLINICAL RESEARCH DEFINED

Scientific research is defined as the systematic collection of information to produce generalizable findings. **Clinical research** is a subset of all scientific research and is defined as the systematic collection of information from humans and/or from organic material taken from humans to produce generalizable findings. The goal of clinical research is to accrue knowledge to improve the treatment of human diseases in the future. Clinical research identifies, accumulates, organizes, and interprets information about the function of the human body in health and disease. Clinical research is vastly different from clinical medicine. Although clinical research requires knowledge and skill in the practice of clinical medicine, clinical research involves human participants in the scientific enterprise of producing new information anticipated to benefit future patients. Although some research subjects may benefit directly from their participation in studies, individualized benefit is not the goal of conducting a clinical research study.

II. CLINICAL RESEARCH ETHICS DEFINED

Clinical research ethics is the practice of addressing the ethical aspects of research involving human subjects. Because applied ethics focuses on

3

what "ought" to be done in a particular set of circumstances, clinical research ethics focuses on what "ought" to be done in research involving human subjects. **Each study component has an ethical aspect. The ethical aspects of a clinical trial cannot be separated from the scientific objectives.** Segregation of ethical issues from the full range of study design components demonstrates a flaw in understanding the fundamental nature of research involving human subjects. Compartmentalization of ethical issues is inconsistent with a well-run trial. **Ethical and scientific considerations are intertwined. Failure on the part of investigators, sponsors, and review bodies to recognize this fact leads to ethical problems that have plagued the field of clinical research.**

III. OVERSIGHT: ORIGINS, RELEVANCE, AND FUTURE ROLE

The performance of clinical research is a highly regulated activity. **Virtually every nation that allows research on human subjects has its own set of regulations governing these activities.** Although this network of regulations can often be confusing, difficult to understand, and time-consuming to navigate, the source materials for these various regulations spring from but a few widely respected national and international clinical research ethics guidance documents. The common thread of these guidance documents and regulations is that their creation arose in response to abuses of human research participants (see information provided on Web sites listed in Appendix). The modern history of this codification and the current regulatory climate date to the Nuremberg trials of the Nazi doctors (Annas and Grodin, 1992). The atrocities committed by Nazi physician/investigators during World War II resulted in **The Nuremberg Code** (Appendix, No. 12), which requires the voluntary consent of the research participant.

The Nuremberg Code's apparent prohibition of research with children and adults incapable of providing their own consent, however, was viewed by investigators around the world as too restrictive. To provide guidance for research involving subjects unable to provide their own consent and to provide more detailed guidance than in The Nuremberg Code, the World Medical Association issued their clinical research ethics code that became known worldwide as the **Declaration of Helsinki** (Appendix, No. 13). This codification, and continuing revelations of abuse, led many nations to produce their own regulatory systems. The concerns raised by Henry Beecher (1966) about the ethical standards of clinical studies published in the medical literature and the recognition of the abuses in the United States Public Health Service syphilis study in and around Tuskegee, Alabama (Jonsen *et al.*, 1998), led to the formulation of uniform regulations for federally funded human research in the United States. These regulations have also come to apply de facto to non-federally funded clinical research.

Regulatory differences among nations, agencies, and branches of federal, state, and/or provincial governments have produced regulatory complexity (Emanuel *et al.*, 2003). In turn, the growing appreciation of problems concerning such regulatory complexity has led to harmonization of some sets of international regulations (Appendix, No. 21). Nonetheless, regulatory constraints can be expected to increase. Each time a research participant is harmed as a result of flaws in the research process, the ensuing intense public scrutiny fosters an environment of public debate and education, usually leading to a tightening of the oversight process and creation of mechanisms to make the process more transparent to the public as well as sanctions for the investigator and institution. An example of legislative response to public concern about the quality of clinical research review is recently passed Maryland State legislation requiring that Institutional Review Board (IRB) minutes be made available to the public upon request (Maryland Code, 2003).

When looking to the regulations for guidance, it is important to remember that regulations are rarely detailed enough to provide specific answers to specific ethical questions. Regulations are like the foundation and framing of a new home. If the builder has cut corners, the structure will forever be flawed. But even when a builder has taken great care to adhere to all building codes, perhaps has even overbuilt to ensure sturdiness and sound construction, a family would never move into a house with only the foundation and framing completed. It takes further ethical analysis to generate the plan that will complete the building of the walls, wiring of the electrical system, installation of the plumbing, and arrangement of furniture in ways that maximize the appropriate use of a space.

Such refined ethical analysis consists of an appreciation of regulatory requirements coupled with thoughtful consideration of the specific ethical issues raised by a particular study. Thoughtful consideration requires vigorous discussion with colleagues and involves the determination of the subtle differences in ethical perspectives that influence study design, risk assessment, depth of information to be disclosed, and creativity in shaping protective strategies and mechanisms.

IV. How to Use This Book

This book is designed to increase the skill of clinical researchers and research sponsors to identify and address the ethical considerations inherent in each section of a clinical research protocol. Our objective is to impress on clinical researchers that the ethical and scientific considerations of a clinical research study are inseparable. **The goal of this book is to assist in the design of a clinical research study by guiding study sponsors, principal investigators, and their colleagues through the process of writing a clinical research protocol. It is also hoped that providing this information will assist those responsible for the review, administration, and oversight of clinical research in becoming more familiar with ethical considerations raised by the various parts of a clinical research study.** The protocol template, which is shown in full at the end of this chapter, provides a sample outline. Depending on the kind of study being designed, only some of the sections in the protocol template may be needed. This book's chapters are organized, roughly, to follow the sequence of the protocol template. Several of the chapters focus on one segment or part of the template, and take the reader through many of the ethical considerations that go hand-in-hand with the scientific considerations of the related protocol section.

We do not claim to cover the universe of ethical issues and/or protocol sections. Each protocol is different, raising its own set of ethical considerations and requiring its own specialized headers and sections. Moreover, clinical researchers should also remember that an ethical analysis can never produce a fixed set of ethical considerations. Ethical norms evolve. This does not mean, however, that ethical standards are simply relative or subjective. What this means is that how ethical norms and values are interpreted and how regulatory requirements are to be applied will mature. What we try to provide in this book is a substantial overview of the range of ethical considerations raised by the usual components of a study involving human participants and/or human biological materials. In addition, this book provides a glossary to assist clinical researchers with their research ethics language skills, and the index at the end of the book can be considered a quick reference for reviewing specific issues.

Sample Protocol Template

Title Page
Table of Contents
List of Tables
Prècis: Scientific and Lay Summaries
Time and Events Schedule
Abbreviations
Investigator Agreement(s)
Investigator Disclosure of Conflicts of Interest
Any Protocol Amendments

Protocol Body
1. Introduction
    1.1   Purpose and Justification for the Proposed Study
    1.2   Literature Review
    1.3   Objectives, Questions, and Hypotheses
2. Study Design
    2.1   Overview of Design Characteristics: Qualitative/Quantitative, Blinded, Randomized, Drug/Device, Social Science/Medical, and Phase I, II, III, or IV and Others
    2.2   Rationale
3. Study Subjects
    3.1   General Description and Rationale
    3.2   Inclusion Criteria—Medical and Demographic/Socioeconomic
    3.3   Exclusion Criteria—Medical and Demographic/Socioeconomic
    3.4   Potential Risks, Discomforts, and Inconveniences
    3.5   Potential Benefits
    3.6   Recruitment Procedures
    3.7   Consent/Assent/Surrogate Permission
            3.7a   For Potential and On-Study Subjects
            3.7b   For Family Members of the Index Subject
            3.7c   Community Consent
    3.8   Medically Indicated Procedures While on Protocol: Consent/Assent/Surrogate Permission, Payment, and Follow-Up
    3.9   Premature Study Termination and Withdrawal: Monitoring and Criteria
    3.10   Rescue End Points
    3.11   Rescue Interventions
    3.12   Completion of Study and Follow-Up
    3.13   Research-Related Injuries
    3.14   Compensation for Study Participation
4. Ethical Considerations Raised by Study Design and Subject Population
5. Study Procedures
    5.1   Drug or Device Study
            5.1a   Administration, Dosage, Storage, and Other Management Information About Drug(s) Used in Trials, Both Standard and Experimental Agents
            5.1b   Concomitant Therapies
            5.1c   Techniques and Other Technical Information About Device(s) Used in Trial, Both Standard and Experimental Agents

    5.2   Molecular Study
        5.2a Tissues to Be Taken
        5.2b Procedures for Taking Required Tissue(s)
    5.3   Social Science Study
        5.3a Explanation of How Experimental Design Is
              Operationalized
6.   Study Evaluations
    6.1   Overview
        6.1a Specifics per Stage of the Study: Prerandomization,
              Pretreatment, Screening, and Others
        6.1b Specifics per Each Experimental Treatment Stage:
              Washout, Double-Blind, Open-Label, and Others
        6.1c Specifics at Premature Withdrawal
        6.1d Specifics at Primary Study Completion
        6.1e Specifics at Completion of Each Substudy or Any Add-
              On Studies
        6.1f Specifics During Open-Label Extension Phase
        6.1g Specifics Throughout Referral and/or Follow-Up
        6.1h Molecular Tests to Be Run on Tissue(s)
        6.1i Physical Description of Study Drug and/or Device
             6.1i.A Description of Packaging
             6.1i.B Labeling
             6.1i.C Preparation and Handling
             6.1i.D Drug and/or Device Accountability
    6.2   Pharmacokinetics
        6.2a Sample Collection and Handling
        6.2b Analytical Procedures
        6.2c Pharmacokinetic Parameters
    6.3   Pharmacogenomics
    6.4   Pharmacodynamics (Efficacy) Evaluations
    6.5   Efficacy and/or End Point Criteria
    6.6   Safety Evaluations
7.   Statistical Methods
    7.1   Sample Size Calculation and Determination
    7.2   Applicable Pharmacokinetics
    7.3   Applicable Pharmacodynamics: Efficacy, Analyses, and Others
    7.4   Safety Analyses
8.   Adverse Event Reporting
    8.1   Definitions
        8.1a Adverse Event Definitions and Classifications
        8.1b Attribution Definitions

8.2   Procedures
    8.2a   All Adverse Events
    8.2b   Serious Adverse Events
    8.2c   Expected Versus Unexpected
    8.3d   Pregnancies
8.3   Reporting the Adverse Event
    8.3a   Contacting the Appropriate Officials
    8.3b   Different Time Frames for Different Reporting Sources
9. Compliance
9.1   IRB and IEC Requirements According to Regulatory Monitoring Agencies
9.2   Informed Consent and Assent Documents
    9.2a   Required Elements: What They Are and How Much of Each Is Enough
    9.2b   Additional Required Elements: When These Are Required
    9.2c   Presenting Information in Understandable Language
    9.2d   Translations
    9.2e   Shortened Forms
9.3   Protocol Modifications and Amendments
9.4   Regulatory Documentation
    9.4a   Regulatory Approval and Notification
    9.4b   Required Prestudy Documentation: Correspondence with Regulatory or Other Oversight Agencies Needed by the IRB or IEC
9.5   Applicable Subject Identification Register and/or Subject Screening Log
9.6   Applicable Case Report Form Information
9.7   Data Quality Assurance Procedures
9.8   Conflict–of Interest
    9.8a   Disclosure
    9.8b   Techniques for Minimization
9.9   Record Retention Procedures
9.10   Data Ownership and Future Potential Commercialization
9.11   Applicable Monitoring
9.12   Approval of Amendments
9.13   Continuing Review Procedures and Timing
9.14   Study Completion and Termination
9.15   Applicable On-Site Audits
10. Publication
11. References

12. Appendices
    12.1 Model Consent and Assent Documents
    12.2 Comprehensive Prescribing Information for Pharmaceuticals
    12.3 Investigator Brochures
    12.4 Investigator Curriculum Vitae
    12.5 Conflict of Interest Documentation

2

. . . .

WHAT YOU NEED TO KNOW ABOUT CLINICAL RESEARCH ETHICS

. . . .

I. INTERSECTIONS OF SCIENTIFIC GOALS AND ETHICAL CONCERNS: HOW STUDY DESIGN INFLUENCES EVALUATION OF ETHICAL ASPECTS

Conflicts between the goals of science and the need to protect the rights and welfare of human research participants result in the central ethical tension of clinical research. The goal of clinical research is to obtain scientifically valid data efficiently while protecting research participants. Decisions must always favor the rights and welfare of human subjects rather than scientific ends.

The statement "Bad science is bad ethics" is true. Putting humans at risk if the study design does not permit a reasonable expectation of valid findings is never ethical. Even a study that presents no risk presents at least an inconvenience to subjects and is in that sense disrespectful. The statement "Good science is good ethics," however, is false. Study design may be scientifically valid, yet the risk of harming human participants is too great to accept. Although achieving the appropriate scientific ends is always the necessary goal of a study, protection of the rights and welfare of human participants must override scientific efficiency. Maximizing efficiency without compromising protection of participants is mandatory.

Understanding the ethical tensions inherent in the relationship between the goals of clinical medicine and those of clinical research is necessary to develop excellence in research involving human participants.

Physicians are trained first as clinicians and second as clinical researchers. When a physician is a clinical researcher in addition to being a clinician, his or her traditional obligations as a clinician are unaltered, but new obligations of a physician/investigator are assumed.

A. Distinctions Between Physician and Investigator Roles

The dual obligations of physician/investigators are to conduct scientifically valid research while protecting the rights and welfare of their research volunteers. Protecting the rights and welfare of research volunteers, however, particularly related to provision of clinical care, is not the same as taking care of the clinical needs of a patient in a nonresearch setting. If a clinical investigator fails to recognize the sometimes subtle distinction between clinical care in research and standard clinical care, the consequences can be disastrous. The subtlety is apparent in the shift of the physician's priorities and the strategies that the physician must devise for monitoring influences on judgment of the often conflicting objectives of the goals of clinical research and the goals of clinical medicine. Gone is the physician's luxury of clinical medicine's singular focus on patient welfare. Becoming a clinical investigator means being a master at achieving two goals: accomplishing scientific advancements and protecting research subjects. Differentiating the role of physician/investigator from the role of clinical physician and maintaining a clear definition of those differences are difficult tasks. Appreciating and differentiating the two roles, however, are in large part what characterizes ethical excellence in human subjects research.

Ethically sound clinical research requires understanding the implications of how, when, why, and where there are conflicts between meeting scientific research goals and protecting research participants.

For example, the scientific importance of learning more about brain metabolism in Alzheimer's disease is obvious. Understanding how brain deterioration progresses may be a necessary step for finding treatments that halt the neurological condition. A study of subjects in early, intermediary, and late stages of the disease could contribute to the understanding of the brain deterioration process. The differences in a patient's decisional impairment at each stage of the disease, however, call for the application of different kinds

Continued

of protections to balance the study's objectives and efficiency with the patient's capacity to give an informed consent.

B. Conflicts with Recruiting One's Own Patients

The goals of science also conflict with the goals of clinical care when a physician recruits his or her own patient into a trial in which the physician is also an investigator. The physician's perceived power based on knowledge of disease and treatment options, along with the patient's inherent dependence on the physician for present and/or future care, may make an otherwise fully capable patient vulnerable to manipulation.

Dr. Jones is an oncologist, a doctor who specializes in the treatment of kidney cancer, at a cancer treatment center at a university teaching hospital. Dr. Jones is also an investigator on several protocols designed to study new agents for the treatment of kidney cancer. Mrs. Smith is diagnosed with kidney cancer and referred to Dr. Jones. At first, Dr. Jones treats Mrs. Smith with an approved drug regimen, but Mrs. Smith's cancer fails to respond. There are other approved drugs to try, but there are also two research studies for which Mrs. Smith meets eligibility requirements in which Dr. Jones is involved. On one he is the Principal Investigator (PI) and on the other he is an Associate Investigator (AI). There are also other reasonable options with approved agents that are not yet standard-of-care. How does Dr. Jones prioritize, in his own mind, what he thinks is the best option for Mrs. Smith? What are the ethical justifications for his prioritization rankings? How does he present the options to Mrs. Smith?

Also at risk is a physician's objectivity in decision making. Whether the physician or the patient is conscious of the potential for manipulation or coercion, unethical behavior is possible when a physician also assumes the role of physician/investigator. The Declaration of Helsinki (Appendix, No. 13) addresses this issue specifically, setting guidelines for separation of the roles of physician and investigator when a prospective subject is in a dependent relationship with a physician who also has an investigator's role.

Becoming cognizant of the differences between the goals of clinical medicine and the goals of clinical research is not the same thing as separating these roles. Complete separation of the roles of investigator and clinician may be impossible as well as undesirable (Miller *et al.*, 1998; Miller and Rosenstein, 2003; Morin *et al.*, 2002). Keeping the clinical researcher alert to these differences and potential conflicts is essential.

C. Conflicts of Interest in General

The conflicts posed by the differing roles of physician and investigator are a special kind of conflict of interest that is sometimes called a conflict of commitment (Levinsky, 2002). The more commonly used term, **conflict of interest**, covers these intangible conflicts as well as the more explicit conflicts caused by financial interests. A **conflict of interest**, in general, is a situation in which professional judgment about a primary interest, such as the rights and welfare of human subjects, is unduly influenced by a secondary interest, such as financial gain (Thompson, 1993). A potential or explicit financial conflict of interest, or at the very least, the appearance of such a conflict, exists when an individual investigator is paid to participate in or conduct a clinical research study (Bodenheimer, 2000), when an institution is paid for clinical research being conducted by its investigators (Press and Washburn, 2000), or when clinical researchers receive payment for activities that create problematic relationships (Steinbrook, 2004; Weiss, 2005). Payment can come from a variety of sources, but it is the money from the private, for-profit sector, essentially the pharmaceutical and biotechnology industries, that cause the greatest concern. Although concern about such conflicts has existed for many years, widespread changes in policies and practices can be dated to the 1999 death of Jesse Gelsinger, an 18-year-old research subject in a gene therapy protocol at the University of Pennsylvania (Smith, 2002). In this situation, financial conflicts of interest played a prominent role (see Chapter 15). Since the case unfolded, financial conflicts of interest have received much research community, public, and political attention, which have resulted in policies, guidelines, and regulatory changes by professional associations, funding sources, research institutions, and the federal government that are still in a state of rapid evolution (DeRenzo, in press). It will be necessary for investigators at institutions to be up-to-date on conflict of interest policies, regulatory guidance, and requirements governing sponsors and research institutions. See Chapter 3 for information on disclosure of financial conflicts of interest to research participants.

II. LANDMARK DOCUMENTS IN THE CODIFICATION OF CLINICAL RESEARCH ETHICS: NATIONAL AND INTERNATIONAL

A. What Are Landmark Documents and How Are They Applied?

Several landmark documents in the codification of clinical research ethics provide fundamental guidance for the conduct of researchers involved in ethical clinical research. These resources serve as the primary documents for guidance in clinical research ethics, nationally and internationally, and many common concepts are found in these documents. This consistency provides a well-articulated framework for the ethical conduct of researchers involved in clinical studies around the world and for the development of legislation, regulation, policies, and procedures in each country and organization involved in the clinical research enterprise. All of these documents, however, have subtle and not-so-subtle differences, resulting in debate and controversy within the clinical research and research ethics communities, as well as sometimes within the public and the media, nationally and/or internationally. The implications of having these differences across documents and the debates these differences raise are that investigators, sponsors, and clinical research review bodies need to read these documents and understand them sufficiently to be able to make ethically optimal decisions about design of specific protocols.

B. Controversies Surrounding Each Document

The first landmark document created for the codification of clinical research ethics is the **Nuremberg Code** (Appendix, No. 12). This code consists of ten points that were developed by the judges following their verdict in the trial of the Nazi doctors convicted of committing research atrocities. The core notion set forth by the code is that the voluntary consent of a research participant is essential.

Although the Nuremberg Code was not the first document that required consent by the research subject, its status as the product of an international tribunal set it apart. With its unqualified "voluntary consent" standard the code appears to restrict research to adults capable of making their own decisions as subjects. The implication of this limitation is that all children and those adults who are too impaired to provide their own consent are excluded from research participation.

The need to learn more about diseases that affect children and adults with decisional impairments, and the controversial possibility that the Nuremberg Code's restrictiveness was intended for healthy research subjects, led to the writing of the **Declaration of Helsinki** (Appendix, No. 13). Unlike the Nuremberg Code, which has never been altered, the Declaration of Helsinki has gone through multiple revisions. The core provisions, in the Declaration since the original document was produced by the World Medical Association and adopted in 1964, however, have not changed either. Unlike the Nuremberg Code, the Declaration of Helsinki permits research involving children and adults who are too impaired to make a decision for themselves. The permission to conduct research involving these types of subjects may be the point of greatest divergence from the Nuremberg Code. The Declaration of Helsinki is a more expansive document covering, in greater detail than the code, issues pertinent to research involving human subjects. The requirement for voluntary consent, albeit liberalized, remains in the Declaration. The Declaration, however, permits surrogates to give permission for research participation on behalf of children and adults who are incapable of making decisions for research participation. The requirement for the research participant's or his or her surrogate's voluntary consent marks a shift from previous clinical research practice. The physician or physician/investigator could no longer involve a patient in research without that person's knowledge and consent or without the permission of his or her ethically and legally responsible surrogate.

The 1975 revision of the Declaration of Helsinki added the requirement for an independent review of projected studies, the second revolutionary change in the procedures for human subjects research. Requiring an independent review acknowledged the inherent conflicts between the goals of science and the need to protect the rights and welfare of research participants. The requirement for independent review, however, did not define how such a review body should be structured. Because of this lack of specificity, membership on review committees has been evolving ever since.

These two revised documents, with their requirements for subject or surrogate consent and independent review of a clinical research study, ushered in modern clinical research ethics. All other clinical research ethics documents, national and international, are derived from the Nuremberg Code and the Declaration of Helsinki. Subsequent clinical research ethics documents are clarifications and specifications of the principles and values established in the Code and the Declaration. At least two of these subsequent specifying documents stand out and have been accepted for authoritative guidance in clinical research ethics.

The International Ethical Guidelines for Biomedical Research Involving Human Subjects, prepared in 1993 by the Council for International Organizations of Medical Sciences (CIOMS) (Appendix, No. 14) in collaboration with the World Health Organization (WHO), is the third major international clinical research ethics guidance document. Focused on ethical considerations for performance of clinical research in developing countries and communities, the CIOMS guidelines add to the more general principles contained in the Declaration of Helsinki (Levine and Gorovitz, 2000).

The CIOMS document, like the Declaration of Helsinki, requires subject consent and/or surrogate permission and independent study review. Because the wording in each document is different, however, there is room for interpretation about the intent of each on several issues. For example, the inclusion of a placebo arm in trials with an expectation of direct subject benefit is currently a widely debated issue across investigators, sponsors, research ethicists, and international regulatory agencies. Less contentious, but equally as ethically unsettled, are matters related to the concept of community consent and the involvement of cognitively and psychiatrically impaired subjects in research. The CIOMS document and the Declaration of Helsinki address all three issues to some degree and in different ways. Because all three documents, that is, CIOMS, the Declaration of Helsinki, and the Nuremberg Code, are considered authoritative by most governments, clinical researchers, and ethicists, the idea that there are nuanced differences in ethical thinking across the three can be confusing to clinical researchers, sponsors, and clinical research review bodies. Yet these differences, and the moral confusions these differences sometimes create, underscore the need for discussion and thoughtful consideration of the ethical issues raised by a particular clinical study. These documents provide important guidance. They do not provide specific answers to the many complicated questions of clinical research ethics involved in study design and implementation of a specific protocol. Although it is important that investigators and review boards read these documents, investigators and review bodies still must struggle throughout the development, approval, and monitoring of a protocol. They must decide how to apply generally accepted principles of clinical research ethics and review the legislative and regulatory specifications on how these principles are applied in a particular clinical research setting.

One U.S. document stands out for establishing a description of each basic clinical research ethics principle. This document, *The Belmont Report: Ethical Principles and Guidelines for the Protection of Human Subjects of Research* (Appendix, No. 11), has shaped the way in which these principles have been codified into legislation and regulations around the world. This report was issued in 1979 by the first U.S. national ethics commission, the National Commission for the Protection of Human Subjects of Biomedical and Behavioral Research. Although this commission issued several important reports, *The Belmont Report* has been the most widely and continuously cited. Its primary contribution to the advancement of the protection of research subjects is its articulation of principles central to the ethical consideration of human subjects research: respect for persons, beneficence, and justice. The report's articulation of these principles as central to the moral core of human subjects research has been integrated into virtually every clinical research ethics training program in the United States and has been adopted by many countries around the world.

III. The Basic Principles and Theories of Clinical Research Ethics: Learning How to Justify Study Design

Basic ethical principles and theories serve as the foundation for ethical judgments about the acceptability of any human subjects research project. Ethically designed and conducted clinical research rests on the principles set forth in *The Belmont Report* of respect for persons, beneficence, and justice. The principle of **respect for persons** requires respect for each individual's values, perspectives, and capacities; assisting individuals in exercising self-determination; and the provision of appropriate protections for individuals who have limitations on autonomous behavior. The principle of **beneficence** requires those involved in a clinical research study to promote good practices and to avoid and prevent inflicting harm on others. **Justice** requires a fair distribution of benefits and burdens. The difficulty, however, is not in defining the principles but in ensuring that they are upheld effectively.

The regulations, which are discussed in Chapter 3, are intended to help clinical researchers, research reviewers, and others involved in the clinical research process to apply the principles. Familiarity with the international guidance documents, *The Belmont Report*, and the standard ethical regulations, however, will not be enough to ensure that clinical research will be designed and conducted with acceptably high ethical standards. None of these documents spells out the specific ethical judgments that are needed to design an acceptable clinical research protocol. Regulations are not specific enough to provide a detailed protocol blueprint. Investigators are advised to discuss complex ethical issues with their peers, research ethicists, potential research subjects, and communities as appropriate during the design phase as well as consult with one another in research review groups as the process progresses; the goal of these discussions is to incorporate basic ethical principles into the studies in question. These refined judgments will also be required during design and conduct of the study.

> *It is critical to remember that ethical judgments are integral to scientific judgments about study design.*

For example, clinical researchers should consider the following list of questions:

- How much risk of harming a study participant is too much risk?
- What protections ought to be built into a protocol that involves cognitively or socioeconomically vulnerable research participants?

- How should it be determined whether benefit of the new knowledge to be gained for society is sufficiently important to place research subjects at risk of harm or even at risk of mere inconvenience?
- If a study does not promise potential direct benefits for subjects, will the study's results be significant or important enough for society to counterbalance the risks or inconvenience a subject may experience during this study?
- When designing consent documents, how much information is the "right amount"? In other words, what is considered sufficient and necessary information, and how does this determination allow prospective research volunteers to make an informed choice about whether they should participate?

The questions just listed describe the types of ethical considerations that are required in the design and performance of human subjects research. Answering these questions or others appropriate to a particular study that we have not listed here requires refined ethical judgments that will shape the scientific aspects of a study. These are not judgments that can simply be tacked on at the end of the scientific considerations. Ethics must be considered along with the scientific design to ensure that a study is ethically sound. It is obvious, however, that if the science is not sound, there is no ethical justification for the study. Thus, scientific review is essential.

Investigators must be able to justify the study design, choice of subject populations, and the objectives proposed by the study. Justification demands that investigators appreciate the ethical fundamentals of what to do and how to do it. Justification rests on the evaluation of potential consequences of any proposal within the context of the clinical researcher's duties and obligations. These deeper theoretical notions determine whether the principles of respect for persons, beneficence, and justice are being adequately upheld. For example, when considering the hypothetical Alzheimer's disease study mentioned earlier in this chapter, how does one respect the severely demented, late-stage Alzheimer's victim? Some would say the only way to respect this individual is not to involve him or her in a study. They would base this conclusion on the proposition that without prior consent it is a violation of a person's rights and dignity to involve him or her as a research subject for the benefit of future patients. Others might qualify their consideration based on the degree of potential risk of harm to the subject. It is difficult, however, to assess how people with dementia react to activities that might be of little consequence to a cognitively intact individual, making risk/benefit assessment highly complex. The international guidance documents are not of much help here, either. Although the most recent revision of the Declaration of Helsinki prohibits the involvement of subjects unable to provide their own consent unless the research is asking a question or testing a hypothesis directly related to the subject's condition, the hypothesized Alzheimer's disease study described earlier relates directly to the proposed subjects' impairment. In the end, the ethical aspects of any protocol must be considered on a per protocol basis as the study is being designed and reviewed.

To answer a myriad of ethical questions sufficiently to develop a study design, the clinical researcher has to engage in a substantive analysis of the ethical issues presented by the proposed study. Simply considering how to balance the ethical principles is not sufficient. Rather, the investigator has to analyze how the ethical principles can be upheld within the context of reasonable expectations of the potential consequences of each protocol design component, including an understanding of a researcher's duties and obligations. To perform this analysis, a rudimentary familiarity with the three basic ethical theories is needed. These theories can be referred to as consequentialist ethical theory; deontologic, or duty-based, ethical theory; and virtue ethics.

A. Consequentialist Ethical Theory

Consequentialist ethical theory claims that the rightness or goodness of an action is based on its potential consequences. The most ethically praiseworthy actions, according to this theory, are those that maximize the good for the greatest number. The whole enterprise of human subjects research is grounded in consequentialist ethics. In general, society accepts that it is ethical to place a few research subjects at risk of inconvenience, burden, or even harm so that important information can be revealed about certain diseases. In general, it is considered ethically acceptable that a (relatively) few persons take on the risks of study participation so many patients in the future can benefit from improvements in medical knowledge. Maximization of future social benefit is weighed against the potential for harm to study subjects. When applying a consequentialist argument, the reader can see how beneficence is accrued for future patients and society.

> Taking consequentialist theory to its extreme, however, can lead clinical researchers toward the kind of efficiency that sent Nazi doctors to the firing squad. In one set of Nazi experiments, the physician/investigators wanted to learn more about how cold water affects the human body, a perfectly reasonable question to explore. Many of their soldiers (as well as soldiers of every country) could be exposed to freezing water temperatures during combat. Thus, gaining such knowledge could have highly beneficial

Continued

outcomes for a wide range of persons. But in the Nazis' rush toward efficiency, they came up with an ethically indefensible study design. They threw humans into cold water and timed how long it took them to die and experimented with different ways of reviving them. One serious problem with the uncritical application of consequentialist theory is that in maximizing future benefit for the many, the rights and welfare of the few can be ignored.

The other serious weakness of consequentialist analysis is that the prediction of consequences is imperfect. Many people start the day by checking and updating a "to do" list of activities they plan to accomplish by the day's end. At the day's end, however, often the original list of items has been lengthened with additional, unexpected tasks, and the final list may not even closely approximate the original "to do" list. Inadequacy of short-term prediction should give the careful researcher pause. A person's inability to predict long-term consequences is reason for grave concern.

Think of a physician who recruits his or her own patient into a study in which he or she is the investigator:

- What if, during the course of a study, the research participant experiences an adverse event?
- What if that person learns afterward that his or her treating physician had a financial interest in the study?
- What might be the effects of this information on the doctor/patient relationship?
- What might be that person's lingering impressions of the medical profession?

If discord between the patient and the recruiting physician occurs, that patient may not only switch physicians but may be disinclined to seek needed medical attention in the future. In addition, that patient might share his or her unsatisfactory experience with others in the community, sowing mistrust of that particular physician/investigator as well as of clinical researchers and the medical establishment in general.

In clinical research, investigators and sponsors need to avoid focusing too heavily on the potential for positive consequences and/or skimming over the potential for negative consequences. Moreover, it is prudent to assume that there will be unintended consequences that cannot be anticipated.

Although it is necessary to predict potential beneficial and harmful consequences of each component of study design as fully as possible, doing so is not sufficient. The risk of trampling research participant protections in the rush to gain new knowledge to help others along with a limited ability to predict outcomes requires that investigators have exquisite appreciation of their duties and obligations. Exercise of these duties and obligations serves as the counterweight to the pursuit of efficiency run amok.

B. Deontology, or Duty-Based Ethics

Deontology claims that the rightness or goodness of an action is based on the degree to which a person meets his or her duties and obligations. The ethical complexity of a person's multiple duties and obligations is its central conflict. It is difficult enough in clinical medicine to know how to meet the obligation to provide patient care. In oncology, for example, what does it mean to meet obligations to the late-stage cancer patient? How much should a physician push an aggressive, interventionist approach, and when should a shift to comfort care begin? Research makes such decisions considerably more complex.

Consider a physician/investigator at a large academic medical center. This institution has an active oncology research program that includes multiple phase I, II, and III trials. It also has a state-of-the-art clinical palliative care unit. A patient volunteer has had disease progression through two different phase II trials. She is young and has small children and a desperate husband at home. Her cancer has metastasized. You are the investigator of one of the phase I trials for which she is eligible. She has started making comments that indicate to the research and clinical nurses that she is tired; she understands that her disease is incurable; and she is ambivalent about whether to try yet another phase II trial, to try a phase I trial, or enter the institution's palliative care unit. How do you advise her? Are you counseling her or subtly recruiting her? How do you know the difference?

Caring for the specific needs of sick patient/subjects or healthy normal volunteers while meeting obligations to conduct scientifically valid science are influenced by how you, your colleagues, and your research review bodies think about the duties and obligations of clinical researchers. The difficulty here, of course, is that each party can be expected to address these duties in slightly different ways. Some may believe that clinical researchers meet their duties and obligations to subjects through the informed consent process, a process that upholds the principle of respect for persons. That is, the investigator need not be overly concerned about risks to subjects as long as these subjects are fully informed. On the other hand, certain individuals—the authors of this book being among them—believe that given the weaknesses of the informed consent process, the ultimate responsibility for subject protection should not rest with the subject but with the investigator and the review bodies that approve clinical research.

> *What is central to the skills of the clinical researcher is to be self-monitoring and to learn how to identify the subtleties of this complex balance.*

All individuals have blind spots. The performance of clinical research takes time and perseverance. Researchers' enthusiasm for their work is needed to sustain them through the inevitable dead ends of science. But this enthusiasm to advance medical progress coupled with a person's blind spots may lead to the possibility that duties to protect subjects may not be fulfilled. Involvement of persons in study review who lack an intense personal interest in seeing that any particular study is performed or completed will help increase the possibility that the researchers' and society's obligations to protect the rights and welfare of human research subjects are met. It is for that reason as well that the initial and continuing review of the study by persons other than the investigator, including nonscientists and those persons unaffiliated with the research sponsor and institution, is essential.

C. Virtue Ethics

The final theoretical perspective discussed in this book evaluates the "good" in clinical research a bit differently. **Virtue ethics** claims that the rightness or goodness of an action is based on the character of the person performing the action. To be ethical, claims virtue ethics, the person must have virtuous intentions. Virtue ethics goes directly to the core of the tension that we as the authors have underscored thus far in this book. The notion presupposes that the virtuous researcher, regardless of the importance of the information being sought, would never place a research subject at risk of unacceptable harm. This ethical grounding comes from some of the earliest writing on clinical research ethics. Claude Bernard's groundbreaking book *Introduction to the Study of Experimental Medicine* (Bernard, 1865) called for putting the practice of medicine on a sound scientific footing. In the book, addressing the need for human subjects in this effort, Bernard identifies the obligations of the virtuous physician as follows:

It is our duty and right to perform an experiment on man whenever it can save his life, cure him or gain him some personal benefit. The principle of medicine and surgical morality, therefore, consists in never performing on man an experiment which might be harmful to him to any extent, even though the result might be highly advantageous to science, that is, to the health of others. (Dover trans., 1927, 101–102.)

Unfortunately, Bernard painted the picture of the virtuous physician/ investigator with the same brush as that of the virtuous physician. In doing so, Bernard started research down the path that confuses the goals of clinical research with the goals of clinical care. Research exposes humans to risk, even if the risk is merely an inconvenience. Risk is present because, by definition, research is the investigation of something that is yet unknown. Reducing clinical research risk to zero effectively eliminates research. The raging debate about the safety, scientific need, and ethical acceptability of placebo-controlled trials glaringly illuminates the flaw in Bernard's dictum. Virtuous investigators expose their subjects to risks by the very nature of the enterprise. It is the investigator's awareness of this fact and of its implications that makes for virtue and integrity in clinical research.

IV. BALANCING SCIENTIFIC EFFICIENCY AGAINST SUBJECT PROTECTION: ENSURING THAT THE BALANCE IS ALWAYS WEIGHTED IN THE RIGHT DIRECTION

However the balance between scientific efficiency and subject protection is struck, the ethical bedrock of human subjects research is that the protection of the rights and welfare of human subjects must take precedence over scientific ends. That conclusion does not mean that studies having no expectation of direct subject benefit ought to be prohibited. This perspective is dangerous to medical progress and may, in fact, put subjects at additional risk.

Investigators have obligations to make scientific progress. Society needs, wants, and calls for such progress. To achieve medical progress, some studies must ask questions and/or test hypotheses that are not anticipated to provide direct benefits to study participants.

A clear example of conducting a study that has no direct medical benefits for subjects is testing pharmacologic properties of a novel agent in healthy subjects before testing that agent in sick patients. To protect subjects of studies

Continued

of a novel agent as it moves through the stages of drug development and approval, the agent will need to be studied and understood to the greatest extent reasonable. It may be simply too unsafe to test a drug in a debilitated, sick patient without having some idea of how the drug works on the human body, even if the sick patient stands the most chance of benefit. The group in which these basic questions can be answered most safely is healthy adults, for whom there will be no benefit from the agent. The authors of this book believe that, provided appropriate protections are in place, no-direct-benefit studies can be ethically conducted and, under certain conditions, are ethically required.

The inviolate rule is that protection of subjects comes first, regardless of whether a study has the potential for direct participant benefit. The Nuremberg Code and the Declaration of Helsinki express this mandate from several directions. Separate from their requirements to reduce risks to the greatest degree reasonable, both documents make clear that the balance must always tip toward participant safety and well-being. The Nuremberg Code's final point states the following:

> *During the course of the experiment the scientist in charge must be prepared to terminate the experiment at any stage, if he has probable cause to believe, in the exercise of the good faith, superior skill and careful judgment required of him that a continuation of the experiment is likely to result in injury, disability, or death to the experimental subject.*

The Declaration of Helsinki states the same conceptual requirement in Point 5 of its introduction: "In medical research on human subjects, considerations related to the well-being of the human subjects should take precedence over the interests of science and society."

Both statements make clear that the welfare of the subjects comes first. But even this universally accepted clinical research ethics maxim cannot be fulfilled without skill in clinical research ethics analysis, which requires practice, time, and intellectual commitment. Fortunately for clinical researchers, research reviewers, and research subjects, rigorous and thoughtful application of the basic ethical principles and theories provides the foundation needed to design and conduct ethically justifiable clinical research.

3

....

WHAT YOU NEED TO KNOW ABOUT THE REGULATION OF CLINICAL RESEARCH

....

I. U.S. AND INTERNATIONAL REGULATORY OVERSIGHT BODIES

A. U.S. Department of Health and Human Services and the Food and Drug Administration

Research involving human subjects is a carefully regulated activity. **Since the publication of the Nuremberg Code, the Declaration of Helsinki, and *The Belmont Report*, most countries in which clinical research is conducted have developed their own legislation and regulatory organizations.**

Primary regulations of the United States are the U.S. federal government regulations promulgated by the U.S. Department of Health and Human Services (DHHS) and the U.S. Food and Drug Administration (FDA) (Appendix, Nos. 15 and 18). The DHHS regulations governing human subjects research are primarily contained in Title 45 of the Code of Federal Regulations (CFR), Part 46 (45 CFR 46) (Appendix, No. 15). First promulgated in 1974, 45 CFR 46 went through revisions in 1994 and 2001. Part A of these DHHS regulations is referred to as the Common Rule, which is shared by 19 U.S. federal agencies. Parts B, C, and D are specific to DHHS. Other departments have other specific rules, such as the Department of Education, which has a specific rule about its own pediatric research. Comparable FDA regulations are contained in the Title 21 Code but are spread throughout several parts of the Code of Federal Regulations, including Title 21's parts 11, 50, 54, 56, 312, and 314 (Appendix, No. 17).

Each set of regulations, as well as those promulgated by other agencies or departments of the U.S. government, establishes the requirements that clinical researchers, review boards, and research sponsors must follow when conducting and evaluating clinical studies. In large part, government regulations have resulted from congressional legislation enacted in response to clinical research scandals and abuses. The present DHHS regulations result from the work of the National Commission for the Protection of Human Subjects of Biomedical and Behavioral Research, which produced *The Belmont Report*. *The Belmont Report* and the subsequent regulations resulted from the public outcry concerning the U.S. Public Health Service's Syphilis Study (Jonsen *et al.*, 1998). The Syphilis Study is, arguably, the most serious known instance of research ethics abuse in the history of human studies research in the United States. In a study run by the U.S. Public Health Service from 1932 until Congress closed it in 1972, poor black males with syphilis were subjects of a U.S. Public Health Service observational study in Tuskegee, Alabama. They were deceived from the outset of the study and deprived of treatment that was discovered during the period of the study. This terrible stain on the integrity of the U.S. clinical research community led to the development of the current U.S. clinical research regulations. Called the Common Rule, these regulations govern human subjects research conducted with support from any of 19 federal government agencies.

1. FDA and International Regulations

The clinical research ethics regulations of the FDA have a developmental path different from the DHHS and cover clinical research from different sponsors, but are consistent in content and intent with those of the DHHS. FDA regulations emanate most notably from creation of The Federal Food, Drug, and Cosmetic Act of 1938, which is commonly abbreviated as FDC. This sweeping legislation extended the scope of the original Food and Drug Act of 1906 that prohibited interstate commerce in misbranded and adulterated foods, drinks, and drugs. The FDC of 1938 extended the FDA's control so that it could also regulate cosmetics, pharmaceutical drugs, and therapeutic devices. This 1938 FDC version required that new drugs be proven safe before marketing, initiating a new system of drug regulation. The FDC of 1938 added the remedy of court injunctions to the previous penalties of seizures and prosecutions. Subsequent amendments required that drugs must be shown to be effective. In addition, the FDC provides for setting toxicity level limits for unavoidably poisonous substances and authorizes factory and laboratory inspections.

The primary U.S. clinical research sponsors are the National Institutes of Health (NIH) and the pharmaceutical industry. The biotech industry and private, not-for-profit health advocacy foundations are also important and growing sponsors of clinical research. As the biomedical clinical research community has grown and expanded, an important portion of human subjects research is performed outside the United States. For example, Europe and Japan are active clinical research sites. As countries have built up their clinical research infrastructures, their clinical research regulatory systems have grown. There are differences among many countries in their regulation of research involving human subjects. These potentially conflicting sets of regulations lead to confusion and impede medical progress. To reduce the complexities of competing and conflicting sets of regulations, the United States, the European Union (EU), and Japan created a process for bringing consistency to this regulatory network. The process is regulated by the International Conference on Harmonization (ICH) of Technical Requirements for Registration of Pharmaceuticals for Human Use (Appendix, No. 21) and connects regulators and industry in the United States, EU, and Japan as equal partners. The ICH focuses on the integration of technical requirements in drug development and new drug registration in the ICH countries.

Harmonization efforts began in the European community (EC) in the 1980s as it moved toward unification of its commercial markets into what is today the EU. The formalized creation of the ICH took place in Brussels, Belgium, in 1990. To date, 45 topic areas have been harmonized, including medical terminology and electronic standards for the transfer of regulatory information. These consensus documents (e.g., ICH2, ICH3) are now the standards for regulatory guidance for trials governed by the FDA.

As regulatory oversight tightens and the level of regulatory specificity intensifies, regulatory compliance becomes more complex. To assist investigators, institutions and other organizations are providing investigator training. Training of investigators in these areas is no longer a choice. **Granting organizations and clinical research sponsors are requiring evidence of investigator training in clinical research ethics and the regulation of human subjects research.** For some, evidence of training is no longer sufficient and certification is becoming the standard. The pharmaceutical industry is moving toward a requirement for certification upon successful completion of an approved training program. The NIH was the first to require investigator training in clinical research ethics. Its Web-based training is required of all NIH-funded investigators (Appendix, No. 2). The pharmaceutical industry is moving to adopt the certification training offered through the Association of Clinical Research Professionals (ACRP) and other similar organizations (Appendix, No. 4). Certification through the ACRP training can be expected to be an industry standard. Because the certification is new, costs are presently negotiable within pharmaceutical industry contracts. After a substantial percentage of investigators have been certified, the expectation is that such training will be at an investigator's expense and necessary for those who are considering becoming a pharmaceutical industry investigator.

II. RADIATION SAFETY COMMITTEES

Radiation safety committees (RSCs) are institutional bodies that are responsible for implementing the regulations of the U.S. Nuclear Regulatory Commission (NRC). The NRC has the authority to withdraw licenses for radiation use from agencies and organizations under its oversight, such as the NIH. Institutions conducting clinical research that involves radiation exposure must have an RSC or its equivalent.

RSCs review and approve requests for radiation exposure for research purposes. Clinical researchers need to differentiate between radiation exposure within a research study that is medically indicated only and/or is specifically for research purposes. The latter does not only mean that radiation exposure is itself experimental. Radiation exposure is ordinarily associated, in the clinical setting, with particular procedures. If such exposure is more or different from that required for standard clinical care, the exposure is considered to be for research purposes.

RSC review is limited to the protocol being evaluated. This limitation means that the RSC has no way to assess safety in terms of accumulated radiation exposure of an individual subject who may be in more than one study simultaneously, may be in several studies in quick succession, or may have been exposed to clinically indicated radiation close to the time of exposure to the proposed research radiation. A subject may be exposed to acceptable levels of radiation in a given protocol, but accumulated exposure may be dangerously high when total radiation in several exposures over a short period of time is considered. To avoid this problem, it would be helpful if eligibility and/or baseline history and physicals include a radiation exposure history and defined limits for accumulated radiation exposure over specified time intervals are included among protocol exclusion criteria.

III. INSTITUTIONAL REVIEW BOARDS AND OTHER ETHICS RESEARCH REVIEW BODIES AND COMMITTEES

A. The Roles of Review Bodies and Their Purpose

Institutional review boards (IRBs) were created by regulation in the United States in 1974 with the promulgation of regulations 45 CFR 46 by the U.S. DHHS (the Department of Health and Human Services was formerly referred to as the U.S. Department of Health, Education, and Welfare). **An IRB is an independent human research review committee.** This committee is responsible for reviewing and approving or disapproving all research involving human subjects covered by The Common Rule (45 CFR 46, Part A) and FDA regulations. IRBs and their international counterparts, commonly referred to as **independent ethics committees** (IECs) or sometimes *research ethics committees* (RECs), represent an important advance in the development, codification, and implementation of clinical research ethics.

1. Evolution of the Peer Review Process: The Qualitative Difference of IRBs and IECs from Peer Review

Early in the history of clinical research, in the mid-19th century and toward the beginning of the 20th century, the only clinical research review was peer review. The 1960s saw this process take a giant step forward toward the system of the 21st century.

In 1964, an NIH committee considering issues in clinical research came to a remarkable conclusion. It determined that "the judgment of the investigator is not sufficient as a basis for reaching a conclusion concerning the ethical and moral set of questions in that relationship" (Livingston, 1975, p. 50). This statement is a formal recognition of the conflicting interests of clinical researchers and makes clear that management of these interests cannot be left to researchers alone.

In 1966, the NIH established a policy requiring independent review for its own investigators and its clinical research affiliates (Jonsen *et al.*, 1998). This policy was followed by a similar requirement in the 1975 revision of the Declaration of Helsinki that set the standard of independent review internationally. In the 21st century, this requirement is codified widely, and independent review bodies review a substantial percentage of human subjects studies.

This important insight, that independent oversight of the investigator is needed to protect human subjects of research, was accompanied by the growing recognition that these bodies need to include persons who do not have scientific backgrounds. To ensure that the needs of human subjects are appropriately met, persons who represent the potential subjects more closely than do the researchers are now routinely involved in the research review process. Thus, IRBs and ethics review committees around the world are composed of a diverse group of people. The U.S. regulations require that each IRB include not only lay members but at least one member who is not affiliated with the institution to distance, even further, the review process from the researchers. Although formalized peer review committees were an improvement over clinical research conducted without review or with review only by one or two colleagues, it took the advent of the IRB to expand the review perspective past that of the researchers.

For example, a clinical study that requires a lumbar puncture (LP) may be viewed quite differently by a physician investigator than by a lay person. Often, the research physician experienced in performing LPs will see the procedure as low risk. But if the lay person on the IRB has or has known someone who has had a severe and/or prolonged headache as a result of an LP, that lay person will bring that experience to review of all protocols including LPs and can be expected to elevate concern about an adverse event from an LP to the attention of the rest of the IRB.

Lay person perspective on potential risks associated with an LP that the professionals may well have missed can be expected to result in assuring both that appropriate protections for such an adverse reaction are in the protocol and that information about the potential risk is delineated in the informed consent process.

B. The Responsibilities of IRBs and Ethical Requirements

Although many human subjects research studies are reviewed by independent committees, some studies are not. Even in the United States, many human research studies are not required by law to be reviewed prior to being conducted. These include studies that are not funded by the U.S. Common Rule agencies or those not funded by pharmaceutical or biotech companies that are seeking FDA approval. One such category is research on *in vitro* fertilization and assisted reproduction. In large part because of the U.S. government's ban on federal funding of research involving human embryos, research studies on technologies of assisted reproduction have been funded by sources that are outside the system of governmental oversight. Other countries, where such research is not prohibited, have developed to differing degrees their own regulatory structures.

Another area of clinical research that is not governed by regulations in the United States involves studies using tissues from the deceased. Because U.S. federal regulations define a research subject as a living human, tissues from deceased persons do not come under the purview of the IRB. This lack of review from the IRB represents an area of clinical research not governed by the clinical ethics regulations that require policy consideration at the institutional level.

For example, genetic studies on tissues from deceased persons may risk breach of privacy and confidentiality for living persons who may become, in effect, research subjects without their knowledge and/or consent. Consider the case of Mrs. Kendal, a mother whose adult son dies of rectal cancer. Mrs. Kendal finds out that her father had died of the same disease, but his diagnosis had not been discussed within the family. Rather, the family, believing there was stigma attached to such a diagnosis, had always told her that her father died of stomach cancer. Now, at the time of her son's death, there is a research study looking for the genetic mutation predisposing persons to rectal cancer and Mrs. Kendal wants to enroll herself and her surviving children. To participate, she wants access to tissue from her father, kept at the hospital where he died. The rest of the family, however, is opposed. That there are no constraints on the researchers does not mean there are no risks posed by the research to other living family members. That is, if one of the primary ethical concerns in clinical research is minimization of risk of harm to human subjects, greater appreciation is needed for the idea that tissue from deceased persons can be linked to living persons, which may introduce avoidable risks. This controversial issue can be expected to receive increasing attention (Annas, 2005; DeRenzo et al., 1997; National Bioethics Advisory Commission, 1999).

It may be wise for scientists conducting research with tissue from deceased persons to discuss such studies with their IRB and/or IEC chairperson and consider submitting a letter explaining the study to the IRB, IEC, and/or to some other clinical research oversight official at their institution.

In the United States, because of these kinds of concerns (i.e., lack of review of studies not under IRB jurisdiction) and other concerns (e.g., variability of review competence among IRBs and resource waste from redundancy of review of multicenter trials), there is a growing consensus that the IRB review system needs updating. A variety of authoritative sources are illuminating these weaknesses and calling for change (Bell et al., 1998; Federman et al., 2003; National Bioethics Advisory Commission, 2001b; Office of the Inspector General, 1998a, 1998b, 1998c).

The two most common responses to this call for reform, still in their infancies, are IRB accreditation (Institute of Medicine, 2001) and the creation of what are called central IRBs and/or regional IRBs (Christian et al., 2002). The methodologies for IRB performance evaluation and the creation of these broadened review bodies are so new in the beginning of the 21st century that more time is required to make any assessment of their utility. It is likely, however, that over the next several years accreditation will become a pervasive addition to the review system and that various experiments with model configurations of IRB-like review bodies will be conducted. The shift from local to regional and/or central IRBs can be expected also. There is no regulatory requirement that an IRB be local and the accumulating evidence of IRB variability in review quality coupled with concerns for review redundancy and better IRB resource utilization can be expected to produce changes in the IRB system in the years to come.

C. Helping IRBs Do What They Do Better

One of the biggest problems with IRBs and IECs is that they waste a tremendous amount of time on inconsequential matters, such as correcting wording and punctuation in the consent documents, and not enough time debating the substantive ethical issues of the study. Another way IRBs and IECs waste time is in trying to help investigators improve their protocols. To avoid these inefficiencies and thereby facilitate substantive discussion during IRB and IEC meetings, **investigators should make certain that they submit only well-written protocols and consent and/or assent documents**. This will require the protocol to undergo rigorous scientific review prior to the IRB and IEC submissions. If a submitted protocol is obviously deficient ethically or scientifically, the IRB or IEC administrator and/or chairperson is advised to return it to the investigator or sponsor for rewrites until it is in suitable condition for thoughtful and substantive review by the IRB (Emanuel *et al.*, 2000).

To avoid the problem of IRB and IEC reviews of scientifically, ethically, or structurally flawed protocols, institutions can establish and require the use of standard protocol formats. IRB and IEC members can thus save time by not having to look for the same kinds of information in different sections of different protocols.

IV. Variability Across IRBs and Other Reviewing Bodies: Those That Exist and Those of the Future

As clinical research has moved beyond the walls of academic medical centers into community hospitals and even the offices of private physicians, IRBs have expanded their reach and support structures as well. In the United States, there are three kinds of IRBs: institutional not-for-profit, for-profit independent, and proprietary IRBs.

Institutional IRBs are found most often in academic institutions, either medical schools at colleges and universities or teaching hospitals, where they are funded from the clinical research overhead budget at the not-for-profit institutions in which they are seated. The **independent IRBs** are set up largely by for-profit companies to provide IRB reviews for a fee. They are heavily used by the pharmaceutical industry but do, sometimes, provide IRB review for academic institutions that want to supplement their own IRB system. Independent IRBs often serve as a central IRB of record for review and monitoring of pharmaceutical company multisite and/or multinational protocols. According to the limited data available (Lemmens and Thompson, 2001), there is little difference between **local IRBs** and independent IRBs in composition of the membership or thoroughness of review. Independent IRBs tend to conduct their reviews more quickly, often because they have several boards that meet more frequently than do academic IRBs. **Proprietary IRBs** are set up by for-profit clinical research sponsors to review specific sponsor's research studies. Little is known about the membership, functions, and processes of proprietary IRBs.

The IRB or IEC, however, is not the only group that reviews clinical research. Although the IRB and the IEC are the only bodies legally allowed to approve a clinical research protocol under their jurisdiction, other groups may review the protocol and disapprove its initiation and/or stop its continuation. Protocols may have to go through several layers of review before or after IRB and IEC reviews to be approved or disapproved on the basis of, for example, consistency with organizational mission or funding. Special committees focused on financial conflicts-of-interest are one such specialized review committee. The multiple layers of review at a particular institution may be spelled out in the institution's assurance documentation. They may not be, however. Investigators will need to make certain they have submitted their protocol to all relevant review committees, a task that they can be assisted in by their IRB administrative personnel.

V. PROJECT ASSURANCES

A **project assurance** is a document that assures how an investigator's institution will comply with the DHHS regulations governing human subjects research conducted with Common Rule agency funding in ways that are consistent with the institutions policies, procedures, and culture. In the past, institutions have held multiple or single project assurances. These are being phased out and replaced with a more streamlined system of federalwide project assurances. These assurance documents are negotiated with the DHHS Office for Human Research Protections (OHRP). The signatory to the assurance is the ultimately responsible individual at that institution. These documents cover the entire institution's research portfolio of Common Rule funded studies. Many institutions governed by a federalwide assurance document, however, agree to review all studies involving human subjects conducted at that institution, regardless of funding source.

A large teaching hospital in the west conducts human subjects research throughout most hospital departments and holds a federalwide project assurance. Within the hospital's clinical research portfolio are many protocols in the area of assisted reproduction because the hospital has an active *in vitro* fertilization (IVF) clinic. These protocols are all privately funded and do not come under the jurisdiction of the DHHS regulations or the IRB's review process. The hospital's policy has been to send to the IRB only those protocols required to have IRB review, but with increased regional media attention to issues such as stem cell research, hospital administrators are now considering amending their assurance to state that any human research project will be reviewed by the IRB, regardless of funding source.

There has been much public discussion of whether or not there should be a federal requirement that any human study, regardless of funding source, receive review and oversight by an IRB. If such federal legislation were to be enacted, this requirement would be integrated into the assurance process. Such legislation has been debated and can be expected to be promulgated eventually. When and if such legislation exists, it will cover all research involving human subjects conducted by a U.S. sponsor, public or private. In the meantime, the existing assurance process is being simplified. On February 9, 2005, it was announced by OHRP that a single Web-based **federalwide assurance** (FWA) will replace the several types of assurances under which research institutions have been functioning. Because of the various types of existing assurance documents, research institutions will have 11 months to transition to the new federalwide assurance. Thus, by December 31, 2005, all institutions conducting DHHS-funded human subjects research must hold an FWA approved by OHRP (Appendix, No. 25).

VI. INITIAL APPROVAL AND CONTINUING REVIEWS

Processes for obtaining initial approval and subsequent review of a clinical study are regulated by law and implemented through institutional policies and procedures. No study that falls under the jurisdiction of federal regulations or that is covered by an institution's assurance agreement can begin until it has been approved by the IRB. This often requires several steps after the IRB has approved a study. Ordinarily, a study cannot begin until the principal investigator (PI) has received a letter confirming that the study can be initiated. A copy of the approved consent/assent document(s) that gives the date of approval often accompanies this letter. As stated before, however, just because the IRB has approved the protocol, the protocol may not be ready to move forward. Each institution and organization has its own final clearance process, which the investigator is responsible for knowing and following. Once a protocol has received all of the approvals required by the institution, the study may start. The regulations require that a clinical protocol that requires IRB approval be reviewed and reapproved at intervals of no greater than 1 year. That does not mean, however, that all studies are reviewed only once a year. Depending on the risk level of the study; the vulnerability of the study population; the complexity of the protocol; the stage of investigation of any experimental drug, device, or other study intervention; occurrence of adverse events; or new information in the literature, as well as other concerns, an IRB may require more frequent reviews. Reviews other than annual reviews may also be set by policy of the institution, depending on the same factors. Continuing review is intended as a substantive safety measure for human subjects. It provides the opportunity to review all aspects of the protocol. It is a mistake to think that the continuing review process is responsible only for new developments in a protocol. Because judgments change regarding such aspects as what is an ethically acceptable risk, what protections might be called for, and what information should be provided to prospective and/or present subjects, it is advisable that at least one member of the IRB/IEC review the full protocol at each continuing review. Doing so increases the probability that a protocol will continue to meet evolving standards for ethical acceptability. Importance of the continuing review equals that of the initial review process.

VII. DATA AND SAFETY MONITORING BOARDS

Data and safety monitoring boards (DSMBs), also referred to as data monitoring committees (DMCs), are a relatively new phenomenon (Ellenberg *et al.*, 2002). Not yet thought of when the regulations were first promulgated, DSMBs are now a review body required for many protocols. At first, DSMBs were created to perform unblinded interim reviews of phase III, blinded, randomized, placebo-controlled trials. The idea was that if an independent body reviewed blinded data in an unblinded fashion prior to meeting study end points, such an interim review might identify substantial risks or be able to document clear benefits before completion of the initial plan. By doing so, a study that had answered study questions about efficacy sooner than anticipated or a study that was associated with unacceptable and/or unanticipated safety concerns could be halted, reducing the number of subjects exposed to risks and/or allowing for more rapid provision of benefits to future patients. Because the utility of having DSMBs perform interim analyses has been demonstrated, an increasing number of studies and clinical research in earlier stages of experimental development have incorporated DSMBs into study oversight. DSMB interim analyses should be planned during design of a study because the number of interim analyses will have implications for the overall statistical demands of the study. In addition, the relationship of the DSMB to the IRB should be defined in advance to the greatest degree reasonable and have completely different membership from the IRB so the two bodies avoid potential conflicts. DSMB reports and evaluations are critical for proper IRB review of a study.

VIII. DISCLOSURE AND MINIMIZATION OF CONFLICTS OF INTEREST: PERSONAL AND INSTITUTIONAL

As a result of disclosure about the financial conflicts of interest in the case of the death of Jesse Gelsinger at the University of Pennsylvania in 1999 (Committee on Assessing the System for Protecting Human Research Subjects, 2001, 2003; Lemmens and Freedman, 2000), intense attention has been directed toward this issue (additional discussion in Chapter 2). The federal government is working on new guidelines, policies, and regulations for financial conflicts of interest surrounding studies and investigators. It is becoming standard practice for investigators to disclose any financial conflicts or potential conflicts to their institution. Many IRBs and IECs require that such information be furnished to them as well. Disclosure of this information to research subjects is getting to be a hotly debated issue about which there is no firm consensus to date. Where a consensus is developing, it is developing around the position that clinical researchers ought to inform subjects of any financial conflict of interest they might have in the conduct and/or outcome of the clinical trial. There are also some IRBs and investigators that disclose investigator's nonfinancial conflict of interest in study outcome. That is, some think it useful to disclose that an investigator's tenure will depend on completing studies and publishing clinical research findings. At a minimum, acknowledgment that any of the investigators has a financial interest in the drug, device, or basic science investigation under consideration should be part of the informed consent process for research participants. No consensus seems imminent, however, about how explicit such disclosure ought to be. Further, what ought to be done to protect subjects from and/or disclose to subjects information about institutional conflicts of interest is still an open and controversial matter. Through discussion, determination of what and how information should be disclosed and what, if any, additional protections for study participants should be added can be made appropriately on a per-protocol basis. What is clear, however, is that conflicts of interest are an area of concern that can be expected to be addressed more fully in future regulations and guidelines. Addressing it explicitly in each protocol and through development of institutional policy is advisable.

PREPARING THE PROTOCOL

4

· · · · · · · · · ·

DESIGNING A CLINICAL
RESEARCH STUDY

· · · · · · · · · · · · · · · · · ·

I. SHAPING THE STUDY QUESTION OR HYPOTHESIS

**The heart of study design is asking a question worth asking or test-
ing a hypothesis worth testing.** Shaping an acceptable question or
hypothesis begins with an idea that interests an investigator or a sponsor.
The idea or interest is ordinarily followed by a thorough literature review.
It is critically important to ascertain that the question has not already been
answered or that the hypothesis has not already been adequately tested.
Conducting a sufficient literature review can be a substantial task.

Although most scientific literature is accessible electronically, the history of medicine is full of examples of important information discovered
and then lost for years, generations, or centuries. Even when searching the
electronically catalogued sources, sometimes data related to a question or
hypothesis are hard to find because they were published in low-visibility
and obscure journals. The core medical and medical research journals may
not include relevant early or obscure data. This problem is not merely academic but is also of grave concern for the protection of human subjects.

The problem of connecting seemingly unrelated and/or temporally dis-
tant literature citations may surface only in the wake of a clinical research
disaster. An example is the research tragedy of the deaths and emergency
liver transplants that occurred in a trial of fialuridine, or FIAU (Straus, 2002;
see also case discussion in Chapter 15). Although the cause of the toxicity

that was finally identified had been reported in the literature before the FIAU subjects became ill, the literature pointing towards the problem was sporadic and not easily understood to predict the adverse events that ultimately occurred. To make the good faith effort needed to review all the possible relevant literature, the responsible investigator will have to reach beyond the electronic citation cataloguing system and scour the records systems for relevant information from multiple related disciplines. Engaging the help of an information specialist and/or pharmacist might facilitate review of the literature. But even after a vigorous and thorough literature review that does not reveal information about the proposed study, other reasons may exist that indicate a proposed question or hypothesis is not appropriate for clinical research. The study may simply not be important enough.

Central to the ethical conduct of clinical research is the requirement that unless important information can be reasonably expected from the completion of the study, it is unethical to subject anyone to even a mere inconvenience. Importance is used in its broadest sense. Adding to the world's knowledge about human and/or animal health, welfare, disease, or suffering and learning more about how humans and animals function in their environment may well advance medical progress. The breadth of important knowledge to be obtained is wide. Nonetheless, justification for the study and the knowledge to be accrued as a result of the investigation is an important part of the process of shaping a clinical research question or hypothesis appropriate for involvement of human research participants.

Answering even an important question, or testing an important untested or inadequately tested hypothesis, does not ensure the appropriate design of a study question or hypothesis. Timing is another critical factor. It may be that extending the research to humans is premature. The risk of harming a subject may be too great because available knowledge is insufficient to ensure a safety level acceptable for human subjects. Balance between the ends of science and protection of the rights and welfare of human subjects must be tipped in the right direction.

A sad example of the perils of attempting to answer research questions with human subjects too quickly is the study of fetal brain tissue transplantation in Parkinson's disease (Albin, 2002; Clark, 2002; London and Kadane, 2002). All one needs to know about the history of this research is that the promise demonstrated in rats in the late 1970s and in nonhuman primates in the early 1980s may have been followed too quickly by the attempted application to humans in the 1990s. The transition from bench to bedside moved so rapidly that clinical trials in the 21st century saw the development of unanticipated side effects in human subjects characterized as catastrophic on the front page of the *New York Times* (Kolata, 2001). The article's conclusion was to return to the bench before considering further fetal tissue research in humans with Parkinson's disease. (See Chapter 15 for a full discussion of this case.)

Moving from bench to bedside must be done carefully and deliberately. Only in this way can the rights and welfare of human subjects be effectively protected. Urgency to find treatments or cures for horrible human diseases is not an acceptable ethical justification for conducting human studies prematurely. The prospect of serious unanticipated outcomes must always be a prime concern of a researcher who is shaping a question or hypothesis for investigation in human subjects. From the very beginning of the development of a clinical research study, the science and ethics of human trials are intricately and inexorably intertwined. Losing sight of this interdependent relationship is a harbinger of disaster.

To craft an appropriate study question or hypothesis, the following questions can be used to guide the process:

- What is it that I want to study? What am I most interested in learning?
- What does the literature say about this topic? How widely has this topic been studied in the past?
- What was the scientific path leading to the current results?
- Logically, what is the next question to be answered or hypothesis to be tested to advance the knowledge and understanding of this phenomenon?
- Does the state of the science justify initiating studies involving human subjects? Are additional animal, bench, and/or computer simulation, and/or modeling studies needed?

By asking these questions, and discussing answers with colleagues, the clinical researcher will be on his or her way to shaping a scientifically and ethically sound question for clinical research.

II. Selecting the Study Design

Study design is a complex process including selection of the optimal population for study, data points for analysis, and analysis strategies. Although selection of a study population ought to be concurrent with considerations of the study's strategy, it is important that the clinical researcher be familiar with the range of study designs from the outset of the planning process.

A. Distinctions Between Hypothesis-Testing and Hypothesis-Generating Clinical Research

First is the matter of whether the study is intended to **test or to generate a hypothesis**. This choice will be determined in large part by findings from the literature. Is the available knowledge about the chosen phenomenon sufficient to shape a plausible hypothesis? Today, the preference is for **hypothesis-testing research—research that is designed to produce statistical support or refutation of a formally articulated research hypothesis.** Funding sources and journal reviewers like to see statistically validated findings. But it is important to remember that a clinical researcher cannot produce theoretically plausible hypotheses if the information available is not adequate. It is just as beneficial to the advancement of science to investigate previously unexplored areas to begin the data accumulation process needed to develop hypotheses. Although some reviewers will consider a study proposal that is not of a hypothesis-testing statistical design as merely a fishing expedition, studies that seek to generate significant new information are justifiable. The justification can be as strong for hypothesis-generating as for hypothesis-testing research.

An investigator is interested in looking for genetic variation or attempting to find genetic markers for diseases of the central nervous system that produce debilitating motor weakness. This is an important area of clinical research that is in its infancy. The investigator decides that there is not enough information to shape an hypothesis on which to focus. Rather, he or she decides to design an hypothesis-generating study in which a genetics component is added to every study at the researcher's institution involving persons with a disease or condition that meets the diagnostic criteria. The investigator obtains permission to take blood or tissue that is left from clinically indicated procedures on the study subjects and is going to scan their genetic material for variations of interest.

Another kind of hypothesis-generating study is demonstrated by the natural history study of patients with a disease for which there is no treatment. As long as there continues to be no treatment, observing their disease course is an acceptable way to learn more about the disease so insights into potential treatments and a cure may arise. At the point at which a treatment emerges, it will no longer be ethically acceptable to conduct a study watching the natural progression of the disease. It will be time for an hypothesis-testing study in which the treatment that is now considered standard-of-practice is tested against other possible interventions.

B. Basic Versus Applied Research

In clinical research, the difference between hypothesis-generating and hypothesis-testing research can often be thought of as the difference between research conducted to understand basic molecular structure and function and what is called applied biomedical research. Research conducted to learn about the structure and function of basic biologic structures, depending on the degree of knowledge about the structure, is often at the stage of **hypothesis-generating research**. Although medical science understands much about the structure and function of human and nonhuman animal physiology, it still has much to learn. By the time research studies have advanced to the point of injecting novel substances into humans or testing new devices on cardiac surgery patients, for example, they have reached the level of hypothesis testing. But human subjects will be needed for both types of testing. It is important to remember that both are clinical research studies. A common mistake is to think that basic research, where there is no human involved and only materials from human beings are studied at the bench, is not clinical research, but that clinical research entails only those studies that involve putting an experimental agent or device into a living person. This is incorrect. Clinical research is research that involves humans or parts of humans. The distinction between basic and applied research is the distinction between early stage human subjects research (i.e., basic), where fundamental mechanisms are being explored and later stage research in which the area of interest is more focused and directed towards some explicit therapeutic intervention (i.e., applied). Examples of basic research include the genetic studies just envisioned as well as brain imaging studies designed to learn more about how the brain functions. Neither type provides information directed towards a specific therapeutic intervention, but both can provide information upon which future therapies are built.

As previously noted, science needs both kinds of studies to move forward. Many important studies cannot be designed to answer discrete, specific questions but are best designed to add to the data pools necessary for creation of scientifically plausible hypotheses. Remember that hypotheses are only as sound as the assumptions built into the hypotheses being tested.

1. Pharmaceutical Industry Research: Drugs, Devices, INDs, and IDEs

After observational research has moved into the applied realm, there are various types of applied study designs. In pharmaceutical industry research, the goal of a study is to bring new drugs, biologics, devices, and/or diagnostics to the marketplace. Such studies have special requirements imposed by regulatory bodies. For example, studies intended to produce data that will become part of a **new drug or device application** will require an **investigational new drug** (IND) or an **investigational device exemption** (IDE) number prior to initiation. Depending on the policy of the researcher's institution, an IRB may review a study while issuance of the IND or IDE number is in process, whereas other institutions require that the approval number be obtained before IRB review. The FDA may require an IRB review and approval prior to assigning an IND or IDE.

2. Investigational Use of Approved Drugs

For the investigational use of approved drugs, an IND number is not always required although prudence dictates that the investigator submit a letter to the FDA requesting an agency opinion. Either the agency will determine that an IND approval number is required, or documentation will be provided indicating that such a number is not needed. If the FDA does not require an IND or IDE number, the FDA letter releasing the investigator from the IND or IDE requirement should accompany the protocol for its IRB review. The FDA letter becomes part of the protocol record and is kept with the original protocol documentation. If the clinical research is externally funded, the sponsor will also want a copy of the FDA release letter.

3. Compassionate and Emergency Use of Investigational Drugs

When new diagnostics or therapeutics or even novel aspects of already approved diagnostics or therapeutics are being tested, there may be requests for compassionate and/or emergency use of the agent or device. **Compassionate use**, emergent or not, represents a request for the use of the test agent or device for an individual outside the inclusion criteria of an approved protocol or within the inclusion criteria of an as of yet unapproved protocol. The first case may be somewhat easier to resolve than the second. An example of the first is that an investigator's institution is conducting a study of a novel agent to avoid toe amputation for drug-nonresponding infection in diabetic patients. The protocol inclusion criteria are for adults, ages 21 and over. A 17-year-old diabetic patient is being treated at the hospital where the study is being conducted who meets all study criteria except for age. Faced with the prospect of amputation, the adolescent and his parents request that the minor have access to the experimental agent as a last ditch effort to avoid amputation. Because there is an institutional policy already in place that provides guidelines for submission of a compassionate use request and specifies the steps for obtaining approval, the child is permitted to enroll in the trial on a compassionate use exemption status.

Ordinarily, approval of the request will have to be obtained at multiple levels. Usually initiated at the investigator level, the request can be expected to go at least from the investigator, to the chairperson of the institution's IRB and/or IEC, and through the medical administrative hierarchy of the institution. Obligations of the sponsor should be clarified as well. Although the terminology *compassionate use* is not regulatory language, it is regularly used and is a *bona fide* avenue to assisting sick patients. Compassionate use exemptions are regularly granted by the institution where the study is being performed when the test agent or device is well along in the research process and the requesting investigator asks for the exemption on behalf of a patient who has failed to respond adequately to all available standard therapy.

The second situation in which requests for compassionate use arise is when a patient meets study inclusion criteria for a protocol that has not yet been approved by an IRB or IEC. Willingness to grant compassionate use exemptions under these circumstances is less forthcoming. Criteria for making such decisions should be set at the institutional policy level rather than on a case-by-case basis. Exemptions of this kind for compassionate use can be expected to be granted with decreasing frequency as regulatory oversight tightens and institutions become increasingly concerned about risk to subjects and institutional liability. The increasing concern about granting a compassionate use exemption of this kind stems from legitimate concerns about risk. For studies that have not yet been approved by an IRB/IEC, one cannot be certain that the protocol will be approved—or if approved—if it will be approved as written at the time this second variety of compassionate use exemption was granted.

Imagine a situation in which a researcher has been working in a particular area, such as eye disease, for many years and is a recognized leader in the field. Over many years of research, this researcher has built up a pool of ready subjects. He or she keeps in close touch with these persons because they have been subjects on previous studies and are eager to enroll when this researcher begins new trials. The researcher has let this group of potential subjects know that a new trial is being designed that will look at a particularly virulent form of visual decline. Of those persons with this condition, they are desperate for anything that might slow the speed of their impending blindness. It is also the investigator's habit to include several members of the community of possible subjects in planning sessions for an upcoming study, to assure that the design is reasonable from the patient-volunteer standpoint. An admirable process, it also produces the byproduct that word of the coming study gets out to the patient community well ahead of the study opening. There is a patient who knows the protocol has been written and is about to be reviewed by the IRB. His vision is deteriorating rapidly and he has failed all standard interventions. He meets all study inclusion criteria in the draft that has been submitted to the IRB and now requests access to the experimental agent prior to IRB review and approval. Should the institution grant his request?

Exemptions for **emergency use** have some regulatory support. The FDA allows for emergency administration of test agents and/or devices under specified circumstances. Some institutions by internal policy restrict the emergency use of test agents and/or devices. Researchers need to familiarize themselves with emergency use exemption policies at their own institutions as well as those of oversight bodies relevant to their research or to those sponsoring research in which they are participating.

4. Outcomes Research or Evidence-Based Research

Another type of study that is gaining increasing attention is **outcomes research**, also referred to as **evidence-based research**. This is clinical research in which already approved drugs or devices or existing standards-of-practice are tested against each other and/or against placebo controls. Design characteristics, which are discussed more fully in Section III of this chapter, similar to those used in drug or device development trials, are directed to a different end. In outcomes research, or evidence-based research, studies are conducted to evaluate established but non-validated treatment practices. Outcomes research is a fast growing area of human subjects research that can be expected to continue expanding. More data from outcomes research will be sought as financial constraints on clinical care increase and evidence-based medicine is practiced more widely.

III. GENERAL DESIGN CHARACTERISTICS

General characteristics of study design include a variety of components with scientific and ethical implications. **Each clinical researcher will have to consider the range of scientific and ethical issues and how the two interact** so that he or she can decide which components ought to be included in or excluded from a particular protocol.

A. Expected-Direct-Benefit Research Versus No-Direct-Benefit Research

One of the most controversial issues in study design relates to the **fundamental ethical premise of clinical research**. The controversy is about the moral differences between studies from which there is a reasonable potential for **direct medical benefit** to individual subjects and those studies with **no reasonable expectation for personal medical benefit** for individual subjects. The claim that it is ethically permissible for individual subjects to place themselves (or be placed, in the case of subjects unable to provide their own ethically and legally valid consent, as discussed in detail in Chapter 5) in harm's way for no medical benefit to themselves but rather for the benefit of future patients is the foundation upon which ethically conducted clinical research sits. Not all accept this claim. There are those who believe that only research that presents a reasonable expectation of direct medical benefit to the participating subjects is ethical clinical research. Others believe strongly that there are instances when clinical research designed with no expectation of direct benefit to participating subjects is ethically acceptable. In general such clinical research is necessary for progress toward clinical studies that afford the prospect of direct medical benefit to subjects and will lead, ultimately, to new treatments and cures for future patients.

This group argues that as long as the clinical research suggests its results will provide knowledge useful to advance understanding of human health and well-being or of human disease and suffering, the study can be conducted ethically. If the clinical study can be expected to produce data that will contribute to society's pool of knowledge, direct medical benefit to individual subjects need not be built into study design.

The ethical acceptability of no-direct-benefit research in the abstract, however, does not clarify which no-direct-benefit studies will be ethically acceptable. There is no formulaic means to ascertain just how much risk relative to how much expected benefit need be anticipated. Each and every protocol balances specific risks for existing research participants against the potential for benefits to society. Individual investigators, reviewers, and IRBs or IECs will come to different conclusions.

Some examples will bring these complex ethical considerations to light. Few would argue that, provided all else about the protocol is ethically acceptable, a drug that has demonstrated efficacy in managing blood pressure with few side effects in a small group of patient volunteers with high blood pressure and heart disease is appropriate to study in a group of patient volunteers with high blood pressure, heart disease, and kidney failure. Both studies hold out a reasonable expectation of direct medical benefit to individual study participants, but let us think backwards about these trials. To be able to ethically run the trial demonstrating efficacy in the high blood pressure, heart disease patient volunteers, previous research would have had to demonstrate that the agent was, at the very least, not excessively toxic to such patients. To obtain this kind of information, the agent would have had to have been given to a group of persons with high blood pressure and heart disease for the very first time. In such a study, where the primary end point is toxicity, not efficacy (see Phases of a Trial section further in this chapter), the reasonable expectation for direct medical benefit to study subjects is greatly reduced. Nonetheless, it

Continued

is not zero, because the agent will have shown some promise in preclinical (i.e., animal) studies, to make it ethically acceptable to bring the agent forward into human trials. More times than not, however, before looking to learn about toxicity of a novel agent in a sick population, it will be ethically and scientifically sound practice to test the agent in healthy persons first. Scientifically, it will be easier to understand how the agent affects the body in a healthy person, whose physiological response is more predictable than is that of someone ill. Ethical reasons for studying a novel agent in a healthy person prior to testing it in a sick person comes from the ethical principles of beneficence and justice that require (i) avoiding doing something to a person in a research setting that might make his or her preexisting burdens more burdensome, even when one's intention is to make things better; and (ii) if the agent proves toxic, a healthy person can be expected to have a better chance of recovering than someone who is already ill. If one accepts these arguments, then in certain circumstances it will be ethically necessary to test a novel agent in healthy persons (see discussion of pharmacokinetics in Chapter 12). Now, however, we have moved to clinical research with no expectation of direct benefit. Clearly, testing new drugs in healthy persons is not for their medical benefit, but for the benefit of society and medical progress. Nonetheless, such studies are important and may be critical to the development of an agent that turns out to be efficacious to many patients in the future. To suggest that such research is unethical *a priori* is a grave error in judgment. Knowing when to move from preclinical studies to humans and from healthy humans to patients, however, is important.

- How many pre-clinical studies will be enough?
- What species need to be studied?
- How much information about toxicity in healthy persons should be accrued before moving from healthy persons to patient volunteers?

These are the kinds of refined ethical considerations that must be made in relation to the differences between direct-benefit and no-direct-benefit research. A blanket condemnation of no-direct-benefit research is not an answer but a demonstration of lack of appreciation of the appropriate and necessary risks that are essential parts of sound, deliberative, measured medical progress.

B. Randomization and Blinding

Randomization is a process of selecting groups for comparison of the safety and/or efficacy of one intervention over another. The randomized trial is considered the gold standard for producing the least biased findings. In a **randomized clinical trial** (RCT), subjects are allocated to the various arms via a random selection process. This might mean that as each participant is determined to be eligible, he or she picks a number from a hat, or chooses heads or tails from a coin toss to determine assignment to a study arm. The most likely method of random assignment today is by computer. Especially for multicenter trials, a group of numbers will be computer generated at the coordinating study site, with each subject assigned a randomly selected, pre-assigned number upon study entry. Randomization reduces bias by reducing the possibility that subjects with special characteristics will be overrepresented in one arm or the other. When there is reasonable scientific uncertainty about which arm of a study might be more beneficial, it is ethically justifiable to run a randomized clinical trial. This equal uncertainty principle is known as equipoise. Only when equipoise exists across arms in a randomized trial is it ethically acceptable to use this design.

Most randomized studies are **double-blinded**. This means that neither the subject nor the investigator knows to which study arm the subject has been assigned. Blinding reduces bias and the possibility that expectations of investigator and/or subject will influence study outcomes. For subject safety, studies that involve randomizing subjects to different treatment interventions are beginning to require a review panel, usually known as a data and safety monitoring board (DSMB), to be formally connected to the trial to break the blind at specified times and to evaluate continuing safety or efficacy. Blinding is a process that maximizes scientific efficiency. Such bodies as DSMBs exist to ensure that scientific efficiency does not interfere with the protection of the rights and welfare of human research participants.

An example of a double-blinded controlled trial with a DSMB attached is one in which drug A is tested against drug B and neither the investigators nor the patient volunteers know which drug the research participant is receiving. Such a trial may be testing a new intervention against an already approved drug for the indication under study. In such a case, ordinarily the institution's pharmacy will participate by providing, or coordinating the obtaining of, study agents in forms that look, smell, taste, and in all other ways, seem alike. The DSMB, at set intervals, will see the data in unblinded fashion to decide if there is an accumulation of adverse reactions in one arm or the other, or if there appears to be overwhelming efficacy in one arm over the other. Evidence of either will be cause for the DSMB to recommend stopping the trial early. If there is no such recommendation, the study will progress to its statistical and/or clinical end points with its double-blinded design intact. The blind will be maintained throughout the data analysis process to reduce, to the greatest degree possible, any bias in the investigators' analysis of the data or of their conclusions.

C. Placebo Controls Versus Comparator Arms

Some randomized clinical trials are designed with only arms testing an experimental agent against one or more approved comparators. An approved comparator is an agent or device that has been approved by a nation's relevant regulatory agency, such as the FDA in the United States, for treatment of patients who have the condition or disease under study. Some randomized clinical trials include a **placebo arm**. A placebo arm is one arm of a trial in which the administered study agent is an inert substance. Others are designed with arms that test experimental agents or test devices against drugs or procedures that represent standard-of-care and include a placebo arm, also. Use of placebos in clinical trials is now highly controversial. Although there is agreement that testing against placebo is the least biased study design, the controversy illuminates the central ethical tensions of human subjects research. When is scientific efficiency too efficient to protect adequately the rights and welfare of human subjects?

There is no controversy in obvious cases. Placebos are not ordinarily used in randomized trials of new anticancer agents. All agree that the risk to subjects of permanent disability or death is too great. At the other end of the continuum, there is also no controversy surrounding the use of placebo when first testing a drug for a disease or condition for which no intervention is known. It is in the grey area that controversy exists. A typical grey area is the use of placebo in testing drugs for mental illness such as schizophrenia or depression. In these therapeutic areas, drugs to treat these conditions already exist, but many patients are not managed by the existing drugs or have unacceptable side effects from them, so new drugs are needed. Withholding ineffective or toxic treatments from subjects with these conditions is not straightforwardly unethical, as it is in such cases as advanced cancer. Persons, unless they are at risk for suicide, do not ordinarily die of schizophrenia or depression, at least not under well-monitored clinical research settings. Data are equivocal about whether or not the long-term course of schizophrenia or depression is made worse by allowing patients to relapse or to go untreated for short amounts of time. Society has not come to consensus about how alike or different physical and psychic pain should be considered and/or treated. Thus, studies in the grey area make answering the following question difficult, "Will placing subjects on a placebo arm pose risk of irreversible and/or severe harm or death?" When this question is difficult to answer and the consequences of approving a new drug present their own set of risks of harm, the ethical tension between scientific efficiency and the need to protect the rights and welfare of human subjects is most pronounced.

Take, for example, the differences among a trial of a new drug for weight loss, a trial of a new drug for depression, and a trial of a new drug for early-stage breast cancer. The weight control and depression trials are both placebo-controlled. That is, both trials have one arm in which subjects receive the drug anticipated to reduce weight without any change in average daily activities and to reduce symptoms of depression, respectively. Each has a second arm in which subjects receive a placebo. But the similarities end here. In the weight loss study, given that there is no drug that will make people lose weight without any change in their other daily activities, including a placebo arm does not place the persons on the placebo arm at any increased risk, nor does it withhold from them anything that would be considered appropriate to their weight loss efforts. That cannot be said for the depression study. Because there are many approved interventions for depression, keeping people from taking such interventions for the benefit of medical progress may be asking too much, an infringement of the principle of justice. Furthermore, having such persons go for the study period without treatment for their depression may put them at a higher risk of harm than would be the case for the average patient outside the clinical research setting, which is an infringement of the principle of beneficence. The counter argument is that depression, although a serious disease, is manageable without drugs. Many people live with depression without drugs. Additionally, depression is a condition (among many) that responds to placebo, making it difficult to know whether or not a drug is better than nothing. Finally, one would be hard-pressed to find anyone who suggested using a placebo in the trial of persons with early-stage breast cancer. Breast cancer is responsive to approved agents, but it is lethal if left untreated. Given these examples, one sees how use of placebo in the weight loss study and no placebo in the cancer trial are judgments easily made, while what to do about a placebo arm in the depression trial is not quite so easy.

The most explicit guidance about use of placebos to date is found in The Declaration of Helsinki, which requires that research subjects should not be denied the best proven therapy for the ends of science. Although explicit in multiple versions, this requirement of the declaration has been systematically ignored for years. The disregard occurs in several ways.

The first has to do with the FDA's preference for placebo controls (Lewis, 2002; Temple, 2002). Consistent with the "grey area" example just given, the FDA position is that placebo controls are ethically acceptable, even ethically necessary. The FDA reasons that when a disease does not produce serious disability or death, especially in diseases where placebos have significant effects on outcomes, it is impossible to know whether a new drug is better than nothing if it is not tested against placebo. Thus, this ethical argument claims that approving a drug for market that is ineffective in large numbers of patients is worse than withholding drug intervention (i.e., including a placebo arm) from a small number of subjects.

Also, specifically related to CNS disease, the FDA contends that a subject who experiences psychiatric symptomatology is not experiencing harm sufficient to make risks of the placebo design unethical. Because this position is understood to be that of the present leadership of the FDA, pharmaceutical companies intending to produce drugs in this therapeutic area for licensing in the United States continue to design studies with placebo arms that are inconsistent with the principles of the most recent version of the Declaration of Helsinki.

Another aspect of ways in which the declaration's constraint on the use of placebo in research is disregarded relates to regulatory agency, investigator, and sponsor interpretation of what is meant by best proven therapy. An argument often made against testing a new agent only against a comparator is that much of what is considered standard practice is not scientifically validated and therefore has never been actually shown to be effective. The often unspoken argument against randomization with comparator arm(s) only, however, is that greater numbers of subjects are required to meet statistical endpoints, making the studies more expensive, longer, and thus harder to conduct and complete.

Yet another related way in which the declaration's prohibition on administering placebo to subjects in certain situations is ignored is based on disagreement about the interpretation of what is meant by drug availability. That is, in drug development trials conducted in countries and communities too poor to have access to interventions proven to be efficacious, the argument hinges on what defines a "best proven and available intervention." Must the best proven treatment be what the scientific community considers best proven anywhere in the world, or may best proven be set in terms of what is available in the country where the study is being conducted? Where no treatment is the answer because the country or community is too impoverished to provide any treatment, most discussions are moving toward a condemnation of placebo use (Koski and Nightingale, 2001; Levine and Gorovitz, 2000; National Bioethics Advisory Commission, 2001a; Shapiro and Meslin, 2001). Nonetheless, because of the regulatory preference for a placebo arm and because of its importance to statistical analysis of research data, the placebo remains a common element of study design.

D. Phases of a Clinical Trial

The clinical trial phase involves the actual stage of scientific development as well as a **term-of-art**, which means that a phase of the research may still be at the observation stage. There may not be enough known about the disease or condition to propose any experimental intervention. Even earlier still, there is confusion about the term *basic*. Some differentiate research into **basic research**, meaning *in vitro* or animal research, and **clinical research**, meaning research involving human participants. Some will talk about basic or basic clinical research and mean bench research with human biological materials. Some think of research involving human subjects as research with living persons only and not involving tissue from living or deceased persons. In this book, we, the authors, refer to **animal research** as research involving whole animals, living or dead, and research on biological materials from animals. When we use the term **pre-clinical research**, we mean research that involves animals or biological materials from living or dead animals. When we refer to **clinical research**, we mean research involving human participants or biological materials from living or dead humans. The meaning of phases I, II, III, and IV clinical trials is much clearer and these definitions are provided in the following section. It is worth noting, however, that studies may merge phases into a single study, such as a study that includes a phase II/III design.

1. Phase I Trials

Phase I trials are the phase of drug or device development studies in which a drug or device is tested in humans for the first time. These trials usually have a small number of subjects who may be healthy volunteers. Starting a phase I trial means there is enough experience with animals and/or computer models to suggest that the intervention may be an improvement over what presently exists in diagnosing, treating, curing, or preventing a particular disease or condition in humans. Phase I trials do not have efficacy end points as primary objectives. Although attempts may be made to document evidence of efficacy, efficacy is never a primary end point. Rather, end points in Phase I trials are safety and toxicity; pharmacokinetics and pharmacodynamics may be evaluated. Many phase I trials include a single group of healthy or patient volunteers in an open-labeled or single-blinded design. **Open-label** means that all participants and investigators know what agent the subject is taking or device the subject is testing. **Single-blind** means that the subjects, but not the investigator, are blinded to the study intervention.

2. Phase II Trials

Phase II trials usually also have small numbers of subjects but have more subjects than phase I trials. Primary end points include efficacy end points. Rather than only involving healthy subjects, the phase II level study may introduce the experimental agent or device to patient study populations. The primary goals of a phase II trial are to begin to accrue efficacy data and continue to identify safety problems. The primary goal of a phase II drug trial is often to define a maximally tolerated dose (MTD). The MTD is the dose just below that which produces unacceptable toxicities. At the phase II level, studies begin to include two or more groups of subjects, usually with randomized assignments. They may be cross-sectional or longitudinal in plan design. Phase II trials may be of parallel or crossover design, the most common choices, or of matched-pair or historical control design. Even less often used, but gaining interest, are sequential and play-the-winner designs and rapid cohort escalation strategies. Each has its own set of scientific and ethical advantages and disadvantages (Fazzari *et al.*, 2000; Hu and Hu, 2000; Knopman *et al.*, 1998; Korn *et al.*, 2001; Lin and Yao, 1996; Montgomery, 1999; Spilker, 2000; Stallard and Rosenberger, 2002; Zhang, 2003).

3. Phase III Trials

Phase III trials involve large numbers of subjects and more groups of subjects than do phase II trials. The study groups will include subgroups representing an ever-widening range of potential patients for whom the drug or device is ultimately intended. Studies at the phase III level include subgroups of patient volunteers, such as persons in extremely old and extremely young age groups, and research at this phase makes vigorous efforts to reach out to ethnically distinct populations. Because the total number of subjects is greater at phase III than at earlier levels, subgroup analyses can be performed. Phase III trials are often multicenter and/or multinational, with efficacy as the primary end point. Phase III trials are the final phase for a drug or device to be submitted to the FDA for approval.

4. Phase IV Trials

Phase IV trials are conducted after an agent or device has been approved for clinical use. Phase IV trials are being scrutinized more closely as human subjects research, in general, is receiving more ethical attention. In phase IV trials, the responsible investigators are walking a tightrope between inconsequential drug company marketing studies and studies that collect important outcome data. Some post-marketing data collection will be required by regulatory agencies. It is up to the virtuous investigator and rigorous IRB and IEC review bodies to differentiate the two.

No approval process for a medical intervention can, or should, require so many studies that data are generated from all patient populations prior to marketing. Further, because so much of clinical medicine is, and will always remain, the art of the skilled physician's educated guess about what might help his or her patient, it is important to the practice of medicine that the law allows physicians to prescribe drugs for unapproved indications as patient need dictates once an agent and/or device is approved for its labeled indications. These prescribing realities of clinical medicine and processes of therapeutic intervention approval mandate research in the post-marketing phase to advance care. When phase IV studies are designed to obtain this kind of information, study questions are important enough to put subjects through inconveniences for scientific progress. If, however, a phase IV study is being proposed that has no substantive scientific merit but is simply a commercial ploy to advance commercial ends (sometimes called "seeding studies"), regardless of how low the risk might be, such a study should not be conducted.

IV. Beginning to Write the Protocol

Beginning to write a protocol for clinical research requires having made decisions not yet considered in this book. Nonetheless, it is not too soon to discuss writing a first draft of the introductory sections of the protocol. Doing so will facilitate clarification of the issues yet to be addressed and allow recognition of many controversies that could be raised by the topic of study.

A. Précis

The **précis** is a brief summary of what the study is about. Sometimes written twice, once as a scientific summary and once as a lay summary, each précis should be approximately 200–400 words. Both briefly state the purpose of the study and why it is needed (i.e., what problem the study addresses and why it is important). Next is a short description of the study subjects, length of study, methods, a short summary of study procedures, and a follow-up. At this stage of study development, it may be possible only to write a rough draft of the last points, to be revised when the protocol draft is completed.

B. Introduction: Purpose and Justification for the Proposed Study

The **introduction** explains the purpose of the study and its scientific importance. The purpose should be a clear statement of the general goal of the proposed study. The introduction should be brief, including only information about what will be done and a short description of the subjects to be studied.

The problem needs to be explained in clinical and scientific terms. A brief statement explains how the proposed study meets existing clinical needs, what scientific debates are related to the question/hypothesis being asked and/or tested, and why/how the proposed study is appropriate given the present state-of-the-art knowledge or practices and/or the literature.

C. Literature Review

The **literature review** presents information to explain and justify the proposed study. This section summarizes relevant studies involving animals, and computer simulation and/or modeling information that are the basis for the study of human subjects that is proposed. In this section, existing data should be included that justify the proposed study and make it the logical next step in expanding scientific understanding of the topic to be studied.

If the study is going to extend work that has already been initiated in human subjects, it is necessary to provide sufficient animal data to assure the reviewers that the animal work has advanced appropriately for the move to human studies in the first place. Do not assume that because there are already human studies in this area that the move from bench to bedside has been appropriate. To be convincing, discuss in the protocol, explicitly, why the animal work is sufficient either to have allowed the use of humans in studies or why the data are sufficient for the proposed study to move toward using human subjects.

If the study is the first to move investigation of the topic from animals to humans, the protocol (and the consent documents) needs to state this clearly and justify why such a move is now appropriate. The justification must stand on scientific reasoning. That is, a convincing argument will explain how all reasonably plausible animal and computer simulation/modeling experiments have been performed and that the only way to advance knowledge of the subject is to begin research involving human subjects.

A clinical researcher writing this proposal SHOULD NOT attempt to ground the justification in terms of human need for the information to be gained. Weak arguments are open to reasonable challenge by thoughtful and skilled clinical research reviewers. It is fair to assume that to be an excellent clinical researcher, a high level of optimism regarding the potential of discovering something of great importance to humankind is necessary. It is important, however, not to let such emotionally driven enthusiasm influence the assessment of justifications of moving research from animals to humans. The potential for failure and, worse still, the potential for unanticipated grave outcomes are too real.

If the proposed study extends work that has already moved appropriately to human trials, a thorough review of the existing clinical data is necessary. If only a small number of human studies have been conducted, all should be cited and discussed in the context of laying the groundwork for a natural scientific progression to the proposed experiment. If, however, the case is a refinement of a still unanswered question or hypothesis requiring further testing in an area in which much human research has already been conducted, clinical data need to be selected carefully. If the field of investigation for this topic has a long history, it is important to cite a few of the seminal clinical studies to set the state of the field. Then the important breakthroughs in scientific understanding of the question and/or problems addressed by the study can be briefly covered. The conclusion to this section can include a substantial review of recent work in the field that directly leads to the reason(s) for proposing this particular investigation.

This literature review is a required step in the approval of a study. The literature review is far more than a recitation of a few studies to give the reader a "feel" for previous work. Instead, this section is the first hurdle in the justification process. This section, if not thorough and convincing, will seriously weaken the protocol. If there are insufficient animal or *in vitro* studies, if computer simulation models are inadequate, or if the proposal is not a logical outgrowth of existing clinical work, the appropriateness of the protocol should be questioned. Reviewers may have concerns about the researcher's capabilities for conducting the study. If this section is inadequate (skimpy) or sloppy, it is fair for the reviewers to ask, "If this researcher is this sloppy about the basis on which this trial is being justified, how careful is he or she going to be in protecting the study's subjects?"

D. Objectives, Questions, or Hypotheses

The **objectives** section presents in clear and concise scientific language the question to be asked or hypothesis to be tested. Unlike the introduction, where the purpose of the study is presented in narrative form, objectives are often written in bullet form. By reading the study objectives, questions, or hypotheses, a reviewer should be able to determine whether study objectives can be met by the methods and analysis strategies to be employed.

5

··········

SELECTING SUBJECTS FOR CLINICAL STUDIES

·················

The appropriate study population for research involving human subjects depends directly on the question(s) or hypothesis(-es) being addressed. In so far as possible, subjects who are fully autonomous adults, with no constraints on their ability to provide ethically and legally valid consent, are most desirable. If such an adult population is not appropriate, the preference, in descending order, is vulnerable, but cognitively intact adults; cognitively impaired adults with an agent or guardian assigned specifically for research purposes; cognitively impaired adults with an agent or guardian assigned for clinical care only; and, finally, cognitively impaired adults with a surrogate. Among adults incapable of providing ethically and legally valid consent, it is preferable to involve as subjects those who are able to provide assent or dissent before choosing those who are not.

The ethically acceptable order to follow when choosing subjects is choosing adults first and then minors. When minors are to be included in a study, the order of preference is minors who are able to provide assent or dissent, followed by those minors who are too young and/or developmentally immature to do so. These general guidelines, however, do not always apply.

An example of an exception to the guidelines for choosing subjects is found in the administration of noxious cancer chemotherapeutic agents. Although

Continued

63

early-stage clinical research might be conducted in healthy adult volunteers, it is just as likely that the phase I trials will be conducted with adult patient volunteers who have failed standard-of-care interventions. Pediatric subjects would be selected to study an agent intended to treat tumors that occur only in pediatric populations. Further, if the pediatric tumor occurs only in newborns, the preference to start with 15- to 18-year-old teenagers capable of giving assent would reasonably be ignored.

Exceptions to the guidelines for selecting candidates are examples of where the primacy of the principle of respect for persons is overridden by justice requirements and the principle to avoid harm. Optimal subject selection calls for an equitable balance of benefits and burdens, minimizing burdens and maximizing benefits while meeting scientific goals. Except for certain studies involving pregnant women or prisoners, there are no U.S. regulatory prohibitions on adult participation in research. The newest revision of the Declaration of Helsinki (2000), however, prohibits research involving any subject unable to provide his or her own informed consent unless the study addresses a matter relevant to the person's disease or condition and cannot be performed with subjects able to provide their own informed consent.

In pediatric research, there are additional regulatory constraints. Although clinical research with no expectation of direct benefit is permitted under certain conditions, ordinarily the knowledge to be gained must accrue to the category of pediatric patients represented by study subjects.

I. STUDY VOLUNTEERS: HEALTHY SUBJECTS OR PATIENT SUBJECTS?

The first consideration regarding subject selection is whether healthy volunteers are appropriate subjects or patient volunteers will be required. Healthy volunteers can be expected to understand most easily the information provided and the consequences of their decisions. Healthy volunteers without any social constraints, such as dependency, poverty, or poor education, are the least vulnerable of possible study populations. Studies exist, however, with scientific ends that can be met only in a specific human disease context. For such studies, patient volunteers are required. Both healthy and patient populations include vulnerable individuals who require additional protections.

Historically, healthy volunteers were considered *a priori*, to need no special protection. By definition, a **healthy subject** has no diagnosed and/or apparent physical or mental disease or condition. Therefore, the presumption has been that healthy subjects are fully autonomous decision makers and present no concerns about vulnerability. As society has become more sensitive to considerations of social injustice and the implications of power differences, however, awareness of limits to self-determination has grown. It is now widely accepted that some healthy adult volunteers may be vulnerable subjects. Healthy adults who might be vulnerable to manipulation in the clinical research setting include individuals who are socially, economically, or educationally disadvantaged. Homelessness, like other manifestations of poverty, makes people vulnerable.

Healthy volunteers who do not speak the language of those conducting the research should also be considered as a special or potentially vulnerable population. Power differences will present concerns about vulnerability for medical students, residents, and fellows who may need recommendations or laboratory personnel considered for studies conducted by their mentors or supervisors. Presently healthy persons who depend on a physician for their future care may also feel unable to decline when asked to participate in research.

On average, when studies call for healthy adult subjects, those healthy people who have constraints on their decision making because of their life circumstances (e.g., imprisonment, social deprivation) ought to be excluded. If, however, the purpose of the study is to examine aspects related to their potential vulnerability and explicit protections are in place, the study may be acceptable. Sometimes standard practices are enough to ensure sound clinical research ethics. In other situations, such as when prisoners are involved, additional protections are required by regulation and ethical practice.

All healthy volunteers, however, are at risk for one problem that is regularly overlooked. **By participating in research, a healthy control subject can find out that he or she is not healthy.** Such a discovery would be made ordinarily during the medical evaluation performed to confirm the person's eligibility and could have serious implications for the person's future. Employment and insurance could be affected and the individual's self-concept may be altered as well. These are not trivial risks and should be explained as part of the consenting process.

II. VULNERABLE SUBJECT POPULATIONS: WHO IS CLASSIFIED AS VULNERABLE AND HOW THIS DECISION IS MADE

What does it mean to be vulnerable in the clinical research setting? Vulnerability, although sometimes objectively identifiable, has a subjective component as well. A late-stage Alzheimer's patient and a 3-year-old child are vulnerable by virtue of their objectively identifiable impaired ability to provide ethically and legally valid consent. But in other cases, vulnerability may have to be more subjectively appreciated. Depression can, but need not, reduce decisional capacity. Yet the depressed patient, who after adequate assessment is determined to be cognitively intact, may still be vulnerable because of other constraints on his or her autonomy. In some jurisdictions, a minor who is married or is a parent might no longer be legally prevented from providing his or her own informed consent. But the legally mature minor may still be vulnerable by virtue of poverty or lack of education. Contemporary appreciation of vulnerability is evolving. Traditionally, adult patients with cancers that do not overtly affect mental status were not considered vulnerable. In current practice, one might be concerned that these patient volunteers are vulnerable. What is it that makes a subject vulnerable?

A. What Makes a Subject Vulnerable?

Vulnerability results from conditions or characteristics that might make a specific subject more susceptible than others to coercion or undue influence. Coercion or undue influence might cause an individual to agree to participate in a study against the subject's better judgment, despite adequate knowledge and understanding of the consent. Any coercion or undue influence that might constrain or limit voluntary informed consent should be avoided.

The common dictionary definition of **vulnerable** includes such words as *weak, unprotected,* and *easily manipulated.* In the clinical research setting, this definition translates into a subject who is unable, for whatever reason, to act in his or her own best interests. In the design stage of protocol development, potential vulnerabilities of proposed study populations must be evaluated. The first consideration might be called the **common sense test**. Ask a few of your colleagues and your next door neighbor if they think people with schizophrenia, a genetic condition that causes premature death or disability, or medical students who work for the principal investigator might be manipulated into study participation. There is probably something about the condition of each of these individuals, medical or social, that opens the door to the potential for coercion. If the subject population you are considering includes people with deficiencies in the ability to reason or people who might have foreseeable pressures on their future careers or home lives, such a population is best considered potentially vulnerable.

B. Distinguishing Between Potentially Vulnerable and Vulnerable

It is important to differentiate between those volunteer subjects who *are potentially* vulnerable and those who *are* vulnerable. A vulnerable population includes subjects who are physically or legally unable to provide informed consent. Young children and unconscious adults are vulnerable subjects. The adult with early stage colon cancer, however, may or may not be vulnerable; that individual is a potentially vulnerable subject. The young child is legally incapable of providing consent. The unconscious adult is physically incapable of providing consent. The colon cancer patient may be psychologically unable to process information adequately or may be so emotionally impaired as to be unable to make his or her own research decisions. Even a healthy volunteer may be vulnerable if he or she is employed in the investigator's laboratory, dependent on the investigator for recommendations, or subject to coercion by the compensation offered by the study.

Frank vulnerability comes from objective barriers to independence. The potential for vulnerability comes from economic, political, and/or social conditions that can constrain freedom of choice or freedom from physical, psychological, or emotional factors that can cloud judgment.

We advise clinical researchers to start from the premise that **all subjects may be potentially vulnerable**. Then researchers can establish that the subject population is not vulnerable, or they can provide the kinds of protections appropriate to address specific potential or actual vulnerabilities.

Ultimately, the IRB and IEC bodies determine how vulnerable, if at all, a proposed subject population is and what protections will be required. Nonetheless, it is the investigator's responsibility to evaluate and define clearly the expected degree of vulnerability, justify the involvement of subjects with such characteristics, and build into study design any additional protections that might be needed.

III. Special Populations and Additional Protections

The term *special population* is synonymous operationally with the term *vulnerable subjects*. **Special populations** include any subject group or community with qualities or characteristics that require specific considerations in addition to those required to protect the rights and welfare of a fully autonomous healthy adult. Most often, the additional considerations will be additional protections. The ethos, until recent years, has always been that clinical research is a burden from which subjects need protection. Contemporary clinical research ethics, however, combine protectiveness with notions of increased access. The need to increase access of women and minorities to research participation has been recognized for well over a decade. This perspective has been extended to include children.

The research field knows that the effects of drugs, devices, and other therapeutic interventions are not necessarily independent of gender, ethnicity, or age. To maximize therapeutic benefit and minimize harmful side effects of an approved therapeutic intervention, research needs to involve subjects representative of those for whom the drug, device, or intervention will be prescribed. If such people (e.g., AIDS patients or women of childbearing potential) view clinical research participation subjectively as more of a benefit than a burden, they ought not to be prohibited from making such decisions. This heightened awareness of the importance of including the full spectrum of human populations does not, however, reduce the need to protect all subjects who are participants in research. Efforts to expand access are supported by all three ethical principles articulated in *The Belmont Report*, but it is important to balance the growing enthusiasm for access with appropriate attention to traditional notions of protection of human research subjects (Appendix, No. 11). In short, contemporary protocol design takes into account both inclusion and protection.

A. Healthy Adult Volunteers

The clinical research least complicated scientifically and ethically involves physically healthy volunteers who are not also economically or socially compromised. The expectation is that such subjects do not need protections over and above the basic requirements of valid study design, including a well-conducted informed consent process, independent review by IRB and IEC bodies, and oversight by a responsible investigator. They are, however, vulnerable to inappropriate financial inducements.

An example is a study in which an investigator is testing a new drug to ward off the common cold. The study is an inpatient study in which physically and socioeconomically healthy volunteers come in on a Thursday evening and are housed in their own private room. The rooms have their own baths, telephones, and televisions; and all meals are brought into the rooms for the subjects. After a subject arrives, is determined to be healthy, and has settled in his or her room, the study participant is given dinner, including a pill that is designed to prevent the subject from getting a cold. Shortly thereafter, the subject is given a mist to inhale that includes the virus for the common cold.

Continued

> The subject is checked every 6 hours, except while sleeping, for symptoms of a cold. If by 8:00 AM the following Monday morning no cold has developed, the subject is finished and may leave. As the subject departs, he or she is given an envelope containing a thank you letter and a check for $25.00.

This study, while it may be quite complicated scientifically in terms of the experimental agent, its formulation, and administration of the challenge virus, it is relatively uncomplicated ethically. Alter any characteristic about the subject and the ethical complexities mount.

1. Socioeconomically Disadvantaged Volunteers

Physically healthy volunteers may present a special population when nonmedical conditions restrict their ability to make choices compared to the average member of an affluent sector of the country or community from which the healthy subject is being recruited. Most often, such characteristics result from socioeconomic disadvantages that can range from joblessness, to homelessness, to social isolation, and to stigma. Any of these can create a situation in which a person lacks access to basic needs, such as food, shelter, and medical services. When studies involving healthy volunteers provide payment to impoverished persons, perhaps for in-patient studies during which subjects will be fed and housed, those components of the study itself could be an enticement too great to forgo, regardless of an individual's inclination to participate without such benefits. Although protective mechanisms, such as recruitment procedures with multiple layers of screening, may aid in assuring researchers that potential subjects will make informed decisions about research participation, this is a controversial area of subject self-selection. **Justice requires that people should not be excluded merely because they are disadvantaged.** A person does not want to disadvantage further the already disadvantaged. Researchers want to be careful, however, that a biomedical study's pool of healthy volunteers is not drawn solely from an impoverished or otherwise disadvantaged group. If it were, equity in subject selection would be questionable.

2. Healthy Volunteers Who Do Not Speak the Researchers' Language

A healthy volunteer subject who does not speak the language of the study environment, or who does not speak it well, will be at a serious disadvantage. This subject will be disadvantaged even if he or she is highly educated, is from a privileged background, does seemingly well with questioning, and is assertive. Justification for involvement of healthy volunteers who do not speak the language of the researchers and the research environment needs to be made vigorously. At the same time, the principle of justice requires that language not present a barrier to clinical research participation. This is a fine balance to strike, and it will be affected by such issues as degree of risk to subjects. **On average, it is prudent to recruit healthy volunteer subjects from populations whose primary language is the language of the investigators and the setting in which the research is being conducted to minimize possible vulnerabilities in subject selection.**

3. Sensory Impairments: Volunteers Who Are Blind and/or Deaf

Categorization of persons with sensory impairments has become controversial. **It is no longer clear that an individual who is blind or deaf is invariably a patient volunteer.** An individual with a sensory impairment, not affecting that person's ability to function in a mainstream environment, may be considered a healthy volunteer. A significant subset of people in the deaf community believe that deafness is an alternative lifestyle and believes those who are deaf do not have a medical condition. Taking this sociopolitical viewpoint into account in determining whether persons with what have been commonly considered medical disabilities might be included in study samples of healthy volunteers is advised. If a study were to include such individuals, it could be argued that the same kind of accommodations would be appropriate as required for such persons in standard employment settings.

4. Volunteers: Women of Childbearing Potential

Nowhere have the moral norms about protectiveness and access for adult subjects shifted as greatly as in the involvement of women of childbearing potential in clinical research. Until the late 1980s, women of childbearing potential were commonly excluded from clinical research participation. Even as the push to involve women and minority populations more fully in research was in full swing, women of childbearing potential were still routinely excluded. This exclusion was no longer true for clinical research studies starting in the late 20th century. Protocols now have explicit requirements for birth control. The implication is that **the clinical research field respects healthy adult women and their autonomy about their sexuality.**

When considering requirements for female birth control, it is important not to ignore such considerations for males. Although the scientific issues may be different (i.e., an experimental drug may have teratogenic effects but no harmful effects on sperm) and, thus, require a prohibition on pregnancy rather than on intercourse, male birth control should be addressed where appropriate. This includes discussion and/or plans for storing sperm and/or eggs and should be clearly explained in protocols and consents as relevant.

5. Pregnant Women Volunteers: Healthy Subjects?

Although liberalizing the constraints in the Department of Health and Human Services (DHHS) regulations on the involvement of pregnant women in clinical research has been discussed, the liberalization has not occurred. Thus, while the social debate about whether a pregnant woman is healthy or has a medical condition continues, for purposes of inclusion in clinical research, she is considered to have a condition over which oversight is required. The U.S. Code of Federal Regulations specifies under what conditions pregnant women may be involved in clinical research (Appendix, No. 15).

B. Adult Patient Volunteers

Adult patient volunteers span the continuum from fully autonomous to completely debilitated persons in clinical research. Many scientific questions can be answered only by investigation of persons with the disease or condition. Involving patients in research, however, invariably presents complexities that healthy study populations do not. Often the very presence of disease makes data analysis particularly difficult. It can be virtually impossible at times to differentiate symptoms of disease and/or disease progression from side effects of the experimental intervention. For ethical reasons, some studies are designed only for persons who have failed all standard interventions, thus restricting subject pools to those with the most refractory disease.

Nevertheless, at times scientific progress can only result from research involving patient volunteers. In this situation, the preference will be first to involve adults who are fully capable of providing ethically and legally valid consent. Doing so, however, may not always be possible. Some studies will have to include populations of adults and/or minors who are unable to provide their own consent. The prudent clinical researcher will consider all patient groups special, or potentially vulnerable, unless the contrary is well justified. Some patient populations, however, can be assumed *a priori*, to be special; some subjects are explicitly designated special by regulation. In either case, special populations ordinarily demand a higher level of protective attention than do fully autonomous healthy volunteers.

Two studies sitting at different points along the continuum of possible patient populations include an open-label trial of a new drug for migraine headaches in a population of otherwise healthy adults with a history of migraines to a randomized, double-blinded, placebo-controlled trial of a new drug for chronic and severe arthritis pain. In the first, there is no randomization at all. Subjects will receive the new drug, they will know they are receiving the new drug, and the outcome of interest is their subjective evaluation of whether or not taking the drug at the outset of their migraine shortened its duration from the time they ordinarily suffer from a migraine. The design calls for them to have timed the duration of their migraines, keeping track of what they took, if anything, for the previous four migraines. They will simply record the time of onset and the time at which they noticed the migraine was gone or the time at which they took an additional medication for four migraines for which they take the experimental drug at migraine onset. Although migraines are complex medical phenomena about which much is still not understood, and persons who suffer with migraines may suffer greatly, this is a rather uncomplicated study—ethically and in terms of its design.

In the case of a randomized, double-blinded, placebo-controlled trial of a new drug for chronic and severe arthritis pain, the chronic nature and severity of the pain adds additional layers of scientific and ethical complexity. Although fully capacitated subjects from both patient populations can be found, the majority of persons with chronic, severe arthritis pain can be expected to be much older than migraine subjects. Older subjects can be expected to have multiple additional comorbidities and can be expected to be on multiple drugs. Some subjects may be depressed from the chronic pain. Sorting through the additional characteristics will add scientific complexity to data analysis. Ethically, randomization itself is not terribly controversial, but the placebo arm will be. Although there are many supposed remedies for arthritis, some are ineffective, meaning that new drugs are needed and a placebo arm, *per se*, can be justified. Withholding beneficial treatment will be difficult to justify, however, so the study may need to be designed for those who have failed all other proven, standard interventions, which would narrow the study population to refractory patients. Showing efficacy in refractory patient populations will have implications for the statistical analysis. Worse still, pain is a condition that responds to placebo, further complicating the statistics. Also, these are only the obvious ethical complexities posed by this trial. Depending on the specific details, there well may be more.

1. Pregnant Women

Pregnant women, as noted previously, are designated a special population by DHHS regulation. According to 45 CFR 46, Subpart B, research is restricted to studies with a goal of serving the health needs of the pregnant woman or the fetus. Risk level is also specified. This means that only clinical research with a valid expectation of direct benefit to the subjects can be conducted in this population. This recently revised Subpart also includes regulations for research involving non-viable neonates.

2. Cognitively Impaired Patients

Patients with cognitive impairments include a wide spectrum of adults and minors and constitute special populations. Unconscious patients; patients with progressive, neurological disorders; stroke patients with residual cognitive deficits; and patients with brain damage from trauma all are special subpopulations of the cognitively impaired. **Each of these patient populations presents its own set of scientific and ethical complexities and may require different kinds of additional protections.** For example, if the adult patient population to be studied is rendered unconscious as a consequence of some unpredictable prior event, the regulations governing emergency research (discussed in Chapter 14) may apply. Another example, however, might be a study of patients who have become unconscious as a complication of drug-resistant infection and sepsis. Then perhaps the study design might be so that all patients admitted to a hospital with a drug-resistant infection would be invited to participate in the study if the clinical course were to develop so that the patient met the eligibility requirements.

For patients with progressive neurological disorders, such as Alzheimer's disease or Huntington's disease, anticipation of eligibility may be relatively easy. For the majority of persons with those, or similar, conditions, there is a long period during which symptoms are present and diagnoses made, yet the patient remains a cognitively capable decision maker. This period is the optimal time to invite persons to participate. Even if the study is designed to investigate something about the later stages of such conditions, when a patient will be beyond the point of self-determination, recruitment may be accomplished while the person is still able to give consent.

3. Psychiatrically Impaired Patients

Psychiatrically impaired patients are one of the most controversial special volunteer populations for clinical research, in part because some of the most vociferous anti-research advocates have focused on psychiatric research. The ethics of psychiatric research is made particularly difficult because of the complexity of the expression of psychiatric disease. Many persons who have a psychiatric diagnosis live fully active and productive lives. One of the hallmarks of psychiatric illness, however, is its variability across patients and within the same individual over a lifetime. Psychiatric symptoms wax and wane over a person's disease course. This is true for diverse diagnoses such as schizophrenia or alcoholism and drug abuse. **Psychiatric impairment and addictive disorders can reduce a person's ability to make sound judgments without clouding mentation.** Some psychiatric illness is characterized by symptoms, such as suspiciousness, that render standard protective measures (e.g., the identification of a clinical research surrogate) therapeutically suboptimal. That is, requesting that a suspicious psychiatric patient assign a research surrogate may result in a potential subject declining study entry and produce clinical harm by increasing the patient's suspiciousness. Adding further complexity are scientific considerations, such as high rates of placebo responses and soft end points. When designing a study of psychiatrically impaired subjects, the researcher is advised to err on the side of conservatism in protecting those who are seriously ill while maximizing their ability to exercise safely the greatest possible self-determination. Although this is not an unreasonable approach in general, it is particularly important in clinical research with psychiatrically ill patients.

4. Patients with a Terminal Disease and/or Chronic Pain Condition

Patients with a terminal disease or a chronic, debilitating illness also constitute special volunteer populations. Until the late 20th century, patient volunteers with chronic debilitating illnesses were not recognized as particularly vulnerable, because they did not have diseases or conditions associated with mental status changes. Findings in the field of cognitive science, however, have demonstrated consistently that anxiety and/or pain can seriously impair the ability of an otherwise cognitively intact individual to attend, process, and comprehend. If a study were to involve persons with anxiety or pain, given the possibility of problems in decisional capacity, it would be important to develop specific strategies for imparting information.

5. Patients Who Do Not Speak the Researchers' Language

A patient volunteer who does not speak the language predominantly used by the researchers and/or in the research setting is doubly disadvantaged. Such subjects participate as patient volunteers because they have some disease or condition that affects their overall health, but they may also be unable to communicate effectively with the researchers and/or research care staff. This situation can be expected only to heighten anxiety, potentially reducing further the subject's ability to comprehend information and make decisions in his or her own best interest. When such persons participate in a study, it is not sufficient to provide them with translated consent documents. **Additional efforts are required to provide translators as the study progresses and the consent process is repeated throughout the subject's study participation.** These additional protections associated with translation assistance are discussed more fully in Section III, F, 6 of this chapter.

6. Socioeconomically Disadvantaged Patients

Economically and/or socially disadvantaged patient volunteers are a special population in multiple ways. Their involvement in clinical research poses complex ethical considerations. A great deal of sociopolitical attention has been paid over the past two decades to increasing the involvement of women and minority populations in clinical research. Within the last several years, this effort has expanded to include increased involvement of minors. These efforts have resulted in regulatory and policy changes that now require investigators to demonstrate their efforts to involve these groups more fully. From a social justice perspective, however, this inclusion adds additional ethical complexity. **Women, minority populations, and children around the world represent the greatest number of individuals living in poverty and are the victims of centuries of discrimination and inequalities.** These population characteristics thus require specific strategies for additional protection of rights and welfare.

In addition, the push to involve these populations more fully coincides with an expansion of pharmaceutical industry–sponsored, multisite, multinational trials. Thus, one philosophical thread in contemporary clinical research ethics calls for greater access to research by often disenfranchised groups while another thread pulls in the opposite direction. This second and traditionally stronger thread requires that such people be protected against undue influence to participate. For clinical research conducted in the United States and sponsored by U.S. entities (e.g., by the NIH or U.S. pharmaceutical companies), the ethical tensions presented are obvious; however, when such research is extended into non-English-speaking and impoverished countries or communities, a topic discussed in greater detail in Section III, E of this chapter, the ethical and scientific complexities grow exponentially.

For U.S.-sponsored clinical research conducted in the United States or other affluent English-speaking countries, the socioeconomically disadvantaged may be included among potential participants. Although it is patently unethical to seek socioeconomically disadvantaged subjects and entice them into study participation, studies will exist in which they are the likely subjects, such as studies of drug abusers or alcoholics. It is a sad by-product of these conditions that many afflicted persons will be found among the society's most disadvantaged populations. In an era when access to clinical research is viewed less as a burden than as a benefit, enrolling only affluent persons with these conditions can be considered unjust. But what may be a non-coercive study benefit to one subject may be an undue inducement to another. Is provision of diapers and lunch too valuable to an impoverished single mother with AIDS to make a voluntary decision unrealistic? Is the promise of food, shelter, and psychotherapy for 6 weeks so enticing that destitute alcoholics will agree to studies that include lumbar puncture but that have no reasonable expectation of direct medical benefit to the subject? An ethical dilemma is an ethical problem about which persons of good will and sound judgment will disagree. For example, whether patient volunteers who are also socioeconomically disadvantaged should be in a study without expectation of subject benefit is, at least to some, an ethical dilemma. Certainly, it is an ethical complexity that the investigator needs to ponder and discuss with colleagues and review bodies when arriving at protections that are neither too restrictive of enrollment nor insufficiently protective of subjects.

7. Research Subjects with Questionable Capacity

Patient volunteers whose capability to give ethically and legally valid consent is questionable present the clinical researcher with an important challenge. It is common that investigators need study subjects from populations in which such capacity may be questionable, either before or during participation in the study. Examples of volunteer subjects with whom the question might arise are those who are psychiatrically ill, are addicted to drugs, are cognitively impaired, or have recently received a diagnosis of terminal disease. Diagnostic labels can be misleading. Some depressed or psychotic patients will be able to provide valid consent, while others will not. Even evidence of moderate dementia should not, categorically, label a person as unable to make decisions. Diagnoses that are characteristically associated with alterations in mental status, however, ought to alert an investigator immediately to the possibility of questionable decision-making capacity. Study designs that require what is referred to as drug washouts, periods when persons will be removed from drugs that treat or affect mental status, can be anticipated to result in subjects who may have questionable capacity. The performance of a capacity assessment is required for all but those at the most extreme ends of the cognitive spectrum. How to conduct a capacity assessment is discussed in detail later in this chapter.

C. Minors

Minors are always considered vulnerable and, therefore, are always a special population. The special status of a minor is formalized in the U.S. research regulations and in regulations and clinical research guidance documents around the world. The DHHS regulations in the United States governing the involvement of minors (Code of Federal Regulations, Subpart D of 45 CFR 46; Appendix, No. 15) have been adopted by the FDA and are being applied globally through the process of harmonizing multinational regulations. Also, the Declaration of Helsinki and the CIOMS guidelines address the special concerns regarding participation of minors in clinical research. The view, however, that children are vulnerable research subjects has not halted the movement towards having more and more children in clinical research, particularly in drug trials. The rationale is that, because children are being prescribed drugs that have not been tested on children, their risk exposure is too high and they are not getting the medicines they need. Because both are true for some children, the momentum to include children in trials to develop new drugs has pushed to the forefront the need to attend to the ethical considerations of having children in clinical research. Examples include studies to test which educational format works best to motivate pediatric asthma sufferers to comply with their medical regimens and behavioral management studies of children with schizophrenia from low socioeconomic families in which at least one parent also has a psychiatric diagnosis. In either case, studies including minors are always complicated by the fact that parents will also be involved, if only to give permission for the child to participate. When a pediatric study poses more than a minimal risk to the child subject and the child is being raised by only one parent, considerations of how to obtain the non-rearing parent's permission, provided that parent is not absent completely or lacks custody rights, can be logistically and emotionally difficult. The process of obtaining assent from a child is often complex and is typically complicated by variability in developmental level in minors not only across the pediatric age spectrum, but also within the same age group, depending on experience with illness and health care professionals. That is, a young child who has been sick and in the medical community since birth may be more capable of providing a meaningful assent than an older adolescent who has been healthy. Processes for assessing developmental capacity to provide an assent related to the specifics of a protocol will need to be planned for and articulated in the protocol. How much about the purpose of the study is explained? How might being told by physician researchers that his or her mother or father is also psychiatrically ill affect a child with a psychiatric illness?

Depending on the age of the proposed pediatric subjects, how might developmentally appropriate magical thinking, coupled with the child's psychiatric and/or physical problems, affect his or her ability to appreciate the voluntary nature of research participation?

The participation of minors in clinical research involves considerations of a minor's developmental stage, the minor's ability to provide meaningful assent or dissent, the capacity of a parent or parents to provide ethically meaningful permission, and, most recently added, the regulatory pressure to involve children in trials more frequently. Like the previously discussed shift in moral assessment of how best to balance benefits and burdens in the inclusion of women of childbearing age or who are pregnant and of minority populations, a similar shift occurred in thinking about the involvement of minors in clinical research. In an atmosphere that is now biased toward their inclusion, the investigator must continue to comply with regulatory protections. The traditional ethical understanding that minors are vulnerable research subjects who require a higher than ordinary level of protection must continue to receive thoughtful attention.

The U.S. regulations and the developing International Conference on Harmonization (ICH) guidelines provide a useful context in which to consider these aspects in the design of pediatric research. The division of pediatric research into categories of direct benefit/no direct benefit, ordered by level of risk, has established a framework in which study design can be set. Like most of the regulations, however, the categories do not provide a formulaic answer to every research design issue. In pediatric research, one of the greatest stumbling blocks is the regulatory language of a "minor increase over minimal risk." Because this concept is not defined, investigators and IRBs or IECs are left to evaluate its meaning within the context of each protocol. The guidance on involvement of minors in the newest version of the Declaration of Helsinki (2000) adds some clarity, but this guidance does not apply to every study. Depending on the age and developmental stage of subjects, severity of the condition afflicting the study population and its other special vulnerabilities, plus the risk level of the study, achieving the appropriate balance between inclusion and protectiveness will always be a challenge in clinical research with minors.

1. Older Adolescents

When a study involves older adolescents, the balancing act can become very difficult. Because Western society has increasingly embraced notions of supporting self-determination over protectiveness, fostering the growing autonomy of adolescents has become an important component of their medical care. **Because the regulations for clinical research do not explicitly address adolescents, investigators and review bodies have to deliberate diligently to find the optimal balance of risks and benefits without such guidance.**

> For example, ought the dissent of a 17-year-old HIV-positive adolescent be honored over the objections of parents who want to enroll their child in a phase II trial of an anti-HIV agent? If dissent is not to be honored, what are the implications for the assent process?

Asking an adolescent, or even a developmentally mature younger child, to volunteer and then overriding that dissent may sow long-standing or permanent seeds of distrust. It might be better, if parental permission is going to govern, to provide the minor with information about what is to happen rather than to seek a meaningless dissent. Further, given that adolescents in many U.S. states can obtain treatment for sexually transmitted diseases or drug and alcohol abuse counseling without parental knowledge, such problems might be treated as private between an adolescent and an investigator in the clinical research setting. If so, what are the implications for separating minors from parents during the permission/assenting process and for record keeping? These are but a few of the issues that involvement of adolescents in research poses for the scientific and ethical design of a study.

2. Young Teens and Pre-teens

The involvement of young teens and pre-teens presents different kinds of scientific and ethical issues in study design. Although, for example, the average healthy young teenager or pre-teen may not be able to provide a meaningful assent or dissent to a complex research study, a teenager who has been ill for some time may be more knowledgeable about the illness and its implications than a healthy adult. There is no regulatory decision-making authority or standardized tool an investigator can employ to assess such understanding. Whereas the balance may now be weighted toward autonomous decision making by older adolescent subjects of research, extension of decision-making authority to young teens and pre-teens will be less easy to justify.

3. Toddlers and Infants

Judgments made about levels of protectiveness for toddlers and infants may be the most scientifically and ethically straightforward in all pediatric research. **These children are the most vulnerable because of their**

inability to understand anything substantive about the clinical research process, their developmental dependence on and need to trust their adult caregivers, the complexities of magical thinking in toddlers, and the desperation of parents of sick infants and toddlers. Their involvement may be justifiable scientifically because children at this stage of life can be presumed to have biologic processes quite different from those of teenagers and adults. Investigators should consider involving infants and toddlers only in studies of diseases or conditions when the scientific ends require their involvement. The regulations do not differentiate among infants, toddlers, and older children. Investigators must consider how additional protections for children and infants need to be customized depending on the risk level of the protocol, the acuteness and severity of the child's or infant's condition, and the level of desperation to be expected in the parents.

D. Fetal Research

In the United States, **fetal research can be carried out only if it is consistent with the health of the fetus, if the risk to the fetus is minimal, and if the research is associated with the least possible risk for achieving the anticipated results.** Investigators are prohibited by regulation from participating in decisions about pregnancy termination in the research setting or in determining viability of the fetus at termination. No inducements, monetary or otherwise, can be offered for pregnancy termination. Ordinarily, research on a fetus can be performed only when both parents provide fully informed consent. The consent of the father can be waived under certain conditions, specified in 45 CFR 46, 46.207.

Because fetal risk is so difficult to assess relative to other risk areas in human subjects research, the number of fetal research studies is very limited. Although scientifically difficult because of the physiological complexity of the fetal environment, the ethics of fetal research is straightforward. Only research with a reasonable expectation of direct benefit to the subject is allowed under U.S. federal law. Fetal surgery, an ethically complicated area of clinical care, is not regulated under these rules unless there is an IND or IDE number.

Much of the ethical complexity in the fetal research field concerns the source of **fetal tissue**, defined as tissue from nonliving human fetuses. But even the definition of the term *fetus* is not without conflict, given that it is not so precise. Although the **fetal period** is often defined as the period of time from 8 weeks after conception until birth, the DHHS regulations define **fetus** as the product of conception from the time of implantation. In

1993, the U.S. congress included in the National Institutes of Health Revitalization Act (Public Law 103-43) language restricting fetal tissue research and extending the previously enacted federal moratorium on such research. That ban was lifted by an executive order permitting research on fetal tissue with federal support. Nonetheless, the issues related to fetal tissue research continue to produce disagreement, which was fueled by the announcement of the cloning of the first human embryo. Since that time, consideration of the issue has most notably focused on the use of cell lines for the creation of cloned embryos and on the differences between research for therapeutic purposes and for human cloning. To date, there is a ban on U.S. federal funding of stem cell research, except that which employs a small number of already existing cell lines. Also, revisions to the DHHS regulations, Subpart B (46.206), require that research involving, after delivery, the placenta, the dead fetus, macerated fetal material or cells, tissue, or organs excised from a dead fetus must be conducted in accordance with any applicable federal, state, or local laws. Additionally, where information associated with any of these materials is recorded in a way that identifies a living person, such identifiable persons are considered research subjects and all relevant regulations apply. Because fetal tissue research is such a fast-moving area of research around the world, because so many persons believe that fetal tissue research holds the promise of producing medical progress, and because this is such an ethically controversial area of medical research, debate around these issues and regulatory and legislative activities can be expected to continue.

E. Special Communities

Consideration of whole communities as special populations is a relatively new phenomenon. Research regulations do not take into account notions of community. The regulatory structure governing human subjects research defines a **research subject** as a living person. The newest revision of the Declaration of Helsinki (2000) and the CIOMS guidelines, however, explicitly consider **communities** as research entities deserving protection. Even though a study may only pose acceptable levels of risk to individual subjects, it is understood that risks to subjects in the study may not be the only ones posed by study performance. For example, sensitivity to this issue evolved from the many studies performed for identification of the BRCA1 genetic mutation, which predisposes a person to breast cancer.

In the BRCA1 genetic research program, the community risk—albeit unanticipated—started when the investigators isolating the gene focused on an Ashkenazi Jewish population. The studies were designed so that samples were taken without identifiers, and so it was assumed that study results posed no risks, because no individual subjects could be identified. As the studies progressed, however, and it was found that Ashkenazi Jewish women had a greater risk of carrying the BRCA1 mutation than women in the general population, Ashkenazi Jewish women were stigmatized, resulting in individual harm.

Another example of risks for subjects developing as a result of a study is found in diabetes research among Native American populations. An investigation of the genetics of diabetes will include having diabetic patient volunteers and other family member volunteers fill out an anonymous, general health survey. The survey may include questions about alcohol consumption. Given that the survey is anonymous, no particular subject would be at risk for any consequence of the study. Nevertheless, because alcoholism is a recognized problem in some Native American populations and because alcoholism carries a stigma, such a study might present a substantial risk of perceived harm to the community instead of to an individual.

A more global kind of concern is the potential harm to communities caused by social inequalities in drug development around the world. As pressure mounts in the developed countries for improved therapeutic interventions, the pressure to run more clinical trials and to run them faster will continue unabated. Patients' and physicians' demands coupled with commercial interests will continue to push trials to the four corners of the world. These demands, together with the requirements of patent law and regulatory compliance in the processes of drug development and approval, plus the incentives for commercialization and profit, will drive trials further into research-naïve and perhaps impoverished populations. The effects that globalization of clinical research have on communities with very different levels of health care or systems for its provision, clinical research infrastructures, and political stability set the stage for potential harm to whole communities and countries. Such harm might take the shape of increased awareness of the inequities being experienced or create new grounds for discrimination based on genetic differences among and within populations. Potential harms have been expressed in terms of community self-rule versus ethical imperialism and the social injustice of exploitation of the weak by the strong.

These issues concerning clinical research's effects on communities as a whole can be considered at several levels. Internationally, the ethical and scientific demands on U.S.-sponsored clinical research conducted in impoverished nations and communities outside the United States are complex. Communities in the United States may be at risk as well. For example, development of drugs for a growing geriatric population who may not be able to pay for them presents its own potential community harms not experienced by individual subjects in a research protocol. Whether the community is a nation of people or subsets of people within a single nation, an investigator's consideration of community coupled with ideas of a special population can add several layers of effort to the preparation of a protocol, as discussed in the following section. Nonetheless, consideration of these effects is an important evolution in sensitivity that demands thoughtful attention. The potential for harm caused to communities by the conduct of clinical research can be expected to garner more attention from research ethicists, regulators, and attorneys in the future.

F. Special Protections for Special Populations

Special protections are needed when clinical research involves special populations. This requirement is articulated in clinical research regulations and international guidance documents. **When all or any of the subjects in a study's research population are likely to be vulnerable to coercion or undue influence, additional safeguards may be needed.** The U.S. regulations specify children, prisoners, pregnant women, mentally disabled persons, and subjects who are economically or socially disadvantaged as special populations. Among the first concerns when an individual in any of these groups, or any other potentially vulnerable subject, is to be involved in research is whether that individual is able to make his or her own decisions about research participation—whether that is about entering a study, agreeing to any particular procedure while on study, or about deciding when and if to end his or her study participation. Children are, by definition, unable to make such decisions. They will require additional protections discussed further in this section. Adults, however, are presumed capable of making their own choices unless evidence indicates the contrary. The ability of an adult at either end of the health spectrum to make his or her own research decisions is usually obvious. But there may be patient volunteers, and even some healthy volunteers, whose decision-making capacity is constrained. When decision-making capacity is questionable, proper assessment is required.

1. Capacity Assessment

The performance of a full and adequate assessment of a person's decision-making capacity in the clinical research setting is the same as it is in a clinical medicine setting (see Chapter 8 for additional information regarding assessing capacity to give consent to participate in a clinical research study). To consider an individual as having, or likely to have, questionable decision-making capacity requires a high level of suspicion on the part of the investigator. **Because consensus is lacking about what constitutes questionable capacity and who might suffer from it, investigators need to be sensitive and alert to its possible existence.** It is prudent to err on the side of caution by questioning capacity in a subject or subject population. Although some might argue that a bias toward persuming impaired capacity is paternalistic, disregard for the decision-making capacity of a subject has contributed to much of the history of research abuse and the residual mistrust of the research community. A high level of doubt about subject capacity upholds the principle of beneficence by protecting subjects from harm. It also upholds the principle of respect for persons. Making a vigorous effort to separate capable from impaired decision makers will protect those with limitations and allow those who have decision-making capacity to exercise it fully.

One of the obstacles to making such refined capacity determinations, however, is that capacity assessment is in its infancy. Some well-tested instruments exist (Berg *et al.*, 2001; Grisso and Appelbaum, 1998; White, 1994), but, for the most part, their use is not yet standard practice in either the clinical research or the clinical setting. Valid capacity assessment can be accomplished without standardized tools, however, by applying sound clinical judgment.

Historically, if a patient could tell the physician his or her name and location, that person was presumed to be capable of making decisions. A more refined appreciation of the differences between lucidity and meaningful decision making resulted in the use of standardized mental status exams to assess decisional capacity. There is now a growing awareness that the ability to pass a standard mental status examination, although necessary, is not sufficient.

Consensus regarding what is sufficient to be one's own decision maker in a clinical or research setting is growing (Chen *et al.*, 2002; Cherniack, 2002; Gill, 2003; van Staden and Kruger, 2003). **Like a patient in a clinical setting, a subject or a potential subject needs to meet four criteria by demonstrating four abilities or capacities:**

- To express a choice
- To understand information
- To appreciate consequences
- To manipulate information rationally (in ways consistent with the individual's beliefs about what is in his or her own best interest)

Expressing Choice

The first and most minimal criterion is the ability to express a choice. Physicians and researchers know that people can express themselves in many ways. Ideally, a person expresses himself or herself without any constraints; with sick patients, however, there are often constraints. For example, patients receiving mechanical ventilation may not be able to express a choice verbally but can still communicate their wishes in other ways, such as with facial expressions or by writing requests on a piece of paper. Paralyzed patients may be able to express a choice even when they are able to move only their eyelids. Research with patient volunteers who are seriously impaired requires additional time and, probably, requires individually designed mechanisms to ensure that they are expressing autonomously desired preferences.

Understanding Information

The second criterion is the ability to understand information. Exchanging and understanding information can be required of research subjects for many aspects of study participation. Understanding is difficult to evaluate. There are no standards for determining whether the depth of understanding is sufficient. Nonetheless, simple techniques can be employed to document that the individual perceives the meaning, significance, and explanation of the study well enough to make a reasoned choice.

One way to assess an individual's ability to understand information is to subdivide a study explanation into small sections. After each section is communicated, the prospective or participating subject can be asked to repeat what was said. Another way to test understanding is to ask the individual to explain, in his or her own words, the information just disclosed. Common sense responses to these tests are reasonable assurance for investigators that a sufficient level of understanding has been achieved.

Appreciating Consequences

The third criterion is the ability to appreciate consequences. Even if an individual can understand information, can he or she appreciate the consequences, or significance, of the choices to be made? As the level of risk surrounding a study rises, how well an individual meets this criterion becomes more important. Determining how much "appreciation of consequences" is sufficient, however, will require thoughtful discussion for each protocol.

Manipulating Information

The fourth criterion is often stated or defined as the ability to manipulate information rationally. Here, the individual is being asked to do more than appreciate potential consequences. This highest level of decision-making capacity demands that an individual be able to evaluate rationally the quality and consequences of his or her choices in a way that makes sense within the context of his or her consistently held beliefs and preferences.

The word *rational* has given philosophers trouble through the ages. Cognitive psychologists have tried to map it to brain activity. Definition is elusive. The ability to manipulate information rationally is particularly difficult to assess. For example, a schizophrenic patient may have demonstrated capacity at the three previous levels; however, when asked why she wants to participate in the study under discussion, she replies, "Because Martians have been beaming messages into my fillings that I am supposed to do this research." The researcher can deduce that a person with schizophrenia who makes decisions based on Martian messages is acting irrationally and lacks ability to make decisions in his or her best interest.

There was also a time when clinicians would have believed that a Jehovah's Witness who declined blood transfusion in the face of certain death was irrational. The refusal of blood products by a Jehovah's Witness is routinely accepted in the 21st century, even if some clinicians do see the choice as irrational and contrary to the patient's best interest. So when does thinking against mainstream beliefs cross the line to irrationality? Although this question has no clear answer, consistency can help in the assessment process. That is, if the belief has been held over a prolonged period of time and is perhaps held by others as well as by the individual being assessed, even manipulation of information in ways seemingly irrational to the researchers may not be considered a manifestation of impaired capacity.

Capacity assessment is complex and includes notions of a sliding scale. The more consequential the decision, the greater the person's capacity to make the decision needs to be, or the greater the need for the person to be protected from having a not-capacitated decision considered valid. As higher levels of complexity in abstract thought are demanded to assure a researcher that a subject has the capacity to make decisions related to research participation, professionals skilled in assessing decisional capacity for research can be usefully added to the assessment process. Traditionally, neurologists and psychiatrists have been asked to perform competence evaluations. Assessment of capacity to provide ethically and legally valid consent as a research subject, however, is not synonymous with competence. Physician investigators of any subspecialty and research ethicists are ordinarily sufficiently skilled in assessing capacity to determine whether or not an individual can provide ethically and legally valid consent.

Competence is a legal status adjudicated only in a court of law. That is, each of us is legally competent until deemed incompetent by a judge. That means, for example, comatose patients who clearly lack capacity to give consent are still competent unless they have been legally adjudicated incompetent. They are, however, not capable of giving informed consent. Any clinical or clinical research professional needs to have the skills to perform an appropriate assessment of capacity for research decision making. Failure to make a good faith effort to determine whether a potential or participating research subject is or is not capable of making his or her own decisions is no longer acceptable.

The following case provides an example of how difficult it can be to make the appropriate assessment. One morning at a major research center, as the bioethicist is coming onto the floor for rounds, one of the research nurses comes running up to her. "Please come into Ms. Wilson's room. She has been trying to leave for the last 12 hours and the principal investigator, Dr. Kelly, has been sitting with her all night trying to convince her to stay until her antibiotics are finished. He's gone home to sleep a few hours and we've been trying to reason with her, but she just keeps insisting that she wants to leave. She's accusing all of us of being racist and sexist for not letting her leave. She says we're just using her as a guinea pig. We keep telling her we won't do any research procedure and that we don't want to keep her here for research, but that she has a serious infection that needs more treatment. Dr. Kelly said to get you involved as soon as you arrived." Ms. Wilson is a woman of color who has just had a bone marrow transplant. She has a fever and infection for which she is receiving intravenous (IV) antibiotics. When the bioethicist walks into the room and sits down with the subject, she finds that Ms. Wilson is fully alert and clearly expressing her wish to be released. The nurse, in front of the bioethicist, tells Ms. Wilson again that there are no research procedures being performed and that she needs to stay in the hospital to finish her antibiotics. Ms. Wilson responds that she does not care what the nurse says and it is her right to leave. The nurse replies that yes, it is her right, but that if she leaves without getting over this infection she may die. Ms. Wilson starts yelling, "I don't care if I die. I want out of this horrible place!" She seems to understand the information she is being given. The bioethicist, however, is uneasy that, although this woman seems to meet the first three criteria for being capacitated, and nobody has questioned her capacity, she simply is not able to meet the fourth criteria. When asked why she wants to leave, she simply says, "I don't have to answer you." When pushed further with, "Are you afraid you might die?", Ms. Wilson responds

Continued

with, "Die, die, die. I want out of here." Given the potentially grave consequences of this decision, whether or not she really is capable of making this
decision is a critical assessment to make correctly. In reviewing Ms. Wilson's
protocol, it is noted that a complication of bone marrow transplantation is
depression. The suspicion that Ms. Wilson may be lucid but not capacitated
is further supported by a slightly pressured nature of her speech and the fast
rate at which she is talking. Even though she seems to be making sense, she
is acting in such a potentially self-harming way, after having agreed to go
through such a difficult procedure, that Ms. Wilson's behavior is simply not
adding up. The bioethicist speaks with the psychiatrist on consultation, who
evaluates Ms. Wilson. In the course of the evaluation it is mentioned that Ms.
Wilson had been given morphine, but that it was discontinued 8 hours ago. A
known side effect of morphine is delirium. The final judgment is that the
patient has a morphine psychosis and, thus, is not a capable decision maker.
Ms. Wilson agrees to stay until her brother can come and get her. By the time
he arrives several hours later, the morphine has worn off, and Ms. Wilson is
no longer threatening to leave. Her antibiotics are continued and she is safely
discharged 10 days later.

2. Non-Research-Affiliated Physicians

The involvement of physicians who are not a part of the clinical research
study is a mechanism for subject protection that is gaining attention.
Participation of a clinician not affiliated with the clinical research study in
assessment of decision-making capacity of subjects adds objectivity to the
recruitment process.

Beyond eligibility, during the study, the unaffiliated physician can serve
as an additional advocate for the research subject. Especially in studies
where the subjects may experience distress or discomfort prior to meeting
off-study criteria, an unaffiliated physician can provide support for removing subjects from the protocol ahead of standardized off-study evaluations.

3. Clinical Research Surrogates and Surrogate Permission

A **surrogate** makes the decision for an individual's participation after the
research subject or the potential subject has been judged incapable of
decision making or makes a research study decision for a minor child. In a
clinical research study, a surrogate decision maker is a person designated
to make decisions for a research subject who is unable to give his or her
own consent. The regulatory descriptor of a surrogate decision maker is a
legally authorized representative. The DHHS regulations do not, however,
specify this term. State and/or local jurisdictions specify who can serve as
a legally authorized, or acceptable, representative. Generally, however,

state and local jurisdictions have not clarified who such representatives might be or for what kinds of research such persons can give proxy consent, which poses problems for clinical researchers and review bodies.

Traditionally, the person chosen to speak for a research subject was identified in the same way as in the clinical setting. In clinical care, a surrogate is most often simply the person who is with the patient when the patient is unable to speak for himself or herself at the time medical care is needed. As long as the surrogate is attempting to make decisions in the best medical interest of the patient, this method is adequate for clinical treatment. This relaxed attitude about who speaks on behalf of a patient volunteer in research has been the common practice. Past research abuses, however, have taught the field that surrogate issues in clinical research are in need of greater attention.

When a study involves a surrogate, provisions need to be made to educate the surrogate about his or her role. In clinical research, the surrogate decision maker has to be alert to ethical complexities that are greater in the clinical research setting than in clinical care. The research surrogate has to understand whether the protocol provides any realistic expectation of direct benefit for the subject. Even in research with direct benefit, surrogates need to be educated that the demands of science require subjects will not be cared for as if they were clinical patients. That is, research surrogates need to understand that subjects will receive care in accordance with the approved protocol. If the research participant's clinical needs fall outside the approved protocol, he or she will not be included in the study and will be transferred to clinical care. This, in itself, means that the research participant does not receive the customized, personalized care he or she would be expected to receive in a clinical setting. The research surrogate needs to understand whether some of the planned procedures are of minimal risk and which, if any, are of greater than minimal risk. The research surrogate is obligated to monitor subject welfare more vigorously than a clinically responsible surrogate might need to monitor the progress of a patient in the clinical setting.

Another concern is that the person who is the research surrogate may also be a burdened caregiver. The surrogate may be an exhausted caregiver of a demented older adult or the parent of a severely and chronically ill child.

For example, a wife who has been taking care of her mentally impaired husband at home would be expected to be his research surrogate when he is invited into a Parkinson's disease protocol. When the protocol involves a long in-patient stay, the wife may be eager to see her husband in a safe setting during which she gets a rest from his 24-hour care.

The same ethical concern applies to obtaining surrogate permission from a single mother of three young children, one of whom is chronically ill. If there is an invitation for the chronically ill child to be in a research study that includes prolonged in-patient stays, the prospect of respite can be a powerful motivator to provide parental permission. The anticipation of respite in both cases may constitute an undue inducement for the surrogate. An investigator will want to be very careful that an exhausted family member is not giving permission for a subject's participation merely so that the surrogate obtains the benefit of relief from the burden of his or her care-giving responsibility.

4. Durable Power of Attorney for Research Participation

A novel protection for adults who lack the ability to give valid consent is the **Durable Power of Attorney (DPA) for Research Decisions**. First developed and still only used regularly at the NIH Clinical Center, the research DPA is a document that should be more widely utilized in clinical research. Similar to the DPA for health care, the DPA for research assigns an agent to be the responsible decision maker at any time the individual is unable to make his or her own research decisions. The document can be drawn up to allow the potential subject to identify the categories and risk levels of research in which he or she would be willing to participate. Like a clinical DPA, the research DPA can be executed only at a time when the individual is a competent and capacitated decision maker. We recommend that such a document be attached to protocols involving persons who are anticipated to become incapable of decision making during a study. We also recommend that research institutions develop policies that incorporate the use of a DPA for research.

Durable Power of Attorney for Health Care Decision Making
in Research

INSTRUCTIONS: You have the right to name someone to make decisions regarding your medical care and research participation if you are not able to make decisions for yourself. Please fill out PART 1 of this form if you wish to name someone to make decisions concerning your clinical care and participation in research in the event you are unable to make your own decisions. You may state in PART 2 your preferences for whether or not various forms of medical treatment including life-sustaining measures should be provided, withheld, or discontinued. This Durable Power of Attorney (DPA) form should reflect (not

---

Continued

replace) the discussion of these and other issues with your personal doctor, your research doctor(s), family, and the person you name. This form must be signed and witnessed in PART 3.

( ) DPA Required for Enrollment on IRB Approved Protocol

PART 1

I, _____ (the patient volunteer), authorize the person(s) named below, in the event that I become unable to make decisions, to exercise power of attorney for health care and research participation over my person for the sole purpose of making decisions on my behalf for my clinical care and participation in research. Unless revoked by me orally, or in writing, the person shall hold the durable power of attorney for health care decision making until I complete my participation in clinical care and research at _____ (name of institution where research is being conducted).

TO: **Person receiving durable power of attorney for health care and research decision making:**

Name:

Address:

       (city)   (state)   (zip)

Telephone: Home: Work:

ALTERNATE: **If the named person receiving durable power to make health care and research participation decisions for me is unavailable, I name this person (optional):**

Name:

Address:

       (city)   (state)   (zip)

Telephone: Home: Work:

Continued

PART 2

STATEMENT OF DESIRES, PREFERENCES, VALUES, SPECIAL PRO-
VISIONS, AND/OR LIMITATIONS: It is important that the person you
name makes health care decisions that reflect your known desires,
preferences, and values. Therefore, you should discuss your desires,
preferences, and values with the person named, your personal doctor,
your research doctor(s), and your family. You are encouraged, but are
not required, to state your desires, preferences, and values in the space
provided below. You may wish to include a statement of your desires
concerning life-sustaining care being provided, withheld, or discontinued. Also, you may ask your personal or research doctor. If additional
space is needed, please attach additional sheets to this form.

[ ] CONTINUATION SHEET ATTACHED

PART 3

PATIENT VOLUNTEER SIGNATURE: You and one witness must sign
this document for it to be valid. This DPA is valid only at _____
(name of institution).

_____ (Patient Volunteer Signature) _____ (Date)

WITNESS SIGNATURE: The role of the witness is to assure that the person who signed as "patient volunteer" is the individual who appointed
the person named in this document. The witness may not be the person
receiving the durable power of attorney or the physician who is directly
responsible for medical and/or research decisions involving the care of
the patient volunteer.

(Witness Signature)   (Date)

5. Consent Monitors

The concept of consent monitors was established in the first human subjects regulations formulated by DHHS but has never been widely used.
Section 46.109 (C) of the DHHS regulations 45 CFR 46 gives the IRB the
authority to observe or have a third party observe the consent process
and the research. Rarely does an IRB exercise this authority. This is
partly because IRBs trust investigators to carry out their protocols as
approved, because the IRBs are overworked, and because the process of

such monitoring is logistically difficult. Nonetheless, consent monitoring presents the possibility of an important additional protection. It might be a part of a clinical research training program for novice investigators, or consent monitoring might be applied to the first five or six subjects for a highly complex, high-risk, no-expected-direct-benefit study. Although unlikely to be widely employed, consent monitors are an additional protection that might well be employed judiciously.

6. Language Translation and Interpreters

When study subjects speak different languages, translation of documents and the incorporation of translators into the clinical research setting are important protections for subjects. When a multinational or a multicenter trial that crosses language boundaries is designed, all written material relevant to a research subject (e.g., consent/assent documents, educational information, referral sources) needs to be translated into as many languages and/or dialects as are needed to ensure that study subjects can read them. What may not be so obvious is that one-way translation may be inadequate. Optimally, material requiring translation is best checked through a process of back-translation (i.e., the translated information is translated back into the original language) to help ensure that idiomatic aspects of either language do not result in distortion of the meaning of the document that was approved by the IRB and/or IEC. The IRB and/or IEC of record must approve the original documents and will also have to approve the back-translations of those documents.

Translating documents, however, may not be sufficient protection. If, for example, a non-English-speaking subject comes to the United States to enter a study, he or she may need assistance with more than just consent issues and other paperwork. The sicker the patient volunteer, the greater the need for assistance in communication, either directly or with family or friends who have accompanied him or her. Researchers often rely on an accompanying family member or friend to serve as a translator. This may not be a satisfactory situation. Family or friends, for reasons related to cultural difference, emotional attachment to the patient volunteer, or constraints of hierarchical family and/or social structure, may consciously or unconsciously alter or distort the meaning when translating to or from a foreign language. **It is best, therefore, to have an objective translator present at agreed upon times throughout the day so that all communications can be as clear as possible.** The patient volunteer, his or her family or friends, and the investigative and care-giving staff can establish a schedule to optimize communication with and on behalf of the patient volunteer.

An example of how such cultural norms can present problems for communicating relevant research information is the case of a wealthy foreign family that comes to the United States so that the wife of the most senior male in the family can be on a protocol of a new treatment for a chronic and lethal disease. Because women from this community do not make their own decisions about many things, including research participation, her husband and eldest sons insist on being in the room when anyone seeks consent from the subject or wants to convey substantive information to her. Because the middle son is the only one who speaks English, he has to be present at all such times too. The problem is that because the middle son is culturally trained to defer to his older brother, they both defer to their father, and their father constantly speaks for his wife, it is impossible to know what the patient volunteer wants and what her husband wants. At first, the research team attempts to work within the family's preferred mode of communications, but things quickly break down. The research team is uncomfortable about whether or not research participation consent is being voluntarily given. They also suspect that the translating son is not providing a full translation and is translating information in a far more positive light than it is being conveyed to him. It is clear to everyone on the research team that the present situation cannot continue, and they obtain the services of a disinterested translator. Once the researchers are confident that information is being accurately conveyed, they are torn about their own unease with the cultural status this patient volunteer has within her family, but they are unsure how to manage the issue. Should they attempt to force the family into complying with the cultural norms of the environment in which the research is taking place? Should the research team accept the differences in cultural norms and attempt to do the best they can given the cultural differences? Should they decide that the patient volunteer is simply not an appropriate research subject, terminate her research participation, and transfer her back to the care of a physician in her own country?

7. Community Input into Study Design

Community input into the study design of U.S.-funded emergency medicine research is regulated. These requirements are discussed fully in Chapter 14. Emergency medicine research, however, is not the only kind of clinical research for which it might be prudent to involve the community in which the study is to take place or that is representative of the population to be studied. **Community consultation** is the consideration of protecting whole communities when planning and conducting clinical research and is a relatively novel notion/development. This type of consultation, however, has been used for some time in research involving Native American populations. Because Native American populations have tribal structures with identifiable community leaders, investigators have sought community input and approval for many years. The idea is that when clinical research is to be conducted in identifiable communities, especially communities that may be vulnerable because of problems such as poverty or gang violence and can be expected to have an interest in research performance and results, the community under study ought to be part of the clinical research process.

The common but unsophisticated approach to community involvement in clinical research is that once a study is designed and protocols are approved, researchers attend community events to present the research project to the community before formal subject recruitment begins. A more refined approach, albeit inherently more time consuming and logistically complex, is to include the community in the study design team from the outset. Positive outcomes can be that the community supports the project by assisting, or at least supporting, subject recruitment and retention. Research needs bridges to be built between community and researchers. To build trust from the outset is optimal. There are, however, problems to this approach. Most notably, it is often difficult to define just what is a community and even more difficult to identify the appropriate community leaders with whom to consult. If the community is outside of the United States, where ethical standards may differ from those of the investigators (e.g., foreign communities in which women do not make decisions independently), it can be difficult to ensure that community leaders are not making decisions for individual subjects. Nonetheless, acceptance of the concept of community consultation appears to be growing. Researchers can expect more questions about community involvement by protocol reviewers as this trend progresses.

IV. WRITING THE PROTOCOL SECTION ON SUBJECT SELECTION

The section of the protocol on **subject selection** should include justification for the proposed subject population as well as the inclusion and exclusion criteria.

A. Characterization and Justification for the Proposed Population

Justification for selection of the proposed study population includes **a description of specific characteristics of subjects who are required and why these subjects are optimal for the proposed study**. This section is not the place to explain in depth the vulnerabilities of the study population, but it is useful to refer to special concerns presented in the population. This section might also conclude with an explanation of specific ethical considerations presented by characteristics of the study subjects that will be fully addressed in the ethics section of the protocol.

B. Inclusion Criteria

In the inclusion criteria section, medical, demographic, and psychosocial conditions or characteristics of subjects should be specified in precise detail. Given that recruitment can be a prolonged process, exclusion of any appropriately eligible subject is undesirable. On the other hand, inclusion criteria that are too broad can result in a degree of variability among subjects that makes interpretation of data difficult or impossible.

C. Exclusion Criteria

Immediately following the inclusion criteria is the section on exclusion criteria. Notions of safety and risk are also to be considered in the **exclusion criteria** section, but they will be addressed from a slightly different perspective. In this section, it is important to **identify those characteristics that would disqualify potential subjects and/or necessitate removal of a subject if the characteristics happen to appear during the study.** If the medical inclusion criteria are thoroughly defined, the first group of exclusions is essentially the inverse. Here, however, instead of thinking expansively, the researcher will have to narrow the subject population. Although difficult, and sometimes impossible, the researcher should attempt to anticipate all medical conditions that might interfere with the interpretation of scientific findings or might compromise subject safety. The researcher should exclude the individuals with these conditions or characteristics from enrollment.

RISKS AND BENEFITS IN CLINICAL RESEARCH

· · · · · · · · · · · · · · · · ·

Balancing risks and benefits is the core ethical responsibility in clinical research. This responsibility is shared among investigators, oversight bodies, and any professional and/or surrogate involved in the performance of a research study with human subjects. The responsibility, however, falls most heavily on the shoulders of the principal investigator (PI). Meeting this responsibility begins with study design.

As already mentioned in previous chapters, when thinking about risks and benefits, **expected benefits must outweigh risks**, whether those are benefits to individual study subjects or to society. **The balance between risks and benefits must always be tipped in favor of protecting the rights and welfare of individual study participants.** Tipping benefits in favor of research subjects means that

- No matter how important the potential benefit may be to a specific subject (e.g., tumor shrinkage in a patient with cancer), a study must not place subjects at unreasonable or excessive risk, and
- No matter how important the information to be gained could be to the progress of medicine, individual study participants must not be subjected to unreasonable or excessive risk.

In the abstract, these constraints on risk seem straightforward; however, shaping the appropriate balance of risks and potential benefits in a

97

specific protocol is often highly complex. That is, finding the ethically optimal tipping point between potential risks and benefits can be a very difficult task. There is no consensus about the meaning of terms such as *excessive risk* or *unreasonable risk*. Although there are some attempts in the literature to describe excessive risk as risk of irreversible disability or death (Temple, 2002; Temple and Meyer, 2003), even setting these boundaries will not clarity all possibilities.

Attempts to define terms related to quantification of risk are a bit more successful at the low end (i.e., minimal risk) of the risk spectrum. The only risk term that is defined in U.S. regulations is *minimal risk* (45 CFR 46; Appendix, No. 15). **Minimal risk**, according to DHHS regulations (46.102), means that the probability and magnitude of harm or discomfort anticipated in the research are not greater in and of themselves than those ordinarily encountered in daily life or during the performance of routine physical or psychological tests. This definition has been consistently interpreted to refer to risk that is inherent in the daily lives of healthy individuals. The ability of review bodies to assess risk becomes more complex as risk rises. For example, regulations in the United States specify that to be approved by an IRB, pediatric research with no expected direct benefit to the subject must not present any risk greater than a minor increase over the minimum risk. What a minor increase over minimal risk might be, however, is not defined. This leaves IRBs, IECs, other reviewers, clinical research ethicists, investigators, and sponsors to estimate what might be only a minor increase above minimal risk in any specific protocol.

The most clear regulatory language relevant to this issue is that the risk must be justified by the anticipated benefit to a subject or society. In the pediatric research field, it is specified that, "the relation of the anticipated benefit to the risk is at least as favorable to the subjects as that presented by available alternative approaches" [Appendix, No. 15, Common Rule, 45 CFR 46, 46.405, (b)]. Otherwise, the U.S. regulations require that (i) risks be minimized and that (ii) risks to subjects be reasonable in relation to anticipated benefits to subjects or society.

In the matter of benefits, the regulations are instructive but are not a blueprint. The IRB is required to consider only those risks and benefits that may result from the research, not the risks or benefits subjects would receive even if they were not participating in the study (Appendix, No. 15, Common Rule, 45 CFR 46, 46.111).

Thus, concerning risks and benefits, regulatory language does not provide the investigator with a formula to compare risks against benefits. The assessment of risk and benefit is an essential component of the design, review, and monitoring phases of each protocol. This includes monitoring and evaluating how study procedures may produce actual risks to individual subjects throughout the course of the study.

I. WEIGHING RISK OF HARM AGAINST POTENTIAL FOR BENEFITS

Balancing risk of harm against potential for benefit is made complex by the differences between subjects and society in their needs to be protected from harm and to benefit from the research. Patients and clinicians need new and improved medical diagnostics and therapeutics. Patients and the public need to know that approved medical interventions are safe and effective. New, safe, and more effective medical interventions are the benefits society reaps from the clinical research enterprise. These social benefits, however, are often, but not always, consistent with potential benefits to research participants. Willingness to serve as a clinical research participant includes altruism mixed with additional motives, such as human hope and desperation. Altruism of investigators and sponsors mixes with drives for fame and profit. The complex combination of potential benefits for society and subjects can push the clinical research process forward in ways that can undermine balancing risks and benefits in ways that appropriately protect the rights and welfare of subjects. When the balance tips in the wrong direction, disaster strikes. Then revelations of abuse produce public outrage that the risk-to-benefit balance has been inappropriately weighted against subjects. These revelations often cause clinical research to temporarily slow down. Eventually, corrective actions are taken through legislative, policy, and/or professional practice changes, and the clinical research engine picks back up. Finding the optimal balance between risks to individual research participants and the pursuit of the research benefits is complex. The optimal balance point is not static. Ethical standards evolve with time. The evolution of ethics, however, has largely favored increasing the protection of individual study subjects.

A. Benefits to Society

The earliest stages of investigation of new treatments or cures will often be clinical research that benefits society through the production of new knowledge but does not directly benefit subjects. As already mentioned, there are those who advocate the abolition of all clinical research with no expected direct benefit. Such thinking may be dangerous to medical progress and, worse, does not serve to protect research subjects. Clinical research that moves too quickly will eventually do harm to others. Instead, clinical research, to be sound, must not skip any of the necessary developmental steps from bench to approved therapeutics. In this process, there are times when a researcher cannot simply get from point A to point B without performing human studies that present no reasonable expectation of direct benefit for the subjects.

Equally problematic is the perspective that the lion's share of the responsibility for study participant protection should be in the hands of the individual research participant. This view claims that as long as a subject is able to provide ethically and legally valid informed consent, each person can weigh for himself or herself the risks and benefits. When an individual is unable to do so, the surrogate performs this function.

Certainly, the informed consent process is one important way in which the individual research subject weighs the risks and benefits of a particular study. **Informed consent is necessary. It is not, however, sufficient.** Informed consent never should be the sole or even the primary approach to the balancing of risks and benefits. The primary means for assuring an appropriate balance between risks and benefits is a well-designed protocol that is followed punctiliously. Responsibility for designing, approving, and monitoring a protocol is held jointly by those who sponsor and/or develop the protocol; by the investigator who brings the protocol forward for review and approval; and by those who approve, conduct, and oversee the performance of the protocol. When each of these entities meets its obligations of alertness to potential risks; minimizing them where possible, protecting subjects from them when risks cannot be avoided, and assuring that the study is designed to produce useful scientific information, then an appropriate balance between risks and benefits begins.

Clinical research designed to benefit only society presents a special set of ethical concerns. **The central question is, how much risk should an individual accept on behalf of the benefit of others? In other words, what level of risk is considered reasonable, fair, just, or ethically acceptable for the subject?** Questions that naturally follow focus on differences among subject populations. What are the morally relevant differences in answers to this question when a subject is a healthy adult who is capacitated; an adult who is capacitated but ill; an adult who is not capacitated; a child who is healthy; or a child who is sick?

In the preceding chapter on selecting human subjects for clinical research, Chapter 5, some morally relevant differences across study populations were highlighted. In the present chapter we address vulnerability to coercion. **The less able a prospective or participating subject is to make his or her own decisions, the more vulnerable he or she is to undue influence.**

As discussed in Chapter 3, regulatory guidance exists for some specific situations, such as research with children, prisoners, or pregnant women. The international guidance documents are increasingly specific about such matters. Moral norms continue to evolve in ever more restrictive directions. Added to the existing regulatory restrictions on pediatric research, the disinclination to involve adults who are incapable of making their own decisions in high-risk research is growing more pronounced, as is evidenced by the most recent changes to the Declaration of Helsinki. Nonetheless, there is still no consensus in the fields of clinical research or clinical research ethics about the best way to balance risks against potential benefits for the almost limitless variations in subject populations. These evaluations continue to have to be made on a protocol-by-protocol basis.

Some in the patient advocacy community wish to exclude any subject who is unable to give his or her consent when the research is to benefit society only. This position is slightly different from that of the Nuremberg Code, which excludes decisionally impaired adults and children, who are unable to provide their own consent, from all participation. The notion that only clinical research promising direct medical benefit should be permitted for the latter groups may put ethically unacceptable blockades in the road of medical progress. To exclude decisionally impaired adults or child subjects from no-direct-benefit research may mean that information needed to move to direct-benefit research is unobtainable. These complexities can be adequately addressed by introducing appropriate risk minimization strategies and mechanisms to ensure that subject dignity and all other rights remain intact.

The Declaration of Helsinki was a liberalizing response to the Nuremberg Code. For participants in research with no expectation of direct benefit to the subjects, increasing layers of protective oversight is the remedy proposed. The protections most frequently considered are discussed in Chapter 5. One level of protection is the delegation of decision making to a responsible surrogate or guardian. Another is the assent/dissent process. Adding unaffiliated physician advocates for research subjects is another. But, as with all else, **determining the acceptable level of risk for a subject to take for the good of another must be addressed early in the protocol design phase.** The investigator/sponsor, perhaps with assistance from members of the potential subject populations, develop their answer to this core question concerning what is an acceptable risk for a subject to take. Once the investigator and sponsor have made their decision explicit in the study design and justification(s) presented in the protocol, it is up to the IRB/IEC to decide whether or not it agrees.

One final point of controversy about research with no expectation of direct benefit to the subject concerns altruism. Altruism, although frequently cited as a potential benefit of research participation, is difficult to measure. Some doubt that altruism exists. Rather, if a protocol does not hold out the prospect of direct medical benefit to individual subjects, the study is considered a no-direct-benefit study. Nonetheless, altruistic reward can be of value to subjects, and important lessons about altruistic behavior can be learned by participation in research.

B. Benefits to Participating Subjects

When research indicates a realistic prospect of direct medical benefit to a subject, it may be quite difficult to keep separate the goals of clinical research and the goals of clinical care. Expected-direct-benefit research is often a last-ditch effort at potentially useful medical intervention in the face of life-threatening or chronic disease. For this reason it may be more difficult to find the optimal balance between risks and benefits than it usually is in a study with no expected benefit to the participants. Addition of the hope of helping sick individuals introduces an urgency that can push the limits of risk taking too far, too fast.

In research that is designed with a reasonable expectation of direct medical benefit to individual subjects, the core ethical question is, **what is an acceptable level of risk that a subject should take in the quest for a theoretically plausible, personal medical benefit**? For those incapable of making this decision, the question to be answered by the responsible surrogate is, **how much risk ought one accept on behalf of another in the quest for a theoretically plausible medical benefit for the individual research participant**? Answers to these two questions reside in the study design process.

Some areas of medical research have standards of practice regarding acceptable levels of risk. For example, the field of oncology research has standardized toxicity staging guidelines that are applied by researchers around the world. That is, when certain specified toxicities occur, regardless of how much risk a subject is willing to incur, the subject will be removed from the study. Specificity of this kind in communitywide standards-of-research practice is, however, rare. Rather, the specification of risk levels in research with expected benefit to the subjects will be developed through the formalization of the inclusion and exclusion criteria of each study.

The gravest ethical concern about research with the expectation of direct subject benefit is that the sick patient's and/or their surrogate's desperation will combine so intensely with an investigator's enthusiasm for a particular intervention that research will rush forward too quickly. The brain tissue transplantation in Parkinson's disease research (Freed *et al.*, 2001; see case discussion in Chapter 15) is a quintessential demonstration of this problem. Nowhere has there been any hint that anything but altruistic motivation played a role in the rapid advance of this line of research.

Unlike the Jesse Gelsinger case (see case discussion in Chapter 15) that was tainted by the perception of financial conflicts of interest, the brain tissue transplantation work in Parkinson's disease was a model of the altruistic pursuit of medical progress at its most pristine. Nonetheless, that work, too, suffered a serious setback because it moved too quickly from bench to bedside and produced a research tragedy. Subjects were harmed. Although this research was charted with the best of intentions and without any obvious errors in either scientific or ethical judgment, one wonders if the adverse outcomes could have been avoided.

Examples of studies in which the only benefit anticipated is to society and studies that extend the prospect of a direct medical benefit to the study participants highlight the differences and the difficulties in evaluating how much risk is too much when compared to the potential benefits. Consider a study that falls into the first category. Huntington's chorea is a terrible disease. It is a dominantly inherited neurological condition that produces motor and cognitive deterioration but does so at a heartbreakingly slow pace. The Huntington's patient ordinarily declines over a period of 10–20 years. The most frequent time of onset is mid-life, in the 30s and 40s, after the individual has had children, but before having the opportunity to watch one's children grow and mature. Additionally, because the age of onset is usually past prime childbearing years, the ability to decide not to have children to avoid passing the genetic mutation on to one's offspring is past. Because Huntington's is a brain disease of the basal ganglia that most severely affects the caudate and putamen, it is important to learn more about how these brain structures function in normal persons and in Huntington's patients. One of the best ways to study these structures is with the use of advanced technology imaging techniques. Unfortunately, many of these techniques require injecting research participants with radio-labeled substances to be able to see the body parts of interest—in this case various parts of the brain. Gaining this kind of information is critically important to the advancement of medical knowledge needed to develop future treatments and, one hopes, eventually a cure for diseases such as Huntington's.

It is up to the investigator, however, to shape the specific research questions needed to produce these therapeutic advances. First, one needs to better understand fundamental, normal brain chemistry and physiology. To do that one has to study brain activity in persons with healthy brains. This means injecting healthy persons with small amounts of radiated material. Even though the amounts needed for the scans are equivalent to a tiny fraction of the radiation everyone is exposed to daily in the general environment, less radiation is surely better than more radiation. How much additional radiation, that is how much radiation used strictly for research purposes, ought a healthy person be asked to have over and above normal daily experience? Is the amount equivalent to a standard set of dental X-rays reasonable? How many scans might it be reasonable to ask a healthy research subject to have—only one per some specified time period or some number greater than one but less than four or six or eight? In the face of no or little data indicating that some amount of research radiation exposure produces measurable harm, on what basis does an investigator, sponsor, or review body decide how much radiation exposure is too much for a healthy subject to accept?

Changing this study example slightly, let us consider the same brain-imaging study, but this time let us have persons with Huntington's chorea be subjects, rather than healthy volunteers. What morally relevant difference, if any, does the switch in subject population produce? Given that the scans will be considered greater-than-minimal risk in either study, might it be acceptable to allow risk to float a bit higher in the sick subjects rather than the healthy ones? If so, what would be the ethical justification(s)? Given that Huntington's causes mental deterioration, should such a study be restricted to only those person's with Huntington's who were still sufficiently mentally intact to provide their own consent? What if the goal of the study was to learn more about how the brains of Huntington's patients change over time? Is this even a question that can be ethically pursued? If so, what kinds of additional protections would need to be put in place to protect Huntington's subjects who were unable to make their own decisions?

Are the questions any easier to answer if the study was designed to provide some direct medical benefit? In brain imaging studies, findings that might be of clinical utility to the subject might emerge. In the studies considered here, however, such findings would only be incidental. When the intent is to explore fundamental brain activity, the study is in the no-direct-benefit category. What if there were a study of a novel agent to treat Huntington's? Although promising, the agent is known to produce serious adverse reactions in some persons and there is presently no way to predict who will have such unpleasant reactions. Also, although the experimental agent is promising for the newly diagnosed, still decisionally intact Huntington's patients, the real promise is for use in advanced-stage Huntington's patients. Ought the study only test the agent on early-stage patient volunteers who can still give their own consent, even if the agent has the possibility of making the little quality time they have left worse if any particular subject has an anticipatable adverse event? Should the study include late-stage patient volunteers, those for whom the agent has the most promise, but who will no longer be able to provide their own consent? These are complex and difficult questions that require investigators, sponsors, and review bodies to think hard and discuss the implications of those questions at length. Once the decisions about the design have been made, reviewed, probably amended, and finally approved, close monitoring of study and individual subject progress will be needed to determine if adjustments are needed as the protocol progresses.

II. REGULATORY REQUIREMENTS FOR MINIMIZATION OF RISK

There are two widespread and universally accepted risk minimization strategies well established in regulation. One is the **voluntary consent of the informed research participant or the permission of an informed surrogate**. The second is the **independent review and approval of a research study by an IRB, IEC, or equivalent body**. These two processes, which are required by regulation in most countries where human studies are conducted, serve as the baseline for risk minimization for subjects. Beyond this, other regulations and documents provide explication of these requirements with varying degrees of specificity and clarity.

For example, although the Nuremberg Code demands voluntary consent, external review was an international innovation of the Declaration of Helsinki. Whereas the code excludes children and adults who are too impaired to make decisions about research participation, the Declaration of Helsinki permits participation by these groups under specified conditions. When a subject is in a dependent relationship with a physician/investigator, that investigator should not be the person to obtain consent for research participation.

The U.S. regulations, extended internationally through the FDA and the ICH, require that IRBs and IECs minimize risk by ensuring that additional protections are in place when subjects may be vulnerable. Also required is that research procedures should be performed as part of those already required by clinical care where possible and that the preparation of data management plans should be made to enhance subject safety and protection of confidentiality. Risk level is limited in pediatric research by established regulatory risk categories. If pediatric subjects are wards of the state or the research involves incarcerated individuals, subject advocates are required. In the case of prisoners, children, or adults who are too impaired to provide consent to research participation, risk is minimized by prohibiting their involvement in clinical research unless it pertains directly to their medical or social condition (depending on which document or set of regulations are applied to the study).

III. STUDY PROCEDURES FOR MINIMIZATION OF RISK

Each study will have procedures specifically designed to minimize risk, depending on the characteristics of subjects and nature of the experimental plan. These procedures are integral, not merely adjunctive, to a study. They should be explained in the protocol and perhaps also in the consent/assent documents.

A. Inclusion and Exclusion Criteria

Inclusion and exclusion criteria should allow for the largest pool of potential subjects that is possible with safety as the defining factor. Exclusion criteria are selected to avoid, from the outset, as many potential safety problems as possible. Inclusion and exclusion criteria are best crafted so that only the least vulnerable individuals in the subject pool will be included in so far as possible. Subjects with concurrent illnesses or conditions that might place them at increased risk for harm from experimental procedures or agents should be excluded. Safety parameters, such as cutoff values for laboratory measurements and clinical indicators, need to be specified.

B. Rescue End Points

Rescue end points need to be clearly delineated. **Even in medical conditions with imprecise and/or soft clinical end points, rescue end points need to be formalized.** When end points tend to be vague, it is optimal to specify standardized measurement and clinical end points. For example, in CNS research, it is common that end points are set to correspond to certain cutoff values on any number of different mood and/or symptom rating scales. Waiting until a subject meets a rating scale cutoff, however, may not be adequately protective. Discomfort or distress may be experienced before formal off-study criteria are met. Thus, in addition to measurably designated end points, clinical end points may need to be specified.

Situations may exist for which specification of clinical end points will be difficult. In these instances especially, but as prudent practice in many protocols, provision for withdrawal of a subject from a study without his or her consent will be needed. The explicit allowance for withdrawing a subject from a study, regardless of subject preference and based on the opinion of the investigator that continued study participation poses too great a risk to the clinical status of the subject, will need to be explained and justified in the protocol, specified in the exclusion criteria, and made clear in the consent/assent documents.

C. Premature Withdrawal of Study Subjects

Formalized procedures for premature withdrawal of individual subjects need to be included in the protocol as it is developed. Investigators and other research team caregivers should understand that clinical end points can be critically important for purposes of risk minimization. When there are concerns about subject safety, researchers need to be trained to act on clinical judgment as much as on more quantifiable data end points.

Investigators may hesitate to remove a subject prematurely because of the loss of data and/or disruption of the study that may result. Subjects to whom research participation presents the last possible therapeutic intervention for a life-threatening or chronic disease, or to whom it represents the best hope for decent medical attention, may be disinclined to be withdrawn. Nonetheless, investigators are obliged to withdraw subjects when the subject's clinical need requires withdrawal. Subjects' awareness that they can be removed from a study prematurely and without their consent is an important safety protection for both subjects and investigators. Appreciation of the need to withdraw subjects from a study prematurely is recognized in U.S. regulation. Also, subjects must be informed appropriately in the consent process of orderly termination procedures.

1. Monitoring and Safety Parameter Criteria

Criteria, even clinical criteria, should be set during the design for use at implementation of the study to monitor subject safety. Safety problems include medical as well as non-medical, psychosocial problems. Monitoring for medical problems requires tight surveillance. As was previously discussed, some studies may need a physician who is not affiliated with the study to serve as a medical monitor and additional advocate for the subjects. This additional level of protection might be appropriate for studies of diseases or conditions with symptomatically vague or surrogate end points, with subjects who might not be able to articulate discomfort effectively, or for initial investigation of agents or devices where risk of toxic and/or unanticipated side effects is high. Thoughtful attention to the level of training for research caregivers that is needed to monitor a subject's clinical status should be part of the protocol development process. For large, multicenter, multinational trials where data are blinded and sent to central data evaluation centers, a protective mechanism is gaining interest: sponsors are hiring a research clinician who will not be part of the research group and who will not benefit academically from the study completion; he or she will be responsible for monitoring the data coming into the data center on a real-time basis in unblinded fashion.

2. Rescue Interventions

Protocols should also include information about rescue interventions, when appropriate. For studies of healthy volunteers, this information may be minimal or may not be needed at all. When subjects are ill (depending on the disease studied, the clinical condition of the subjects, and the study procedures), consideration of rescue interventions can be substantial. For example, in studies of antihypertensive agents, subjects are often required to go without any antihypertensive medication before administration of the study drug is begun. This process, referred to as a **washout period**, will place subjects at risk of experiencing potentially dangerous hypertension. Minimization of risk will include detailed specification of requirements for blood pressure monitoring and explicit instructions for antihypertensive treatment as needed.

Provision for **rapid rescue interventions** is an important part of considering whether, and if so, under what conditions, a placebo arm can ethically be included in a study. Cancer and hypertension are disease examples that illustrate these issues. Because it is most likely that no rescue intervention will be available, placebos are rarely used in oncology research. The knowledge that a rescue intervention can be quick and is usually fully effective in hypertension has been sufficient to satisfy reviewers that the use of placebo arms in trials of antihypertensive therapy is acceptably safe. Schizophrenia research is an example of the issues being less clear. In schizophrenia research rescue intervention can be expected to quickly quell any psychotic symptoms that might arise during the washout period or while a subject is receiving a placebo, thus averting serious harm. Concern remains, however, that the lifetime course of schizophrenia is adversely affected by psychotic breaks. If this is correct, the risk of disease progression despite rescue intervention resembles that of cancer more than hypertension. This highly controversial point will, perhaps, be settled with the accumulation of more data. More data, however, will not settle the question of how similar medical pain and suffering are to psychic pain and suffering. For those who believe that psychic pain and suffering can be severe and permanently debilitating, psychiatric studies that set end points at psychotic relapse will look more like cancer studies than like antihypertensive research. For those who believe that psychotic symptoms, at least in those who have experienced them previously and who can be medicated, are not permanently harming or excessively risky, allowing such symptoms to occur for research purposes will be an acceptable risk of ethically acceptable science. These disagreements may be settled over time. For now, an investigator will have to be as precise as possible in evaluating the severity of the condition of the study subjects, the short- and long-term effects of relapse, and the availability or effectiveness of rescue interventions to minimize risks appropriately. Once the sponsor and investigator have made their decisions, it is advised that the basis for the decisions be made explicit and be well defended in the protocol.

In addition to considering medical rescue interventions, investigators need to consider non-medical kinds of rescue interventions as well. For example, whereas it is true that a cornerstone of voluntary research participation is the ability to withdraw at any time without penalty, the fact is that times may exist when a subject cannot withdraw without serious risk of harm. The U.S. regulations that address the need to inform subjects of procedures for orderly termination of a study apply not only to conditions in which the investigator deems it necessary to remove a subject from study prematurely, but also when a subject decides he or she has had enough and just "wants out." **The essence of the ethical standard of voluntary research participation includes the notion that subjects ought to be able to leave at any time. The ethical requirement for risk minimization, however, in some instances, indicates otherwise.**

In a bone marrow transplantation study, there is a time beyond which a subject can simply withdraw without risk of grave harm or death. Although experimental interventions can be stopped and the patient volunteer can be treated as a clinical patient, leaving the research unit may be life threatening. Bone marrow transplantation protocols are harrowing and prolonged. It is common for subjects to become dejected and want to leave the research unit before it is safe to do so. Investigators need to anticipate such problems and build protections into their protocols.

Assuring subjects the ability to obtain one-to-one nursing, establishing a collaboration with a psychiatrist who can provide emergency capacity assessments, as well as obtaining the subject's permission to contact family members or friends to address the problem of a dangerous withdrawal are all potentially useful additional protections.

D. Premature Study Closure

Premature closure of a study presents different kinds of concerns and approaches to risk minimization than premature withdrawal of a single subject. **Safety concerns are the primary reason for closure of a study before it meets its statistical end points.** The advent of serious, unanticipated adverse events can signal a risk to subjects so grave that the study must be terminated prematurely.

Premature closure can also be appropriate, under certain circumstances, on the basis of **efficacy findings**—that is, in a study of two or more arms, it may become evident before study end points are met that one arm is benefiting study participants substantially more than the other(s). The problem with using efficacy as a reason for premature closure of a study is the difficulty in being very sure that the decision is scientifically unbiased. Bias can lead to a type 2 error that is declaring one intervention efficacious when in fact it is not. Such a scientific error results in the ethical error of having placed subjects at risk of harm for no useful outcome. Blinding systems in expected-direct-benefit trials are intended to avoid this kind of investigator bias. On the other hand, if the effectiveness of an intervention is demonstrable before study end points are reached, it is not warranted to expose additional subjects to ineffective intervention. That is why data and safety monitoring boards, as discussed in Chapter 3, were developed. Their unblinded interim reviews permit the investigator to remain blinded while assessing whether the study should be terminated prematurely or continue to reach its original end points. Because interim reviews have implications for statistical analyses, they should be part of the statistical design of the original study.

Many clinical investigators believe strongly that recognition of a serious safety problem is the only ethically acceptable reason to close a study prematurely. Studies are closed prematurely, however, for a variety of other reasons. A commercial sponsor may close a study for business reasons. An academically sponsored study may be closed prematurely when the investigators leave the institution and there is nobody to continue the study. This is an issue that has not been extensively discussed in the published literature (Ashcroft, 2001; Lievre, 2001), and it is an area ripe for future inquiry. Nonetheless, investigators ought to plan for the possibility that a study might close prematurely, regardless of the reason for the closure. Such planning includes informing subjects of this possibility in the consent process and providing referral plans where appropriate. Established procedures for transfer of subjects to appropriate facilities and/or providers for clinical care minimize risk by assuring patient volunteers the continuity of medical attention.

IV. COMPLETION OF A STUDY

Minimization of risk should continue throughout study completion and follow-up. At completion of a study, the patient volunteer should be provided with referral information so that a smooth transition to community clinical care can be made. It is all too common that patient volunteers get to the end of a study and are simply discharged from the study. Too frequently there is insufficient effort made to connect them to community services. This is an example of the confusion between the goals of research and the goals of clinical care in reverse. Now, rather than confusing the patient volunteer with a patient, the patient volunteer is treated as an object, leaving research participants feeling like they have been treated as laboratory animals. **What is required, instead, is a plan for transitioning patient volunteers back into community care if such care has been decoupled or they lacked such care coming into the study.** If patient volunteers are being treated in the community, concurrently, some form of communication to the subject's health care provider, with the subject's permission, is ordinarily sent. Included in this information is at least that the subject has completed study participation and is being returned to the provider for care needs.

A. Follow-Up

After a subject has completed all study procedures, follow-up may still be needed. **Follow-up may involve a single return visit for minimal evaluation or it may involve a series of regularly scheduled visits for extensive follow-up well into the future or for the subject's lifetime.** Follow-up to meet scientific goals and for clinical care of subjects is an integral part of a study and needs to be well designed and fully described to subjects during the initial informed consent process.

B. Sponsor Obligations After Study Termination

Whether sponsors of a study have obligations to the subjects after the study's completion is an issue that is gaining attention. Related to the social justice debates about research sponsors of affluent countries conducting clinical research in impoverished countries and communities is the question of whether these sponsors have obligations after the studies have terminated. **Common practice has been that sponsors and investigators**

have no obligations to subjects or subject communities once studies are concluded, provided that appropriate referral has been made. The ethical acceptability of this practice is now controversial and evolving. More discussion is needed about whether clinical research can be conducted more justly by adding mechanisms to maximize post-study benefits. Possibilities include community benefits, such as a commitment to increase a country's medical or medical research infrastructure through provision of equipment and/or training.

The idea of possible obligations at the end of a study to the study population or population from which the study group was selected is not the only area of controversy about post-study obligations. The degree to which a particular subject has claims post-study is also a point of controversy. For example, where a study is an expected-direct-benefit study and a subject is receiving measurable benefit, what is the sponsor's or investigator's obligation to continue providing that benefit to that particular subject once the study has met its scientific end points? What might be the harms of removing that benefit, even if the subject had been told in the consent process that no intervention could be anticipated past study participation? As part of the original study design, providing a post-study, open-label trial of the experimental agent to benefitting subjects is already becoming frequent practice. Such post-study, open-label extensions are included to maximize benefit (for subjects who may not be able to obtain the drug off-study because of access problems) as well as to continue collecting data. Post-study concerns about individual subjects and the study's broader population-based concerns are controversial, and they are an area of clinical research ethics that can be expected to garner increasing attention.

A drug company is conducting a trial of one of its approved drugs in a pediatric population. The drug is approved to treat chronic and severe bone pain in adults. The study is to determine if the drug is also effective in young children and adolescents. The drug is expensive and the company is going to be testing it in parts of the world where adult patients have little ability to pay for it, although patients have access to other, less expensive pain medications. The study design is a two-arm, randomized, double-blinded trial of the company's pain killer versus the pain killer that is affordable and accessible to the study population. This drug is approved in both adult and pediatric populations. Bioethics consultants to the sponsor recommend that if the company's drug produces benefit, at the end of the trial, all subjects be allowed to switch into an open-label extension of the company's drug until they can be transitioned onto equally effective medication that is affordable and obtainable.

V. RESEARCH-RELATED INJURIES

Handling of research-related injuries is one area in which there are sizable differences between the United States and other places. **In Europe, there is virtually full coverage for research-related injuries—in the United States there is virtually none.** In the United States, it is standard practice for subjects to pay for care required as a result of research-related injuries. Some institutions, such as the NIH Clinical Center, will cover short-term medical needs. An occasional U.S. academic institution or pharmaceutical company sponsor will commit to paying any medical bill that results from a *bona fide* research-related injury. Ordinarily, however, U.S. research subjects can expect to have to rely on their insurance companies, if they have private coverage, for medical care resulting from a research-related injury. Progress has been made in this area, however, with Medicare coverage being extended to many procedures provided within the context of the clinical research setting. Many private insurers will cover any costs covered by Medicare.

VI. MAXIMIZING BENEFITS

Although the international clinical research ethics guidance documents and regulations governing human research focus more heavily on minimization of risk, there is also a mandate to maximize benefits where possible. **For all clinical research, and especially for research with no expectation of direct benefit to the subjects, the traditional assumption of those in the research community is that reward to participants is altruism.** Altruism refers to a person's unselfish regard for the benefit of others. The expectation that information gained from study participation will benefit society is considered by some as the altruistic motivation for study participation. The only problem with assuming that subjects participate in research for altruistic reasons is that most persons participate in clinical research with the expectation of personal medical benefit, whether the study is designed to provide the possibility of personal benefit or not. Thus, perceived potential for benefit, real or not, is an inducement for many persons to join studies. Because it is important to avoid turning an inducement into an undue inducement, the shaping and explanation of study benefits is an important ethical component of study design.

A. What Constitutes a Benefit?

Where benefits are possible, vigorous efforts should be made to provide them. **The problem is that what constitutes a research benefit is**

highly subjective. Although it is a maxim of ethically conducted clinical research that benefits to subjects should be maximized, this maxim is somewhat platitudinous. Certainly one wants to maximize benefit in the face of an endeavor that presents risks of harm. There is the ring of justice to such a goal. What constitutes a reasonable benefit, as opposed to an undue influence, however, is not easily identified. Although some consider the intrinsic reward for an altruistic act a benefit, many do not. Diagnostic or expected-direct-benefit studies, well along in the development process, may reasonably expect to provide direct medical benefit to individual subjects, but many studies do not. Ought the excellent medical attention that a research subject ordinarily receives be considered a study benefit? Alternatively, **should a direct study benefit be only that which can be reasonably anticipated from participation in the experimental aspects of a study?**

Studies with placebo arms are not necessarily no-direct-benefit research. When study subjects agree to participation in a randomized trial, the prospective subject may be randomized to any trial arm, including an experimental agent or device arm, placebo arm, or standard-of-care arm. This provides the subject with the possibility of being randomized to an arm from which the subject might obtain direct personal medical benefit. This is not the same kind of potential benefit, however, as that given to all subjects in the form of sound medical monitoring throughout the course of study. We consider the latter merely a requirement of ethically acceptable research and not a benefit of study participation. Additionally, physical examination may not turn out to be a benefit if there are unanticipated findings that cause the subject concern, or worse, to produce the need for medical care that they cannot obtain.

We exclude such medical attention from benefits, including state-of-the-art diagnostic procedures, because people with means can obtain such care outside the research setting. To deem study clinical care a benefit may be thought of as an exploitation of social inequities. This is admittedly a controversial point and one that investigators will want to consider and discuss with their colleagues and review committees in designing the benefits sections of a protocol. The issue is raised here because it is a common point of discussion among investigators and IRBs or IECs that reflects the subjective nature of determination of study benefits.

An inner city university medical school wants to increase its inclusion and retention of poor women and minority populations in its studies, particularly its HIV/AIDS research program. To do this, the medical center is setting up an HIV/AIDS clinic that will provide both standard clinical care and the opportunity to participate in research studies. As the organizing group is

Continued

developing the project, discussion turns to concerns about providing benefits that might turn out to be undue inducements for clinic patients to participate in research. It is an expectation that women who come to the clinic for their own care will have to bring their children with them. Given that patients can expect to be at the clinic for many hours on their appointment days, lunch will have to be provided to the women and their children, and when there are babies, diapers will have to be provided as well. Might these basic needs act as an undue influence for impoverished women when it comes to asking these patients to participate in clinic studies? How free will these women feel to decline research participation invitations when they are dependent on the clinic for medical care and given a day's worth of meals and diapers?

B. Compensation Versus Payment

Compensation for study participation is another issue related to study benefits around which there are differences of opinion. **When subjects are paid, either with money or other kinds of compensation, the question arises about whether such money or compensation is payment for labor or for mere inconvenience.** This issue has received increasing attention (Anderson and Weijer, 2002; Dickert *et al.*, 2002; Menikoff, 2001). If one takes the position that subjects should be paid as if they are performing work, which is a shift from traditional notions that subjects ought to be motivated by altruism, the basis for payment may be determined by considering the following questions:

- Should research payment be based on a minimum wage basis because research participation is to be considered unskilled labor?
- Or should payment be based on risk: the riskier the protocol, the higher the payment?
- If researchers should not be paying patients for their labor, should subjects at least be compensated for their time and/or inconvenience?
- If patients should be compensated for their time, how does one judge the value of a subject's time and the inconvenience incurred? How should researchers account, if at all, for disparities in income and life circumstances across subjects?

The answers to these questions have important implications for avoiding coercion or undue influence. For example, payment of $50.00 per hour to a research volunteer who is CEO of a Fortune 500 company would probably be considered trivial by the recipient. But $50.00 per hour for a subject who is homeless and unemployed may be considered an undue influence. For an impoverished single parent, would lunch and diapers for her baby be an undue influence?

Discussion is complicated because there is a seeming discrepancy between the motives attributed to research subjects by researchers and the motives expressed by the subjects themselves (Cogneau *et al.*, 2002; Cunny and Miller, 1994; Hercberg *et al.*, 1995; Pentz *et al.*, 2002; Warner *et al.*, 2003). Researchers tend to attribute research participation to altruistic motives. It has been assumed that healthy research subjects or subjects participating in phase I clinical trials volunteer for the greater good because these studies are designed to benefit society only.

It is clear, however, that a primary motivator for clinical research participation, at least for healthy volunteers, is money. For poor parents of healthy children, the implication is alarming. For patient volunteers, even in phase I trials, the primary motivation appears to be the expectation of personal medical benefit. Although there is evidence that some patient volunteers do participate in clinical research for altruistic reasons, the majority of patient volunteers participate with the expectation of medical benefit. What is worse, even where studies hold out the potential for medical benefit, the whole process of scientific study and the differences between anticipatable benefit in the clinical setting and the potential for benefit in the clinical research setting seems beyond the grasp of many study participants. Known as the **therapeutic misconception** (Fried, 2001; Dresser, 2002; Lidz and Appelbaum, 2002; Williams and Haywood, 2003), this phenomenon is explained as subjects consciously or subconsciously ignoring information regarding a study regardless of how well study procedures are explained (e.g., randomization, blinding). Many subjects believe that the research arm in which they participate is the optimal clinical intervention for them, personally.

This subjectivity, and in some circumstances frank error, about what constitutes a research benefit demands consideration and attention by investigators and review groups. Although efforts should be made to maximize subject benefits when possible and reasonable, care should be taken to how such potential benefits are presented to subjects. It is important to avoid overselling clinical research benefits.

VII. WRITING THE PROTOCOL SECTION ON RISK, BURDEN, AND DISCOMFORT

The **risk, burden, and discomfort section** may take up as much space as any other section in a protocol. **When experimental agents, devices, or diagnostics are being tested, the known risks need to be detailed thoroughly.** Although risks of clinically approved interventions need not be elaborated, information about the comparison interventions, if any, will need to be provided in a general way. If interventions are being compared, any additional risks to subjects by not receiving the standard intervention must be explained and justified. This includes the risks of study procedures themselves, such as randomization and blinding. In addition, if a subject is to undergo more numerous or frequent standard-of-care procedures as part of a study, this also needs to be explained and justified. If it is theoretically possible that death could result from research participation, the researcher must also state this possibility very clearly to the subject.

In addition to physical risks, psychological risks need to be considered. Common examples include anxiety provoked by placement of a subject in the small space of an MRI scanner or boredom resulting from long periods of confinement as an in-patient.

Psychosocial risks and burdens need to be addressed in this protocol section as well. For example, fatigue so severe that it prevents normal daily activities can be a burden of participation in an oncology protocol. Although fatigue in the face of life-threatening disease is unlikely to be thought of by a researcher as a serious deterrent or risk of harm, a patient whose disease has progressed through several trials may feel that the time left is valuable and the ability to perform daily functions between treatment cycles is of utmost subjective importance.

The social risk of participation in genetics research is another area of potential risk of increasing importance. The substantive risks of genetics research are not the blood drawing. Employment and insurance may be threatened by a breach of confidentiality. If the study involves family linkage, encouraging other family members to participate in the study may cause stress and friction. Risks to family dynamics need to be anticipated and minimized as vigorously as medical risks. Prudence dictates that the possibility for unanticipated risks should be addressed as well.

In short, the full range of potential risks posed by study participation needs to be explicitly articulated in the body of the protocol and any consent/assent documents. This includes the risk of a subject being removed from the study when, in the judgment of the principal or medically responsible investigator, continued study participation would not be in the best interest of the subject.

VIII. Writing the Protocol Section on Benefits

The risks, burdens, and discomforts section of a protocol can be long, but the **benefits section may be brief.** When the goals of the study are to unveil knowledge to advance medical progress, a researcher must explain this succinctly. It is important to make clear that no direct benefits are anticipated for individual subjects. Something like, *You will receive no direct health benefit from participation in this study. It is anticipated that the knowledge gained from this research may help others in the future,* may be adequate. When there is a potential for direct medical benefit to subjects, researchers should state this fact in the most neutral language possible. Something like, *It is possible that you could receive a health benefit from participation in this study, but none can be predicted. The primary goal of clinical research, however, is to produce new knowledge that will help others in the future,* may be most accurate.

c h a p t e r

7

· · · · · · · · · ·

RECRUITING SUBJECTS

· · · · · · · · · · · · · · · ·

Recruiting subjects is the first step in the informed consent process. Any provision of information by the investigator to a potential subject or source of subject referral begins the informing process and shapes expectations about the clinical research project. It is important to plan this part of the study in a way that maximizes potential for subject accrual. Recruitment should employ strategies most likely to identify, engage, and enlist eligible potential subjects. Recruitment strategies that produce a large fraction of inquiries from ineligible individuals suggest that the recruiting net was spread too widely. Although recruitment needs to be efficient, recruitment strategies must avoid employment of coercive elements in subject accrual.

The **recruitment section** of a protocol needs to begin with **an explanation of how, when, and where subjects will be recruited, including a thorough rationale for the proposed recruitment strategies.** Copies of print advertisements and/or scripts for television or radio advertisements should be attached to the protocol for IRB and IEC review. Attention should be paid to gender, race, ethnicity, and any other potential sources of subject vulnerabilities. An explanation of how recruitment procedures will not serve as an undue inducement to study participation can be included. In this chapter we discuss only those aspects of the recruitment process that precede the formalized beginning of the informed consent process.

I. WHO IS RESPONSIBLE FOR RECRUITING SUBJECTS?

Although the **principal investigator (PI)** is ultimately responsible for recruitment, just as he or she is for all aspects of a study, others on the research team often carry out many of the recruitment activities. A **clinical research coordinator** will often be responsible for overseeing and conducting recruitment activities. Sometimes this process includes implementing recruitment strategies up to the final discussions and signing the informed consent/assent/permission documentation. Protocols with complex recruitment strategies (discussed later in this chapter), however, may call for distancing the research team from prospective subjects. In such cases, the research coordinator and **study investigators** may be only peripherally involved until eligible subjects have been identified and screened. It is advisable to specify in the protocol which member(s) of the research team will be involved in and/or oversee recruitment activities.

For many clinical trials, **the actual primary recruiter is a physician who is treating potentially appropriate patient subjects**. Many trials are not advertised to the public. Rather, recruitment is started by sending a letter to physicians who treat patients with the condition to be studied. In this case, the referring physician may not formally recruit a patient, but only provide information about the trial and refer the patient to someone on the research team.

When the treating physician is also the physician investigator, however, he or she will actually recruit the patient onto the trial. This is a common subject recruitment pathway for many studies, but this method causes ethical concern. Most notably, this method has the potential for coercing patients into trials. In the physician-patient relationship, the patient is always in a dependent position and, ordinarily, will not want to displease his or her physician. Even a neutral presentation of recruitment information, when provided by a patient's physician, can be interpreted by a patient as the physician's preference to have the patient enroll. When the treating physician is also the physician/investigator, it is prudent that someone other than the treating physician initiate recruitment. Although the Declaration of Helsinki requires use of this strategy to reduce the influence of patient dependence on a treating physician in the recruitment of research subjects, it is a requirement consistently ignored or overlooked.

> A study of blood transfusion and blood transfusion products in hemophilia is being proposed. Subjects will be recruited from across the country through a letter sent to relevant treating physicians. The PI anticipates conducting the informed consent processes herself. There is a Center for Excellence in Care of Patients with Hemophilia at the university at which the PI is a faculty

Continued

member, and she expects to recruit many of the patients from this center. Although the PI does not regularly see patients because her area of expertise is blood products transfusion, she works at the center two days a week as a consultant to the medical director and staff. In this capacity, she sees some of the patients and reviews the charts for all patients. Because she will be at the center regularly, she plans to recruit there herself. During the IRB review of the protocol, one of the IRB members suggests that, for potential subjects from the center where the PI assists, an associate investigator (AI) should be responsible for the consent process. The PI and AI look uncomfortable. The PI responds that she really does not have a professional relationship with any of the patients that would compromise their ability to decline and wonders out loud how the logistics of having an AI engage in the formal consent process might work. Should the IRB insist on separating her recruitment efforts from the consent process? What would be the ethical justification for such a requirement?

Another autonomy concern when using referring physicians as the primary recruitment strategy relates to gatekeeping. Researchers have been disinclined to recruit patients without including the patient's physician for reasons of professional etiquette. This practice, however, makes the physician a gatekeeper who can block subject entry. That is, if physicians contacting their patients is the primary means by which subjects are recruited, then physicians have the power to select which patients they will inform about a study. **A protocol needs to justify any recruitment strategy in which physicians act as gatekeepers controlling access to study information or participation.**

A study of women with late-stage breast cancer is being proposed and the recruitment strategy is going to be a letter to physicians who treat women with the disease. It will be up to each physician receiving the letter to provide the information to his or her patients who meet the study criteria. The protocol is approved, and the physician letters are sent, but accrual is much slower than anticipated. In calling a few of the physicians and asking about whether their patients seem interested in the study, the study team realizes that patients are not being given the information. Many of the physicians indicate that they believe their late-stage patients ought not be burdened with such information when they are coping with their impending death. Because of this view, the physicians are not giving their patients any information about the study, which is effectively blocking study participation for the patients without the patients' knowledge.

The matter of physician payment, if any, needs to be addressed if treating physicians are involved in the recruitment process. The common belief of patients is that their physician's behavior is based only on patient care needs. If a patient's physician is paid to assist in recruitment, even if the payment is contractually specified for administrative costs, **prospective subjects ought to be fully informed of such payment as part of the recruitment information.**

Recruitment of patient volunteers should avoid use of information or actions that might "oversell" potential benefit of a study. **Potential for direct medical benefit to sick patients ought to be avoided as an inducement to participate.** When recruiting healthy volunteers, it is important that study personnel realize that physical health is not the only consideration in ensuring sound recruitment methods of healthy populations. Physically healthy volunteers can be vulnerable for non-physical reasons.

II. WHEN DOES THE RECRUITMENT PROCESS BEGIN AND END?

Recruitment starts only after the protocol has been approved by the IRB and/or IEC and all institutional requirements have been fulfilled. Investigators cannot proceed with advertising, referral letters, or presentations about the study before all necessary protocol approvals have been obtained. Once the study has been approved, recruitment can begin. Recruitment has started when information about the study is disseminated.

Any advertisement, whether in print or broadcast media, should be reviewed and approved by the IRB or IEC of record. In countries where regulations are not clear on whether IRB or IEC approval is required, formalized approval is encouraged. Content of advertisements should be neutral. Information concerning the study needs to state that persons are being recruited to a clinical research protocol. Even if free treatment will be provided, it should not be highlighted. It is best if the word *free* can be kept out of advertisements.

Some of the large, multisite, multinational trials have started the trend of using catchy acronyms as names. Trial names such as *affirm, hope,* and *miracle* are designed to send a message about the agents being studied. These acronyms are themselves part of the recruitment strategies. Whether they present an undue influence on prospective subjects by attempting to manipulate expectations of benefits requires greater consideration (Hochhauser, 2002).

When protocols involve potentially vulnerable subjects, such as studies focused on substance abuse or studies involving the economically disadvantaged, recruitment strategies that distance the researchers from prospective subjects during preliminary recruitment and screening phases may be wise. The natural enthusiasm of researchers for their work and their eagerness to recruit subjects can influence how they nuance provision of information. Even if the information is essentially scripted, voice inflections have a subtle influence if subjects are highly vulnerable because of a life-threatening disease, dependence, poverty, or another desperate situation.

One distancing tactic is to hire a recruitment firm to conduct the initial conversations that result from queries generated by print and broadcast advertising. For example, the firm might perform telephone screening, or the firm may lead the process from telephone screening through initial face-to-face conversations and additional screening before a prospective subject speaks with a member of the research team.

The advantage of such layered and distanced recruiting is that prospective subjects are not biased by overly enthusiastic investigators. Outside recruiters, however, may not be neutral either. Such groups are paid to recruit subjects and may, therefore, employ tactics that are coercive. It is the researcher's responsibility, if others are involved, to review all scripts, informational brochures, and other such information that will be a part of the recruitment plan. Incentives to complete recruitment quickly should be avoided. The researcher is also responsible for monitoring and supervising the outside recruiters to ensure that their presentations or other recruitment procedures are not coercive. During and at the end of recruitment, the principal investigator is responsible for ensuring the confidentiality of records as specified in the protocol.

III. RECRUITING SUBJECTS FOR MULTIPLE STUDIES

While participating in one study, a subject may be asked to participate in another study. Although this may be a convenient and an efficient recruitment strategy, it presents some ethical concerns. **The participation of subjects in more than one study is least problematic when add-on studies are built into the original protocol.** For example, many studies add genetics components to their protocols, which become additional parts of the study. Supplemental studies may have separate consent documents, or the additional information required for the consent process may be integrated into a single consent document. In either case, the subject can be recruited into the primary study, agree to the primary study, and decline or accept the supplemental study during the informed consent discussions or subsequently, which should not affect the individual's decision to participate in the original study.

The integrity of independent decision making is also maintained if the study involves both required and optional components

as part of the same protocol. For example, some studies involve optional procedures. The optional aspect of the procedure is explained as part of the initial information-providing process, differentiating it clearly from declining a study procedure that would lead to the subject's removal from the study. A subject recruited into the primary study who does not want to go through the optional procedure can decline without difficulty, and the recruitment process progresses without discomfort.

The situation of declining a particular procedure may be different, however, after a subject is enrolled. Once a subject has become a part of the study, he or she will develop a relationship with the investigative team. This relationship entails a power differential that favors the researcher. If, for example, the subject is a patient volunteer in a study that has potential direct medical benefit to the participants, the subject may not want to displease the researcher by declining participation in optional parts of the study. Even if a subject is invited to participate in a protocol not conducted by the PI of the primary study but by an AI on that protocol or one conducted by an unassociated colleague in the same institution, the subject may still feel that his or her autonomy is constrained.

That the autonomous decision making of an otherwise autonomous subject may be constrained does not mean that the subject ought not, *a priori*, be invited to participate in another current or future study. It does suggest, however, that such an invitation be offered with attention to any circumstances that might limit autonomy. Such subjects may be vulnerable, and, thus, consideration of additional protections is advised. It may be useful to have an objective physician or other relevant professional who is not affiliated with the research act as a witness throughout the recruitment process and attend the signing of consent documentation for a new protocol. The prohibition in the Declaration of Helsinki of physicians seeking research consent from their own patients might well be applied to this situation. PIs and AIs intimately involved with management of patient subjects might be excluded from recruitment of their own subjects for other protocols while these investigators are participating in the primary study.

> Mr. Richards is a research participant in a study of persons who have had appendectomies. The study requires a two-day inpatient stay at a university teaching hospital near Mr. Richards' home. After Mr. Richards' protocol was approved by the IRB and Mr. Richards consented to participate, the investigative team amended the protocol to include an optional genetics component that involves a single additional blood draw and storage of the blood for future genetic analyses. Now Mr. Richards is in the hospital for his 2 days of scans and study procedures. He is approached to consider participation in

Continued

the genetics add-on study. Does it make an ethical difference if the invitation comes from the PI or an AI? Why might the process be improved if the investigator making the invitation involves a non-research-affiliated hospital staff member during the consent discussion?

IV. THE PROFESSIONAL RESEARCH SUBJECT

Occasions will exist when a particular subject is well known to a set of researchers or a research institution. Colloquially referred to as **professional research subjects**, these persons volunteer for many clinical research studies. The individual may be a student or indigent, both conditions associated with having flexible schedules and a need for money. Although there is no reason, *a priori*, to suggest that persons should not be frequent research participants, a responsible investigator needs to be careful when recruiting these subjects. Some people who volunteer frequently for biomedical research are merely good citizens motivated by altruism; others, however, may volunteer out of desperation for income or attention.

V. WRITING THE PROTOCOL SECTION ON RECRUITMENT

The section on **recruitment** should include **a brief, but complete, description of the subjects to be recruited and a thorough description of recruitment procedures**. When subjects are from vulnerable or potentially vulnerable populations, processes to protect them against undue influence by recruitment procedures should be described and explained in the protocol. The document needs to specify who will be involved in recruitment, identifying persons by name and/or professional title and category. If persons or companies other than the clinical research team members will perform recruitment activities, they should be identified, and their involvement justified as well. Procedures for oversight and monitoring of outside recruiters should be included. In addition, an explanation of how privacy and confidentiality of records will be kept by outside recruiters should be explicit. If and when such records will be destroyed should also be recorded. Mention should be made of any print or broadcast advertisements, referring the reviewer to ad samples included in the appendices section. Samples of any recruitment scripts should also be included in the appendices section.

c h a p t e r

8

· · · · · · · · · ·

INFORMED CONSENT

· · · · · · · · · · · · · · · · ·

Informed consent can be described as permission given by an individual or someone acting on behalf of another individual for a procedure or set of procedures in clinical medicine or in clinical research. The practice of obtaining informed consent for research participation comes more from the courts than from clinical medicine. Practically speaking, **informed consent is a 20th-century legal construct that has been incorporated into medical and medical research practice**. Scholars looking for historical evidence of informed consent find it in 18th- and 19th-century clinical medicine (for an expanded historical account of informed consent, see Faden and Beauchamp, 1986). Where such evidence exists, it is weak and demonstrates an ethical basis for informed consent different from that which exists in both clinical and research medicine of the 20th century. In clinical medicine, considerations of disclosure and honesty grew from a concept of beneficence, whereas the courts shaped contemporary notions of consent as a right of self-determination.

I. TRADITIONS AND PURPOSE OF INFORMED CONSENT

The purpose of informed consent is to ensure that **(i) a patient or research subject understands relevant information and explicitly agrees with the intervention or activity requested** and that **(ii) the agreement is voluntary.** Contemporary notions that a patient or research subject should provide an informed agreement are based on individual rights of autonomy. This rights-based justification differs from the motives of the earliest inclinations to inform patients (Doyal and Tobias, 2001). For the most part, 18th- and 19th-century efforts to inform patients were not part of an attempt to engage them in making decisions about their own care or clinical research participation. Earlier evidence of disclosure in clinical care shows informing patients was meant to promote patient compliance. The beneficence model, grounded in ancient Hippocratic notions of acting in the best interest of the patient and the primary model of medicine used until the mid-20th century, viewed informing patients as useful for promoting their compliance with medical recommendations.

Approach to patient care changed around the middle of the 20th century. General speculation is that multiple broad social changes came together to produce the shift. Increasing strength of the civil rights and the women's movements focused legal and political attention on rights of self-determination that permeated all layers of society. The challenges to authority during the Vietnam War era along with decreasing trust of individuals in positions of authority and of social stature may have accelerated these social changes. Regardless of what were the many threads of social change in the clinical arena, the model of patient autonomy replaced the model of physician beneficence.

The term *informed consent* was introduced in the Salgo versus Leland Stanford, Jr., University Board of Trustees case in 1957. In this landmark case, Martin Salgo, paralyzed from a translumbar aortography, successfully sued his physicians for negligence in performance and in failing to warn him of the possibility of paralysis. The court found in favor of Salgo by stating that "any facts which are necessary to form the basis of an intelligent consent by the patient to proposed treatment" should be disclosed (Faden and Beauchamp, 1986, p. 125). In the decision, the court used the term informed consent, first used in an Atomic Energy Commission memo in 1947 (Moreno, 2001). In its discussion of this new duty, the court implied that physicians are obligated to disclose risks and alternatives to subjects, and in addition, physicians should disclose the nature and consequences of a procedure.

Until well into the mid-20th century, there is virtually no evidence that consent for research participation was ever considered or sought. Although there were contracts with research subjects since the beginning of the 20th century, the Nazi atrocities and, subsequently, revelations of clinical research abuses in the United States, such as in the Tuskegee Syphilis Study (Jones, 1992; Reverby, 2000), led to international and national clinical research ethics guidance documents and regulatory structures that established the requirement for informed consent of research subjects.

II. WHEN DOES THE INFORMED CONSENT PROCESS BEGIN?

As noted in Chapter 7, the informed consent process begins with the first exchange of information between the researcher and a potential subject. The process can be thought of as having four separable, but linked, phases.

A. The First Phase of the Informed Consent Process

The first phase of the informed consent process includes activities designed to provide potentially eligible persons, or their referral sources, information designed to encourage study participation. This phase includes all recruitment and any screening activities that take place before a potential subject meets a member of the research team. The process may start when a treating physician informs his or her patient that a potentially interesting study exists. When the physician is the first provider of information and the patient shows interest, the physician may give the patient the contact name and phone number of a member of the research team.

When the patient follows through and calls the research team, he or she usually receives additional information about the study and goes through initial screening activities. A research nurse or coordinator often conducts such screening sessions, but sometimes the researcher of the actual study performs this task. This initial screening is usually done over the phone; it not only provides more information to the potential subject, but it may also be a preliminary screening device for the researcher.

Other possible activities during this early phase are those related to studies designed with secondary recruitment strategies. For example, some genetic studies require the involvement of multiple family members. Usually, there will be an index subject, often referred to as the **proband**. In some study designs, the proband provides information to other family members, including a name and address card to be sent back to the researcher to permit contact with the family member.

Any information about a study received by a potential subject initiates the informing process. This includes print and broadcast media advertisements, letters to referring physicians, presentations made by researchers to the public and other audiences, and word-of-mouth advertising. It is critical that this preliminary printed and broadcast information is balanced, does not overstate potential benefits, and has a clear identification of the activity as clinical research. Presentations by clinical researchers should also be balanced and should not oversell potential benefits to subjects or society.

B. The Second Phase of the Informed Consent Process

The second phase of the clinical research process gives substance to the initial information given to prospective subjects. **Whereas the first phase is a one-way provision of initial and usually incomplete information, the second phase is an exchange of information, an evaluation of the potential subject's understanding, and an active discussion between researcher, or designee, and potential subject.** This phase of the process provides a prospective subject with detailed information. There is a full disclosure of what will be involved. This includes informing potential subjects about the purpose and nature of the study as well as the potential risks and benefits of the research. The subject is given all other facts needed to make a considered, thoughtful decision about participation. Investigators are also responsible for ensuring that prospective and/or already enrolled subjects understand the information and that their consent is voluntary (not coerced) and free of undue influences.

C. The Third Phase of the Informed Consent Process

The third phase is the **documentation of informed consent**. This is the part that many mistakenly consider the sum total of informed consent. Thinking in this manner, however, leads clinical researchers down dangerous paths. Rather than viewing informed consent as a process, the researcher may focus on obtaining a signature. Obtaining the signature, however, is the least ethically substantive part of the process and is best thought of as a procedural aspect of regulatory compliance. Under most circumstances, the signature of a capable adult, or of a parent, guardian, or other legally and ethically acceptable person on behalf of a minor or incapacitated adult, is required before clinical research can proceed. Under the worst of circumstances, the signature is thought of as the sum total of a merely regulatory checklist. Under the best of circumstances, the signature is emblematic of a substantive and continuing ethical process of sound decision making.

D. The Fourth Phase of the Informed Consent Process: When Does It End?

Some make an additional error of assuming that once the consent form is signed, the consent process is over. Little could be further from sound practice. **The fourth phase of the consent process comes after the** consent form is signed. **This fourth phase encompasses the subject's study participation and ends only when the study is concluded.** This phase may be at the end of the subject's active study participation when he or she terminates involvement with the researcher. If involvement continues, however, as long as the protocol specifies (i.e., through whatever kind of follow-up procedures are included in the study), a process of ongoing consent is taking place. If there are to be follow-up visits or contacts between researcher and subject, this fourth phase can stretch out for the rest of the subject's life.

The fourth phase of informed consent includes all educational, informational, and explanatory exchanges between a subject and members of the research team for the duration of the study. That is, each time a subject engages in a study procedure, even those explicitly agreed to as part of the early phases of the informed consent process, that subject must agree again to do what is being asked of him or her. Thus, ongoing study participation requires renewal of the subject's agreement. Willingness to continue participation is a demonstration of continuing consent. Sometimes this ongoing consent will be made explicit, such as for procedures that require a specific consent just before the test is performed. Examples include surgical procedures such as lumbar puncture or magnetic resonance imaging (MRI) scan. Ongoing consent can also be implicit, such as when the subject has blood drawn, for which there is no additional separate consent. In either case, the subject's continuing cooperation in the completion of study procedures represents a continuation of the consent process. This process ends only when the subject is no longer called upon to do something or the subject asks to have his or her samples or data removed from further investigation related to the study.

III. The Difference Between Process and Product

It is important to remember that **informed consent is a process, not a product**. Informed consent is not a verb: researchers do not "consent" subjects. **Informed consent is a noun: it is a process that takes time, effort, and multiple iterations and is best approached through varied formats.** At the very least, the informed consent process requires thoughtful conversation, questions, and answers from researchers and prospective or present subjects as well as information in printed form and hard copy documentation. More complex protocols and informed consent processes may include electronic media. Some studies use interactive videos to augment the person-to-person consent process as well as electronic documentation of the actual process and its result, such as whether the subject has agreed or refused to participate.

Information provided to subjects, in any format, should be in language understandable to the prospective or present subject. Medical language should be translated into lay terminology. That does not mean that either spoken or written communications should avoid using medical language. Expunging medical terminology and other technical language is not recommended because the subject, throughout the study, will be hearing researchers speak to each other using technical language. Clinical researchers can be expected to unconsciously use technical terminology when speaking with subjects during the study. Familiarity with technical terminology is advantageous for study subjects. The process of informing subjects is optimized when technical terminology is accompanied by explanations that are understandable to the nonscientist. Documents are best written at an 8th-grade level.

Time is a critical component of the informed consent process. Frequently, if the consent process is not well handled, a researcher may give a consent form to a prospective subject, directing the individual to read it and then asking him or her to sign it. This procedure is unacceptable. Instead, researchers need to accept the fact that a sound informed consent process takes time. Time is required to work through the information with a potential subject and to assess the individual's understanding and quality of decision making. The process also includes the time the prospective or present subject needs to consider the information provided and seek counsel of persons outside the clinical research setting. Depending on the study, a prospective research participant may want to, or will need to be advised to, consult family and friends and medical professionals who are not part of the research team, which can be expected to delay the individual's decision. Such delays can be anticipated in the design phase of the study to aid in estimating with reasonable accuracy how long recruitment and consent processes will take. Time devoted to the consent process can have implications for scheduling such things as inpatient beds, acquisition of equipment such as MRI and PET scanners, and hiring of research and monitor staff. It is absolutely essential to allocate time for the process sufficient to ensure that decisions about research participation are made autonomously by subjects or surrogates.

Regardless of how sophisticated the approach, how many persons are involved, or how much time it takes, the PI is ultimately responsible for ensuring that an agreement to participate has been made in a thoughtful, knowing way, free from pressures that interfere with the individual's capacity to decline. Such assurance can only come after a sound process has been implemented.

IV. REQUIRED ELEMENTS

A. What Elements Are Required by Law?

There are eight elements of consent required by DHHS and FDA federal regulations, with an additional set required as appropriate. The eight required elements are listed here.

1. A statement that the study involves research, an explanation of the purposes of the research, the anticipated duration of the subject's participation, and a description of the procedures to be followed, identifying those procedures that are experimental
2. A description of reasonably foreseeable risks or discomforts to the subject
3. A description of any reasonably foreseeable benefits to subjects or to others
4. A description of appropriate alternative procedures or courses of treatment, if any, that may be advantageous for the subject
5. A statement describing the extent, if any, to which confidentiality of records identifying the subject will be maintained
6. For research involving more than minimal risk, an explanation of whether there will be any compensation and/or medical treatment provided in the event of a research-related injury or illness, and if so, what it is or where further information can be obtained
7. The name(s) and contact information of persons to whom questions should be addressed about the research, the rights of research subjects, and research-related injuries
8. A statement that participation in the research is voluntary and that refusal to participate in the study or discontinuation of study participation after enrollment will not engender/result in penalty or loss of benefits to which the prospective or participating subject would otherwise have been entitled

Additional information may be required in some situations. U.S. federal regulation specifies some of these possible additional required elements. These requirements are as follows.

1. A statement that the particular treatment or procedure may involve risks to the subject (or to the embryo or fetus) that are unforeseeable at the time
2. The understanding that the investigator, without the subject's consent, may terminate a subject's participation in the study
3. A description of any additional costs to the subject that may result from research participation

4. An explanation to the subject of the consequences of a decision to withdraw from the research and procedures for orderly study termination
5. An explanation that significant new findings developed during the course of the research, which could be relevant to the subject's willingness to continue participation, will be provided to the subject
6. The provision of the approximate number of subjects involved in the study

Complying with the regulatory requirements for informed consent requires ethical interpretation. The regulations provide guidance on the content, but in most cases, they are not sufficiently specific to relieve the investigator of judgments about precisely what content to put in and what to leave out. Furthermore, how the content of the required elements are presented and the process this presentation follows is up to the investigator and research review bodies to shape, depending on the particular needs of the study, its subjects, and the research environment. Thus, even though the elements of consent may seem to be explicitly articulated, how they are applied in a particular study will require thoughtful application of the rules.

B. What Additional Elements Are Required by Good Practice?

In addition to what is required by law, additional information may be provided to the potential or current subject as part of good ethical practice. This kind of information includes whatever else might be useful for the individual to make his or her decision about whether to join or continue participation in a study.

1. Full Disclosure, Deception, and Consent Waivers

Under ordinary circumstances, full disclosure of study purposes, procedures, risks, and benefits to a potential subject is noncontroversial. There are times, however, when investigators can make a logical argument that having subjects know everything about a study will invalidate the findings. For example, single-blinded studies withhold from subjects, but not investigators, knowledge of what study intervention the research participant is receiving. Blinding, as discussed in Chapter 4, is intended to reduce bias and thus increase the prospect of valid conclusions. When blinding is a part of the study, subjects should be told that they will not know which intervention they will receive. The process of randomization and blinding will have to be explained. After the blind is broken for the subject, individually or at the end of the study for the study group as a whole, subjects are sometimes informed which arm of a randomized, blinded trial they were in. The consent process should explain the potential risks and benefits for all arms of a trial. Although information regarding which arm a subject is assigned to is withheld, practically speaking this is not deception. Whereas the interventions will, to the extent possible, appear the same, a deception of sorts, no essential information needed by the individual to make a decision about participation in a blinded, randomized study is withheld or distorted. Although randomized, blinded trials, especially placebo-controlled randomized trials, present their own set of controversies, deception is not one of them.

There are studies, however, in which actual deception is required if subjects are to behave in ways natural enough to produce the data sought. The primary ethical concern in these studies is precisely the deception. Some will argue that any deception of research subjects has the potential for harm too grave to justify its use. Any deception, some believe, is an unacceptable affront to dignity rights. Even when there are no physical risks to subjects from the deception, the potential for psychological harm always exists. Simply destroying trust in clinical researchers is a serious negative outcome. A study to examine private, intimate behavior, as in the Tearoom Trade studies (Faden and Beachamp, 1986) of homosexual men, or studies using deception that produce behavior for which a subject might be embarrassed or ashamed, such as in the Milgram Obedience Studies (as discussed in Chapter 15), are cause for concern. Some believe the potential for harm to subjects and society outweighs the usefulness of any information gained, regardless of how important or useful it might be in the abstract.

An example of a study that would require deception is one in which study participants are psychiatrically ill mothers and their babies. The mothers are told that they will be observed playing with their babies to learn more about how babies respond to toys of different colors, shapes, and functions. The deception is that the mothers are really being observed for the presence or absence of nurturing behaviors, such as how often they smile at their baby and tenderly touch the baby or how often they raise their voice to the baby or handle the baby roughly. If the mothers were told why they were really being observed, they would be expected to alter their natural behavior patterns to avoid doing anything that could be construed as non-nurturing, and thus, the data would be skewed. An IRB/IEC reviewing such a study would have to decide first if the question was worth asking at all. If it is decided that this is an appropriate area of study, is the deception necessary, or could the information be obtained without it? If not, what additional regulatory and/or ethical considerations are required to allow the protocol to go forward?

Some consider deception acceptable under certain circumstances. For those who do, there are several sources of guidance. The most thoroughly considered guidelines come from the **Ethical Standards of the American Psychological Association** (APA) (Bersoff, 1995). After consideration throughout the 1940s, the first APA code of conduct for clinical psychologists, adopted in 1952, formalized the notion of informed consent in psychological research. Since the earliest versions of the code, the APA has explicitly addressed the ethical concerns raised by deception in research. The APA has consistently held that there is a legitimate use of deception in research but that such deception must be "managed." Management includes prohibiting deception about critical or "significant" aspects of a study, such as physical risks, discomfort, and unpleasant emotional experiences. The APA code also requires that researchers explain any and all deceptions to subjects either at the end of research participation or at the end of the study (Appendix, No. 22).

Internationally, the Council for International Organization of Medical Sciences (CIOMS) guidelines also explicitly address deception in research. CIOMS calls on researchers to avoid the use of deception unless absolutely necessary for study validity (Appendix, No. 14), but the guidelines do not prohibit it completely. The CIOMS commentary that follows guideline 5 calls for research that (i) allows deception to be permitted only at the minimal risk level, (ii) uses an independent review body that must be convinced that only deceptive methods will work, (iii) is sufficiently important to balance the potential harm of deceiving subjects, and (iv) sets the reasonable person standard for evaluating the appropriateness of the deception and/or information withheld.

Although the U.S. federal regulations do not address directly the issue of deception, they cover it indirectly through the permission for consent waivers. The consent waiver is a mechanism that allows, in some instances, the requirement for consent for alteration of some or all consent process elements to be waived. To obtain a consent waiver, there are four criteria to meet. The four required criteria are the following:

1. The research poses no more than a minimal risk.
2. The waiver or alteration does not adversely affect the rights or welfare of subjects.
3. The research could not be reasonably carried out without the waiver or alteration.
4. Whenever appropriate, subjects will be provided additional pertinent information after study participation.

The fourth criterion is similar, but not identical, to the debriefing requirement of the APA code. The APA code requires a full disclosure, either at the point of termination of the subject's participation in the study or at the conclusion of the complete study. In the U.S. federal regulations, such disclosure is not mandatory, although documentation is. Disclosure is required only, as appropriate, and timing is not specified.

A more substantive difference between conditions for the ethically acceptable performance of deceptive research, as stated in the APA's code, and the regulations governing the use of consent waivers is that use of the regulatory waiver is not confined to deceptive research. The regulatory waiver applies to any research that is covered by the regulations, not only research in which deception is employed; the waiver can be used for any study in which the required process for obtaining a fully informed consent is altered. For example, some research waivers are requested for studies in which the need to obtain consent is avoided altogether, such as research involving stored samples (an issue discussed more fully in Chapter 13) or in some epidemiologic studies.

An example of a study for which an alteration of consent might be appropriate is one in which proposed subjects come from a community that believes signing their names to enter into an agreement is disrespectful. In such a community, signing a consent document would violate community moral practice. For such a protocol, an allowance of an alteration in standard consent processes would have to be devised. The altered consent process might have the investigator and a non-research-affiliated witness sitting with a prospective subject. The investigator reads and discusses each section of the consent document with the prospective subject. At the end of each section, if the prospective subject consents, the investigator and the witness initial each section, thereby indicating that the prospective subject consented. Perhaps, also, a tape recording of the consent process would be made as a second piece of evidence that the individual appeared to understand and made a voluntary determination about study participation.

Meeting the standard of minimal risk may become more difficult if IRBs and other reviewers become less willing to evaluate various study procedures as low-risk. In deceptive research, it is also becoming difficult to convince protocol reviewers that the risk of producing distrust in the medical and/or medical research community is not more than a minimal risk. Also, risking a subject's dignity rights (Katz, 1997) is more widely appreciated today than in the past as an avoidable, even if an intangible, harm.

2. Medically Indicated Procedures During the Study

A wide variety of medically indicated procedures may require obtaining separate informed consents while a subject is participating in a study. Subjects can be asked to consent to medically indicated procedures for two different reasons. First, some medical procedures are performed as a part of the study itself (i.e., they are designed to obtain data). In addition, standard and approved procedures are used to monitor the safety and/or clinical condition of the subject (e.g., drawing blood, taking X-rays). These procedures are required to ensure that the experimental studies are proceeding as planned and the subjects are not harmed during the protocol. Both types are integral to a study, and their explanation is a part of the initial consent process.

Other occasions that call for medically indicated procedures may be unanticipated, but these are necessary for the safety and appropriate care of a study subject. The need may arise from a problem that is not, may be, could be, or is definitely related to a study intervention.

An example of an unanticipated need for a medically indicated procedure that is clearly related to an experimental aspect of a study might be a CAT scan as part of a diagnostic evaluation. Consider the following scenario.

> An asthma study is testing a new inhalant and, so far, there is no evidence of serious pulmonary problems for subjects. The protocol includes periodic chest X-rays, but with no expectation of a subject's need of a CAT scan, the possibility of a scan was not discussed in the study consent process. During the study a subject becomes ill, and X-rays reveal bilateral pulmonary infiltrates, which require a diagnostic workup that includes a CAT scan as standard of care. Regardless of whether the infiltrates are somehow related to the experimental intervention (an aspect of evaluating adverse events discussed more fully in Chapter 11), the CAT scan was not experimental but was medically indicated for the medical care of the subject. Therefore, the researchers are required to obtain the subject's consent for an unexpected but needed (medically indicated) procedure while the study is in progress.

Other indications for unanticipated medical procedures may be clearly unrelated to the experimental aspects of the study. For example, if a subject slips on a staircase coming into the research building and breaks an arm, it is expected that the subject will be examined and that X-rays will be obtained by the research team although the arm may not be immediately set in a cast. Necessary care for the subject's broken arm will obviously call for this individual's consent to medically indicated procedures regardless of any relationship of the incident to a study intervention.

3. Standard Procedures for Research Purposes Only

Some standard and approved procedures, such as additional blood draws and lumbar punctures, are conducted for research purposes

only. Some of these procedures will be integral to study design while others may be optional. All will be part of the initial informed consent process. Researchers will make subjects aware at the outset that refusal of study-required procedures will result (in most cases) in a subject's termination from the study. Whether refusal of any particular set or type of for-research-purposes-only procedures will result in termination of a subject from the general study will be based, however, on the scientific ends of the study. If such procedures can be refused without compromising scientific validity of the data, subjects should be permitted to decline without affecting their overall study participation. For example, testing cerebral spinal fluid by lumbar puncture might add information useful to a researcher, but the procedure is not required to reach study end points. Perhaps only a limited amount of cerebral spinal fluid is needed to provide the data to answer a significant but ancillary question. In either situation, not every subject would have to agree to the lumbar puncture, or if too few subjects agreed to the procedure, the question could be eliminated from the study without effect on analysis of the data needed to answer the primary study questions.

Prospective subjects, however, need to know what specific procedures, if any, they can decline without being removed from the study. This is especially important for studies in which there is expectation of direct benefit. If subjects do not know that they can decline specific procedures and still remain in the study, they may feel pressured to agree to otherwise unwanted procedures for fear of losing access to the potential overall study benefits.

4. Participation in Substudies

The presence in a study of both discretionary and required research-only procedures differs from the inclusion of substudies. Substudies can be either built into the original design of the major study or added as the study progresses. In either case, participation in the substudies is, for the most part, optional for the subject (i.e., refusal to participate in the substudy will not cause the subject to be removed from the main protocol).

A form of substudy that is common in contemporary research is a pharmacogenomics component. **Pharmacogenomics** is a growing field intended to identify differences in gene sequences that can predict differences in responsiveness or sensitivity to specific drug molecules. The expectation is that by understanding how genetic variations determine differences between populations or individuals in responses to drugs, pharmacologic efficacy will be enhanced and side effects will be reduced. Genetic substudies, however, are not only being added to pharmaceutical trials. Genetics is the "science of tomorrow," and a genetics component is frequently included in a wide range of clinical studies. This interest in genetics and complexities of consent issues are discussed in greater detail in Chapter 14; in this chapter, it is sufficient to include only an example of the interest in genetics research because it is becoming ubiquitous.

A different but typical add-on study that could be expected to be part of a study's original design and has relatively straightforward consent considerations is a **quality-of-life study**. These studies often employ survey questionnaires to be completed by a subject to indicate how his or her quality of life has been or is being affected by either the disease process and/or study participation.

To the greatest degree possible, substudies should be planned at the inception of protocol design and integrated into the original protocol. At this point steps can be taken that will ensure consistency of review, communication with subjects, statistical analyses, and data evaluation.

Sometimes, however, a potentially valuable substudy simply cannot be anticipated when the main study is designed. Perhaps new technologies have become available that could be advantageously employed in the context of an ongoing study, leading to information gained at relatively little additional cost (to patient/subject or investigator). Perhaps the publication of new findings calls for the addition of questions or experiments related to the primary goals of an existing study for similar reasons of efficiency or economy. Moreover, perhaps there is simply a great leap in scientific understanding of a phenomenon that suggests extension of the original and ongoing research. Substudies will be indicated for many reasons and will often be most appropriately appended to an existing ongoing study.

The consent process for a substudy added well after a primary study is in progress is more complex than the consent process for a substudy built into the research from the outset. Again, if a substudy is added to a study in which direct benefit is expected, a subject may feel—real or imagined—pressure to agree to participation. This matter must be handled carefully to ensure that an existing study subject, when asked to participate in a newly added substudy, feels completely free to decline. It is preferable, whenever possible, to add the substudy in a way that does not involve existing subjects but begins with recruitment of future subjects. By engaging new subjects in the substudy, the need to reconsent existing subjects is avoided, avoiding all the problems mentioned earlier related to having subjects already in relationships with researchers. The consent process for the substudy can then be integrated into the updated process for the main protocol.

5. *Follow-up and/or Referral Procedures*

Consent to follow-up is as important to study participation as any other aspect of study involvement. Follow-up procedures or contact by the researcher after completion of a study, may be important for scientific reasons, for safety and clinical care reasons, or for both. The form and schedule of follow-up procedures is integral to study design. For a potential subject who is considering whether to enroll in a study, the follow-up procedures need to be fully specified in the informed consent process. Subjects should be made aware of the importance of and reasons for all follow-up procedures. To the extent that follow-up is needed, mechanisms for maintaining communication with subjects should be planned, explained, and arranged in principle during the informed consent process to attempt to overcome the chronic problem of lack of retention of subjects for follow-up procedures.

Whether there will be follow-up or not, making a good faith effort to ensure that subjects are appropriately discharged requires that sound referral mechanisms are part of the protocol to which subjects agree. Referral of patient volunteers either back to their own physician or to a new community provider for medical care is essential. It is important for subject safety and welfare to have robust referral strategies in place with which subjects have agreed to cooperate.

Whatever strategies are to be employed, involving representatives from the subject population in this phase of study design can provide important information on the feasibility of proposed strategies for ensuring that referrals are completed and, where follow-up is part of protocol design, strategies for maintaining contact with subjects have a reasonable prospect for success and enhancing the potential that patients will participate in follow-up procedures.

V. OBTAINING VALID INFORMED CONSENT

A. Assessing Capacity to Provide Valid Informed Consent for Research

Although it is now firmly established that participation of a human subject in research requires voluntary informed consent (see Chapter 5), the process for evaluating a subject's capacity to provide such consent continues to be quite primitive. Minors are legally incapable of providing their own informed consent, an issue addressed in the following Subsection B. Processes for assessing which adults are capable of providing their own informed consent are at present woefully inadequate. In general, protocols do not specify how capacity to provide ethically and legally valid informed consent is to be assessed. Even for studies involving subjects who can be anticipated to be of questionable capacity, such as floridly psychotic persons, it is a rare and highly sophisticated protocol that explicitly addresses capacity to provide informed consent. Improvement in the practice of capacity assessment is long overdue. For standard criteria required to assess decisional capacity, see Chapter 5.

Readily available and research-focused assistance already exists for investigators moving in this direction. Information provided by the National Cancer Institute (NCI) of the NIH, listed on its Web site (Appendix, No. 26), provides guidance on assessing understanding. The NCI guidance suggests that asking the following questions as part of the informed consent process will assist an investigator in assessing an individual's capacity to provide ethically and legally meaningful consent to the research study under consideration:

- Can you tell me in your own words what this study is all about?
- Can you tell me what you think will happen to you in this study?
- What do you expect to gain by taking part in this research?
- What risks might you experience by participating in the research?
- What are your alternatives (other choices or options to participating in the research)?

Another approach to capacity assessment in research is to talk to the prospective subject about research in more general terms and then go through a similar assessment process. This approach provides a researcher with a more general assessment of an individual's global decision-making capacity while still assessing an individual's understanding of core research concepts. We suggest that a sense of this global capacity is important, if only to provide a researcher insight into a person's interest in and prospects for completing complex clinical research activities. The capacity assessment needs to be research-specific—how specific, however, is unclear. The NCI guidance and other capacity assessment instruments developed for use in clinical research call for the capacity assessment to use the precise information relevant to the study being considered. A slightly broader exploration of research concepts, however, prevents an individual from appearing to be capable of meaningful decision making on the basis of repeated presentation of study-specific information. Nonetheless, the assessment of capacity needs to be tied to the ability of the subject to provide ethically and legally valid decisions about research with a design similar to that of the study under consideration to ensure that the person has a grasp of the full range of study components.

Any question about a person's capacity to provide ethically and legally valid informed consent to research, or any disagreement of the research team about a person's capacity to provide such consent, should occasion serious consideration of whether inclusion of that person in the study is advisable. If a study involves groups of such persons, justification for the study of subjects with questionable or clearly impaired decision-making capacity needs to be presented in the body of the protocol. The newest Declaration of Helsinki (2000) (Appendix, No. 13) prohibits the involvement of such persons in a study that does not pertain to some aspect relevant to their limitations on decision making. This heightened attention to the vulnerability of such subjects further strengthens the opinion that it is long overdue to improve radically and rapidly clinical researchers' ability to differentiate between those who can from those who cannot provide their own ethically valid informed consent; this differentiation should occur through an explicit, well-designed process of capacity assessment.

B. Assent for Adults and Minors Who Are Unable to Make Decisions

A range of protections apply to individuals who lack capacity to make their own decisions either because as minors, they are legally prohibited from doing so or because as adults, mental or physical limitations render them incapable of making decisions. Inclusion of these protections in protocol design upholds the second half of the definition of the principle of respect for persons that calls for protections for persons who have limitations on their autonomy. Appropriate protections depend on what is being asked of each person, the level of risk of the protocol, and the degree of the individual's impairment.

It is important to remember that the Nuremberg Code (Appendix, No. 12) excludes individuals unable to provide their own ethically and legally valid consent from research. That is, the Nuremberg Code makes voluntary participation of the subject an absolute requirement, which excludes all children and adults with impaired decision-making capacity. It is important to remember, also, that the response of the international clinical research community was to liberalize this strict interpretation of the Nuremberg Code. Creation of the Declaration of Helsinki and subsequent preparation of the CIOMS guidelines were international research community responses, making the absolute requirement in the Nuremberg Code sufficiently elastic to allow research with subjects who are unable to provide their own informed consent. The ethical justification for introducing this elasticity into the Nuremberg Code is grounded in a consequentialist argument. That is, this perspective holds that the risks of performing research that can help us better care for children and adults who lack decisional capacity are outweighed by the good anticipated to be gained by the research knowledge to be accrued.

Some accept this consequentialist argument, and others do not. Those who do not most frequently express their objections in duty-based terms. They claim that the duty to respect the rights and welfare of individuals is too gravely threatened by involving subjects unable to provide their own consent to research. Some prefer to take a position of compromise, considering the consequentialist argument as sufficiently compelling as long as the risk of harm to a subject is not too great. But when the risk rises, individuals taking this midway position may put increasing layers of restrictions on the involvement of subjects unable to give their own consent, setting outright prohibitions when risk rises and the studies lack potential for direct subject medical benefit. The new restrictions in the most recent Declaration of Helsinki (2000) are an example of such a position of compromise. Another example is the DHHS regulations Subpart D adopted by the FDA. These regulations pertain to research involving children, providing for increased levels of protective restrictions as the risk level increases.

After these conditions are met, however, and study design justifies adequately the involvement of individuals who are unable to provide their own consent, all ethical norms of research and regulatory requirements call for the studies to include protections beyond those expected for adult subjects with intact decision-making capacity. The first, and almost universally applied, protection is the mechanism of research assent. Regulations in the United States require assent only for research involving children. According to these U.S. regulations, assent is not mere acquiescence, but it requires positive and explicit agreement to research participation. The U.S. regulations specify that provision of assent can be accomplished in two different ways. The assent process must be explained in the body of the protocol, or there must be an assent document attached to the protocol. Where assent is to be used, we recommend strongly that both the explanation and document be included (unless the study involved only children unable to read).

Assent, however, is not universally required. The obvious exception is when subjects are simply too impaired or too young or both to be able to provide meaningful assent. In such studies, the fact that assent will not be sought can be explained in the protocol quickly by reference to the condition, age, and/or developmental level of the proposed subjects. When subjects are children, the IRB bases its determination of whether meaningful assent can be obtained on the basis of the age, maturity, and psychological state of the children participating in the research.

Assent from adult research subjects who are unable to make their own decisions is not required at all by regulation. It is required, however, from an ethical perspective. To the greatest degree reasonable, researchers are bound to support self-determination for every subject. The principle of respect for persons demands it. **Assent, as defined in the pediatric regulations, is a fundamental step in meeting this ethical requirement for persons unable to provide their own legally and ethically valid consent.**

Seeking assent, whether from adults or children, implies that dissent will be honored. For an adult, honoring dissent should always be the default position. If a potential adult subject dissents from initial cooperation in some aspect of the study, it would be prudent not to enroll that subject. Even if the study has the expectation of benefit to participants, it is still research. Benefit is not assured to a subject, and, thus, there is no overwhelming medical reason for the individual to be enrolled, regardless of how much a surrogate and/or the researchers expect that benefit may result.

If an already enrolled adult subject dissents from cooperation in a research procedure, the procedure should be halted. That does not mean that a researcher should terminate the subject's study participation altogether. A subject may be approached at a later time to participate and may then be willing to proceed. There is no guidance, regulatory or otherwise, about how long or often researchers might reasonably attempt to get an enrolled subject to agree to participate. Such repeated attempts, however, may at some point place inappropriate pressure on a subject with impaired decision-making capacity. A complete research team, with additional consultants as warranted by the situation, can make this judgment for each subject. Nonetheless, a point in time will come at which all agree that the subject should be dismissed from participating in a particular procedure or should be removed from the study altogether. There must be a strong ethical justification for permitting a surrogate to override the authentic dissent of an adult research subject, regardless of how severely his or her decision-making capacity is impaired.

Whether the view to always honor the dissent of an impaired adult is justified, honoring a dissent is not the regulatory stance in pediatric research. The U.S. regulations and CIOMS guidelines specifically allow parental permission to override a child's dissent if the research anticipates direct benefit, and that benefit may be obtained only in the research setting. This regulatory and international allowance should not be mistaken for a mandate. Sponsors, investigators, or review bodies can choose to design protocols to make a child's dissent final. When it is agreed that a minor's capacitated dissent is to be overridden, we recommend that rather than seek a meaningless dissent and risk creating distrust, information should be provided to the minor in such a way as to obtain the minor's assent to study participation without giving the child a choice that is merely a regulatory sham.

VI. WRITING THE PROTOCOL SECTION ON CONSENT, ASSENT, AND SURROGACY PERMISSIONS

The protocol section on consent, assent, and surrogate permission is often mistakenly believed to be the major ethics component of the protocol. Investigators need to remember that what makes a protocol ethical is its scientific value and the considerations that balance risk against benefit for society and subjects. The consent, assent, and surrogate permission aspects of a protocol, if designed poorly, can mean that a study is not being conducted ethically. But that is not the same thing as saying that these components of the protocol constitute the sum total of the ethical considerations. Unfortunately, many protocols are written as if the investigators and study sponsors are thinking in this "sum total" manner. They provide a separate section in the protocol entitled "Ethical Considerations," which contains a line or two stating that the protocol adheres to the principles of the Declaration of Helsinki—even though it may not—and then they include copies of informed consent documents, perhaps along with assent documents.

> *Inclusion of consent documents does not in itself meet the ethical or regulatory requirements for covering protocol issues related to consent, assent, and permission. To meet the ethical requirements for consent, assent, and surrogate permission, the protocol needs to explain the processes designed to implement these study components.*

A. Prospective and On-Study Subjects

The protocol section that addresses consent processes for prospective subjects and subjects already enrolled in a protocol (commonly referred to as **on-study** subjects) should start with **an explanation of what will be done to obtain initial consent**. This explanation should include a description of how information will be provided to subjects (i.e., verbal and printed materials only, inclusion of interactive video). The place, timing, and personnel involved in the consent process should also be given. For example, the section describes details such as who will be the first person to contact the prospective subject—will the first person to speak with a prospective subject be a research coordinator talking to the person by phone? The protocol also documents which members of the research team will be working through the major portions of the consent process with the prospective participant, and who will be responsible for obtaining the consent form signature. In sum, the protocol description should be sufficient to provide reviewers with a reasonable appreciation of what a prospective subject will experience in the informed consent process from initial interaction with a study representative or a research team member to the signing of the consent and/or assent forms and additional encounters as appropriate.

Discussion of consent activities during the study also needs to be addressed. The extent to which this is explained in the body of the protocol will depend on how complicated the on-study activities are expected to be. For example, if the study involves healthy adults in a one-time intervention, consent during the study may not need to be addressed at all. Initial consent will be all that is needed to enroll in and complete the study. Studies involving multiple visits over a prolonged period of time with patient volunteers needing various surgical procedures and scans present different issues. The design indicates the requirement for additional consents throughout the course of the study. At the very least, a list of the procedures that will require individual, specific consent should be included in the protocol.

If subjects lack decision-making capacity prior to study entry or if they can be reasonably anticipated to lose or have fluctuating capacity during study participation, researchers should address this during the design phase and should include in the protocol how ongoing consent will be sought. For example, what procedure will researchers use to deal with dissent by a subject with questionable decision-making capacity who does not have an assigned durable power of attorney for research participation? Or in a pediatric protocol, will researchers honor the dissent of a terminally ill adolescent instead of honoring the permission of parents who want their child to continue participation in the study?

B. Family Members of Index Subjects

Another consent issue that will need to be addressed during the design phase and discussed in the protocol is **the concern for index subjects' relatives who may have an obvious role in many genetics research studies.** That is, to what degree and how ought family members be involved in protocol consent procedures when a genetic sample is obtained from a *bona fide* study subject? Although this issue is addressed more fully in Chapter 14, genetics research is not the only research area in which this issue arises.

For many clinical research studies, subjects provide information about family history that can be sensitive information (e.g., related to psychiatric problems, sexual practices, child abuse, drugs, or alcohol consumption). Although such information is routinely collected in the clinical setting without much thought, concern is rising about collecting such information in the research setting (Botkin, 2001).

In the United States, the regulatory definition of a **human subject** is a living individual about whom an investigator obtains identifiable private information. With regard to identifiable private information, the condition is also met when an existing subject gives a researcher identifiable private information about a family member that is recorded in research records. Awareness of a need for consent from such family members is only beginning, but any study that includes the collection of such information is encouraged to indicate clearly in the protocol how consent to collect family member information will be obtained and, if needed, how the decision not to seek consent will be justified.

C. Addressing Assent in the Protocol

When pediatric subjects are involved, considerations relevant to assent should be addressed in the body of the protocol. **This section includes the investigator's justification for either including or not including a pediatric patient's assent. This justification needs to cover not only the standard issues, such as the child's age(s), developmental stage, and psychological state, but also whether dissent will be honored and why or why not.** If pediatric dissent is going to be ignored, this protocol section should include an explanation of how overriding a child's dissent will be addressed with the child. It can be argued that if a child's dissent is not to be honored, assent should not be sought. To ask a child to agree or not agree, then ignore the child's disagreement, has the potential for creating or exacerbating grave mistrust of the medical profession and, by extension, caregivers as well as possibly all adults in the child's environment. If dissent is not to be honored, we recommend that the child be given an explanation of what is going to happen and why, without asking for his or her agreement.

D. Surrogate Permission

Although guardians sometimes act as surrogates offering permission for a child's participation, most often the surrogate will be the child's parent or parents. Whether one parent or both need to provide permission to participate in research is dictated by regulation in the United States. (Generally, the term *consent* is reserved for adults making their own decisions. When one person makes research decisions for another, the correct terminology is *permission*.) The U.S. regulations allow for circumstances in which permission of only one parent is required. The regulatory expectation and prudence dictate that both parents provide consent whenever reasonable. The U.S. regulations also specify that it is unreasonable to expect consent of both parents when one parent is unknown, incompetent, unreasonably available, and, of course, deceased; regulations also indicate that one parent's consent is sufficient when only one has been adjudicated legally responsible for the child.

In cases of divorce, often only one parent has custody. From a regulatory perspective, this situation allows for only the custodial parent to be involved and be the permission-granting surrogate. It is critically important to remember in these cases, however, that research is for science, not for personalized medical care of the child. Given this distinction, it is important to realize that when parents, divorced or otherwise, are in conflict over a child's research participation, excluding the child from study may be the appropriate action to prevent the child from suffering harms that could possibly result from the research. The psychological harms to the child of emotional distress and possibly decreased trust of parents and/or physicians are likely to far outweigh the benefits of knowledge gained from the research or benefits offered to the child for his or her participation.

In studies where the questions being asked pertain to distress in children, the needs of the child also govern considerations of parental permission. When permission of a parent or guardian might endanger a child, such as in neglect or abuse research, permission can be waived if various other conditions are met (DHHS and FDA regulations: Appendix, No. 15 and No. 18).

Minors can make their own decisions under certain conditions (e.g., a child adjudicated to be a "mature minor" in a court of law). Minors are sometimes allowed this autonomy if they have a unique situation; for example, an adolescent who is a Jehovah's Witness may be granted the right for religious reasons to refuse a blood transfusion in a research setting. State law often determines minors to be their own decision makers by statute. A common example of this exception involves minors who are married and/or minors who are parents.

As rigidly defined as the permission requirements are in pediatric research, there are no comparable regulatory constraints on research surrogacy for decisionally impaired adult subjects. There are no international guidance documents or U.S. federal regulations that address specifically the issue of research surrogates for adults. Research surrogacy is addressed in policy statements of some research institutions or sponsors. Certain state jurisdictions, however, have addressed this issue, such as California and the District of Columbia. Researchers conducting studies involving adults who are too impaired to make decisions should check for any specific state legislation governing such research.

E. Consent Alterations or Waivers

Under limited circumstances, changes in the regulations and ethical requirements for obtaining informed consent may be altered or waived. These alteration and/or waiver mechanisms have been addressed in some U.S. regulations (i.e., those of the DHHS) and not in others (i.e., those of the FDA). For example, the DHHS regulations allow for an alteration or a waiver when the research involves only minimal risk for the subjects, when rights and welfare of subjects are not adversely affected, when the research could not be practicably carried out, and if it is appropriate, when subjects will be debriefed (Section IV.B.1 and Appendix, No. 15). These regulations also allow for standard consent process alterations if the only risk of study participation is breach of confidentiality because of a signature on consent documentation. Such elasticity does not exist within the U.S. FDA regulatory framework. An area of research where the application of consent waiver allowances has been the practice but where the practice is being ethically challenged is epidemiological research. As ethical thinking evolves in epidemiological research and the research community grapples with the ethical obligations for use of samples from long-established tissue banks, determination of appropriate application of consent waivers and alterations can be expected to be in flux.

F. Community Consent

Community consent is an innovation that has received substantial attention in the research ethics literature. Except in emergency medicine research (discussed in Chapter 14), the U.S. regulations are silent on this issue, at least in large part, because when these regulations were promulgated, research was not considered as involving or affecting communities. Rather, the U.S. regulations were written to protect individual human subjects. Today, however, there is an appreciation that research subjects are members of communities and that communities, as well as individuals, can be harmed by clinical research. Appreciation of this point has led to growing attention to the protection of communities from harm, with one of the strategies being community consent (Bayoumi and Hwang, 2002; Fisher and Wallace, 2000; Foster *et al.*, 1997, 1998; Norton and Manson, 1996; Sharp and Foster, 2002; Strauss *et al.*, 2001). **Community consent** is most commonly understood as consent by the leadership of an identifiable community.

On the face of it, obtaining community consent sounds admirable. The difficulties, however, are numerous:

- Who is the community?
- Do individuals with a disease or condition under study characterize a coherent community?
- Even if the boundaries of a community can be reasonably identified and set, who might best speak for the community? (Just determining what groups of individuals reasonably represent potential subjects is often a serious stumbling block.)

In the case of research involving Native American populations, answering the last question in the previous list can be a reasonably simple task. The tribe from which subjects will be recruited is the community. The tribal elders speak for the community. But what if the proposed subjects are drug addicts from the south side of Chicago? One might be able to describe the universe of potential subjects both by geographical area and kind of addiction, but who speaks appropriately for such a community?

Employing the concept of community consent presents hurdles but should not prevent researchers from integrating community members into the research process from the outset.

For example, HIV research has routinely involved members of the homosexual male community who are infected with the HIV virus. One would not suggest, however, that American gay males with HIV can or should be representative of the universe of persons with HIV infection. Having many individuals with HIV from different backgrounds, such as American heterosexual college students with HIV or impoverished Hispanic mothers with HIV, involved in the design phases of a study can only be expected to strengthen the study. It can also be expected to slow down the process of study design and development. But what is lost in speed of protocol development may be gained during performance of the study. Such community involvement may assist researchers in recruitment, which can be expected to produce larger numbers of eligible and eager subjects. Thus, although the notion of community consent needs additional conceptual and practical attention by researchers and research ethicists, it is an important and novel concept.

VII. WRITING CONSENT, ASSENT, AND SURROGACY PERMISSION DOCUMENTS

Writing consent, assent, and surrogacy permission documents takes thought and skill. These documents should not be afterthoughts, thrown together by junior team members or assigned to writers without extensive knowledge and experience in the clinical research setting. They should also not be written by lawyers. Knowing the regulations is insufficient for producing well-crafted documents. **Deciding on what is the optimal amount and kind of information for a particular protocol, given the subject population proposed and the risk level, is complicated. Crafting this information into written documents that are meaningful and useful for subjects and/or surrogates is the goal.**

A. The Basics

To produce useful consent or assent documents, writers/researchers should start by constructing a format that enhances readability and the understanding of important points. Headings help the reader to digest complex, technical information; white space between paragraphs improves readability. Language needs to be clear, accurate, and understandable by the average 8th grader.

An excellent model is provided by the NCI and available on the Internet (Appendix, No. 23). The format and headers of this consent form can be adapted to fit any study with little conceptual change no matter what kind of protocol is being designed.

For protocols that involve both healthy and patient volunteers, we recommend two separate consent documents to avoid the necessity for the reader to move back and forth between information that pertains only to one type of subject or the other. Having to sort through a combined document only adds confusion and exhaustion to an already confusing and exhausting process. If there are substudies, such as pharmacogenetics studies, additional consent and assent documents will need to be attached to the protocol. It may be preferable to have multiple documents for prospective subjects to follow sequentially with investigators than to have a single document that is excessively long and packed too tightly with information.

The best that can be hoped for is that a research subject and/or surrogate and investigator will use a consent form as a reference document and as a blueprint for the subject's study participation, and that this person(s) would refer to the document repeatedly as the study progresses. Do not expect prospective subjects and/or their surrogates to read, remember, and digest a consent document at a single sitting. It is a rare person who is able to do so in any meaningful way. Remember that reading and signing a consent, assent, or permission form is only one piece of a process that starts long before anyone looks at the paperwork.

A consent or assent form starts with an invitation to participate followed by an explanation of the purpose(s) of the study. In general, writers should avoid jargon. For example, in a complex protocol involving a cardiac stent, the consent document might say that the purpose of the research is to learn which type/form of stent works better at keeping heart vessels open.

The purpose and objectives of the study is often described first, followed by an explanation of what will happen to a research participant. Often, investigators and reviewers are confused about whether the investigator must include an explanation of every procedure or only experimental ones. Ordinarily, all procedures should be mentioned, differentiating clearly which are experimental, which are approved clinical procedures performed only for study purposes, and which are approved procedures that the research participant would be expected to have outside the research setting as part of standard care for the subject's illness or condition. Only the experimental procedures and/or aspects of the study, however, will be explained in detail. Prospective subjects should be told how long it will take to complete the study. If there are to be follow-up procedures, these too should be included with information on duration of follow-up and differences of procedures from those in the formal study period.

Consent and assent documents need to describe all reasonably foreseeable risks, discomforts, or mere inconveniences. Traditionally, risks and discomforts were thought of strictly in medical terms. This is no longer adequate. Psychosocial harm is as important to anticipate as are physical harms. For example, consent documents from the early days of genetics research list drawing blood as the risk and discomfort. Today, the research field understands that the potential for physical harm is not the substantive risk in genetics research; rather, breech of confidentiality and other psychosocial stressors pose the greatest risks for a subject. Even in such low-risk research as paper and pencil outpatient research, however, the risk section of the consent and assent documents should fairly represent the inconveniences. A potential subject might face additional time during an outpatient visit or the potential for fatigue or boredom.

The consent and assent documents need to indicate whether risks are rare or commonly experienced. Subjects need to know whether harms that occur during study participation can be reversed and/or how long after study participation problems might still arise. In research that poses substantial risk, it is important to include the caveat that there may be risks related to research participation that cannot be anticipated.

The protocol section of the consent and assent document also includes a description of expected benefits that must not be unduly emphasized or oversold, despite any potential benefits of a study. Research is not treatment. Even when research of a novel medical intervention is nearing the end of the approval process, until a diagnostic agent, device, or other intervention is approved and in clinical practice, it cannot be said to be treatment for the subject. Treatment provides fully individualized care. The same statement cannot be made for research. Even at the late phase III level, when it is realistic to anticipate obtaining direct medical benefit, a person's care is not fully personalized. It is personalized only within the specified parameters allowed by the protocol. Any care required that is outside allowed protocol limits will result in the subject reaching off-study criteria. **In short, even studies with a high probability of direct subject benefit will never provide personalized care synonymous with personalized clinical care. Recognition of this difference is emphasized by keeping the benefits sections of informed consent documents neutral and equivocal.** We recommend that anywhere in the consent and assent documents where the word *treatment* or *therapy* appears, it be proceeded by a word such as *experimental* or *investigational*.

For medical research that involves patient volunteers, a section on **alternatives to study participation** is required. Alternative procedures or treatments potentially advantageous to the subject, including those of no further aggressive intervention, should be mentioned briefly as appropriate. Obviously, when a study involves healthy subjects, the only alternative is not participating, and this section is not needed.

The extent to which subject confidentiality will be protected must be described fully. How confidentiality will be maintained and what procedures will be used to protect the subject's privacy and confidentiality should be explained in detail. In addition, to avoid making a promise that cannot be kept, there should be a statement that privacy and confidentiality cannot be guaranteed.

Consent forms need to include a description of payment for any research-related injuries that might occur. Explanation of any payments for expenses or other compensation for the study must be included, also. That means there is a statement telling subjects they will not be paid for their participation if that is the case. If they will be paid, an explanation of the compensation and procedures for compensation disbursement should be included. Payment for study participation is best differentiated from reimbursement for expenses.

Consent and assent documents will also include information regarding whom to contact about a subject's rights, whom to call regarding questions about the study, and whom to call in the case of emergency. In most cases, these names and phone numbers will all be different and at a minimum include contact information for the principal investigator and a regular 24-hour number for emergencies.

Subjects are encouraged both in the informed consent process and in the written consent documents to ask questions not only as they occur during the consent process but at any moment in time. There should be a statement in the consent document that explains that participation is voluntary. From the start of the protocol, the subject can withdraw at any time without penalty or loss of benefits to which the subject would be otherwise entitled. There should be nothing in the consent document that suggests that a subject waives his or her legal rights. Nonetheless, because a subject can withdraw prematurely, it is critical to discuss safe termination procedures with the researcher (when this is applicable). Documents need also to make clear, if it is relevant, that subject participation may be terminated by the investigator without subject consent.

Consent forms need to include a statement that significant new findings arising during the study will be transmitted to the subject as such findings may relate to a subject's willingness to continue participation. Depending on the study, some investigators will include a statement that if clinically relevant findings emerge after the study is completed, then the investigator will make a good faith attempt to find the subject and provide that updated information.

Finally, among the standard elements included in a consent and assent document is the number of subjects to be included in the study. If it is a multisite trial, this section may include how many sites there will be, how many subjects will be participating at each site, and, if different, how many subjects will be at the site where the particular subject is considering participation. In addition, if appropriate, a consent document includes information regarding risks to an embryo or fetus for pregnant women and information about the need to protect against pregnancy.

B. Debriefing for Altered or Waived Consent Processes

Under some circumstances, written informed consent may be altered or waived, as discussed previously in this section. If, for example, the signed consent document is the only record that links the subject to the research, and a breech of confidentiality poses risk of harm, written informed consent and/or assent should be waived. In such a case, an information sheet might be provided for subjects. A process for debriefing subjects, if appropriate, should be spelled out in the body of the protocol. When research involves deception, as discussed previously in this chapter, debriefing is important to disclose aspects of the study that were omitted or that differ from the consent process and documents.

When a protocol including subject deception is approved, we recommend that in addition to the protections in the Ethical Standards of the American Psychological Association and the CIOMS guidelines, the consent and assent documents state, *"This research includes purposes or activities, and other such points or procedures that are not being disclosed to the subject."* This lack of full disclosure is needed to ensure reasonable expectation of obtaining valid information from the information collected but informs the potential research participant that he or she is agreeing to be in a study in which some relevant information about study participation is being withheld. The consent language may go on to state:

> *What is not being disclosed to study participants, in the evaluation of the investigators and approval groups responsible for this research, does not present a serious threat to the physical or psychological well-being of study participants. At the end of either the study or the subject's participation, all aspects of the study that were not fully disclosed will be explained.*

C. Written Informed Consent in Health Services Research and Quality Improvement Projects

The need for written informed consent has become an important consideration in the health services research (HSR) and quality improvement (QI) projects research area. HSR and other kinds of epidemiologic studies have historically been granted consent waivers. There is growing concern that many of these studies may pose a greater than minimal risk for a subject and, therefore, fail the criteria for waiver of consent. Much of this research, however, cannot be practicably done without the waiver. Because society continues to believe this research is important, review bodies continue to give waivers. As scrutiny of medical research tightens and discussion about the boundaries of minimal risk continues, researchers can expect greater constraints on research that had previously been permitted to proceed without written informed consent.

This expectation seems reasonable, also, in the area of **quality improvement/quality assurance** (QI/QA) projects. Historically, such projects have not been reviewed. Now, there is substantive discussion in the literature (Bellin and Dubler, 2001; Casaret *et al.*, 2000) about what the criteria should be to tip a QI/QA project into the IRB-review required category. A part of the discussion is what sorts of consent, if any, ought to be obtained and from whom. Are only patients treated as subjects, or are staff members also treated as subjects? Further, QI/QA projects are no longer considered merely useful for good institutional management, but they are now integral and required. Given this shift, questions are now arising, such as:

- If all hospitals must do QI/QA projects, do these projects involve research of the usual kind in which persons have a right to participate or not?
- Is it the responsibility of all patients and staff to simply be a part of a continuous QI process?
- If patients and staff must be part of a continuous QI process, then how can consent be required if dissent is not a possibility?
- If QI/QA projects are simply part of hospital process, must anyone be told of anything in particular?

There are some who feel that not only is consent for QI/QA projects not relevant, but no information needs to be provided to the subjects. Others think that an infringement of the right to personal dignity results from not telling individuals what is being done to them or with their personal medical information. To prevent this infringement, the protocol would require that written information about any QI/QA project be provided to the patient and or surrogate. This is an area of research that can be expected to have new requirements. There will be an increasing demand for written documentation of formalized project review and approval as well as some sort of information provision.

D. Short Form Documents

There are two types of consent forms allowed by U.S. regulation. One is the **standard consent form**, in which all required elements of consent and any additional elements required by the needs of subjects in a particular study are included. The other is a **short form**, which is sufficient if all the required elements for ethically and legally valid informed consent have been presented orally to the subject or the subject's rightful surrogate. The body of the protocol gives data supporting the use of this consent, and the IRB/IEC accepts or rejects the justification. When a short form is used, there needs to be a witness to the oral presentation. The IRB/IEC also needs to approve a written summary of what is to be said to each prospective subject or the research surrogate. A copy of the summary in addition to a copy of the short form should be given to the subject or surrogate.

E. Translations

When some or many of the subjects in a research study can be expected to speak a language other than that of the researchers and research environment, consent and assent forms need to be translated. Simple, one-way translations may not be adequate. Optimally, when a consent document needs to be translated, one translator can be responsible for translating the form, for example, from English to Spanish. The form may then be back-translated from Spanish to English by a second translator. This process of translation/back-translation means that the researchers will have a greater level of confidence that the content will be properly translated into the final document. All of these copies need to be attached to the main protocol as part of the package reviewed and approved by the IRB and/or IEC.

F. Timing

Regardless of which form is used, the subjects and/or surrogates need time to not merely read the consent document, or have it read to them, but to study it. The subject and/or surrogate need the document for a length of time sufficient to digest it, to re-read it, to ask questions, to have other people review it, and to make a reasonable decision. It is typical in a flawed consent process that somebody sits down, runs through a consent document, and then asks the subject, "Are you ready? Do you want to do this? Will you sign?" Ordinarily, this short time frame for contemplation is not acceptable. It is important to reemphasize that there must be enough time for the subject to have his or her questions answered by investigators and to discuss it with people outside the research setting.

In summary, questions about how much information to convey and how best to convey it are very difficult and have no clear answers. IRBs and IECs spend a great deal of time reviewing consent documents in an attempt to ensure that an appropriate amount of information is presented in ways subjects and surrogates can understand and consider meaningfully. Most persons believe, or at least hope, that consent and assent documents expand on the information exchanges that are at the heart of the informed consent process.

9

PRIVACY AND CONFIDENTIALITY

I. TRADITIONS AND EXPECTATIONS

Privacy and confidentiality are related but different concepts. **Privacy** is a right connected to personal integrity. As a positive right, the right of privacy means that a person has the right to control access to and distribution of personal information, property, and/or knowledge of behaviors. As a negative right, the right of privacy ensures absence of interference or the right to be left alone.

Confidentiality protects the right of privacy. The notion of confidentiality recognizes that personal information is like personal property and that access to a person's information, property, and/or knowledge of behaviors must be protected. Confidentiality is a kind of promise that information and/or access provided by an individual to a professional, within the context of a trusting (i.e., fiduciary) relationship, will not be divulged without permission.

Although distinct and separable, these inherently linked notions of privacy and confidentiality are among medicine's most cherished values. They date back at least as far as the Hippocratic Oath and are central to physician obligations today. Although many modern versions of the Hippocratic Oath exclude the prohibition on euthanasia, abortion, sexual contact with patients, use of knives (i.e., performing surgical procedures), and the covenant with a deity, they uphold the provisions to protect privacy and confidentiality.

The requirement to protect privacy and confidentiality is perhaps even more stringent in clinical research than it is in medical practice. This is because of the inherent ethical tension between the two different kinds of physician obligations that are involved. Given that the primary goal of research is not the treatment of patients but the accrual of knowledge for the future benefit of others, research participants must be vigorously protected from the risks posed by studies undertaken to obtain that knowledge. All international documents that guide research ethics require protection of subject privacy and confidentiality. Research with human subjects needs a well-designed and clearly written plan to protect subject privacy and confidentiality.

Inherent in that plan is the appreciation that although privacy and confidentiality are to be protected to the greatest degree reasonable, guarantees of ironclad privacy and confidentiality cannot be given because they cannot be assured. There will be legitimate needs for subject data to be reviewed by others, such as study sponsors and the FDA and for criminal investigations. When subject data are to be seen by those outside the immediate research setting, the identity of such persons and/or entities should be disclosed to subjects. The possibility of an accidental breach of confidentiality always needs to be made clear to subjects.

The regulations protecting personally identifiable research information have become much more explicit, however, with the advent of the Health Insurance Portability and Accountability Act (HIPAA) (Appendix, No. 27). HIPAA, or the Health Insurance Portability and Accountability Act of 1996, is a major U.S. legislative effort to streamline and reduce paperwork, to make it easier to prosecute for medical fraud and abuse, and to protect patient's personal medical information. Originally planned to cover only electronically managed personal health information, HIPAA covers a wide swath of all personally identifiable information, both in the clinical and research arenas. HIPAA has complex jurisdictional constraints, however, that result in some research sponsors but not others being covered by HIPAA. All researchers are advised to consult their own institutional policies to ensure that they are in compliance with the new HIPAA regulations (Amatayakul, 2003; Dimond, 2002; Durham, 2002; Fox *et al.*, 2002; Maloney, 2001).

II. Management of Subject Privacy and Protection of Confidential Information

Like the concepts of privacy and confidentiality, management of subject privacy and protection of subject confidentiality are distinct but related activities. Consideration of both is part of planning a study.

Protection of subject privacy begins with the first interactions with a potential subject. For example, researchers can consider the following series of questions:

- Is the phone line that prospective subjects call in response to an advertisement only used by the researchers?
- If a member of the research team does not cover this phone line on a 24-hour basis, are prospective subjects directed to leave their name and a number through which they can be contacted?
- If personal information is left on the phone message machine for this phone line, how are names and numbers protected?
- Who picks up messages at the phone number?
- If someone from the research team returns a call, how does that person identify himself or herself when asking for the prospective research subject?

Simply identifying oneself as a researcher to members of a prospective subject's household may be a significant breach of privacy. For example, if the only number to return a call to a prospective subject is his or her home number, simply leaving enough information to inform others in the home about the research approach may present risk of harm to the subject. In the case of research about spousal abuse or teenage sexual activity, the implications are obvious. Even when the research is low risk about non-controversial topics, care needs to be taken from the outset in protecting information about a person's involvement, even mere interest, in a research project.

Once a prospective subject enters the research setting during the process of decision making about study participation, attention to privacy issues is required. Is there a place where researcher and prospective subjects can discuss study participation without being seen or overheard by others? If the person agrees to study participation, and there is any reasonable risk to the subject if he or she is identified as a participant, provisions will have to be made for private entry and exit from the research environment.

In studies in which multiple family members are involved, either as controls or as surrogates and the subject's identity is not kept from them, the subject may still want and/or need privacy from the other family members. For example, it is a common occurrence in oncology treatment trials that a patient volunteer is ready to withdraw from the study or does not want to join another study, but the spouse wants the patient volunteer to continue with the research. At such times, it is necessary for the patient volunteer to have time with the researchers alone and away from the pressuring spouse.

Pediatric research presents even greater barriers to privacy. The presumption, ethically and legally, is that parents have the right of access to their minor child's research records. But what if the research team finds that an adolescent subject has a sexually transmitted disease (STD)? Should they simply treat the condition without informing the subject's parents if the minor requests that the information not be divulged? The clinical practice today, at least in most U.S. jurisdictions, is that older adolescents can be treated for STDs without parental knowledge or permission. If researchers are willing to provide adolescents this measure of privacy, what about more serious and/or less easily concealed and/or treatable conditions, such as pregnancy, HIV infection, or illicit drug use?

Keeping subject information confidential involves complex considerations that are exemplified by the following questions:

- Is sensitive information that might carry the risk of stigma, discrimination, emotional distress, or legal problems for the subject being collected?
- Is such sensitive information being collected only about the subject, or will similar information about other family members also be collected from the subject?
- What special precautions, if any, should be taken to protect that sensitive information?
- How should data be recorded?
- Who can have access to the records? Should they or how should they be coded?
- If coded, who can have access to the list linking the subject name to the code? How and where will the list be kept?
- How secure is the location chosen to secure sensitive information documents? Will the information be in a locked cabinet in an open laboratory or in a secure area with limited access?
- How will records, such as photographs and/or video or audiotapes that are created by the research team, be stored and identified? How long will each of these kinds of research records be kept? Because a researcher needs to plan for the transfer of research data when membership of the research team changes, how does the researcher treat the research data from his or her own studies? Are the data the property of the researcher, the research sponsor, or the institution where the research is conducted?
- May any of the data ever be provided to other researchers?

Answers to the above questions can be incorporated into a protocol as appropriate, and there may be additional protocol-specific considerations. Sometimes the only document that links a subject to the research is a signed consent form. Ethically, and according to U.S. regulations, in this situation, when a breach of confidentiality places the subject at risk merely by being identified as a participant, a waiver of signed consent should be sought from the IRB/IEC.

III. PROVISION TO THE SUBJECT OF CLINICALLY RELEVANT PRIVATE RESEARCH INFORMATION

Some private information about a research subject that is obtained during a study may need to be given to the subject, the subject's surrogate, and/or the subject's community physician. This is usually clinical information that is considered relevant to a subject's immediate and/or future health. During design of the study, the possibility of obtaining such information can be anticipated and plans set for systematically providing the information to the appropriate person or individuals.

A. Provision of Information During Study Participation

Clinically meaningful information, obtained during a subject's active participation in a study, should be provided to the subject, the subject's surrogate, and/or the subject's community physician, as appropriate. **Explicit procedures for providing a subject's personal information to other individuals should be a part of the protocol.** For example, providing information may be as simple as sharing the regularly scheduled scans performed as part of a phase II breast cancer trial of a novel anticancer agent. The protocol ought to contain directions for transfer and disclosure of such information when the subject wants this information shared with his or her own oncologist. In pediatric treatment trials, it is expected that such anticipated, clinically relevant information will be shared with the pediatric subject, as appropriate, the parent and/or parents, and the subject's pediatrician or pediatric sub-specialist. There may be occasions, however, when the subject wants the information but does not want it shared with physicians. That is why a subject's permission is required before information is shared with medical professionals outside the research study.

Researchers may not be able to anticipate all occasions, however, when they discover information that was not expected but that has immediate and/or substantive predictable or future clinical relevance to a subject. This information should be conveyed to the subject and/or the subject's surrogate and, with appropriate permission, to the subject's community physician. The protocol should mention that such a situation might arise and can specify procedures for providing the information. For example, considering these questions may be helpful:

- Will the information only be provided to the subject?
- If the subject wishes to share the information with others, who (subject or investigator) will be responsible for arranging and assuring that the information transfer is performed in a confidential manner?
- If the subject is a minor, will information be provided to both or only one parent?
- In what form, written and/or oral, will the information be conveyed, and by whom (only the PI or other research staff also)?

Deciding what is immediately relevant to a subject's clinical status, or what may be in the future, is not necessarily a straightforward task. It may not be easy to decide which data have immediate clinical relevance. Or the investigator may not be a physician or be a physician but not in the specialty relevant to the subject's condition. Deciding which data a subject might want to know or what information may have clinical importance in the future can be a point of disagreement.

A common area of controversy is the degree to which genetic susceptibility to late onset disorders (those occurring later in life) ought to be considered clinically relevant and in what time frame. Wide differences of opinion exist among investigators and study participants, with no consensus about the best way to handle this information. We recommend that this issue be worked out for each protocol by the investigator in collaboration with the responsible IRB and/or IEC. The possibility of obtaining such information should be investigated during the study design process.

B. Provision of Information at Study Conclusion

Many consent documents inform subjects that information will be made available to them at the end of the study. It is often unclear what information will be made available and whether the end of the study refers to the end of active participation by the subject (including follow-up activities), the conclusion of active participation by all subjects, conclusion of data analysis, or the publication of study results.

At the end of the subject's participation in the primary study activities, he or she can receive much relevant information, regardless of its relation to the subject's medical status. This information could be clinically or psychologically meaningful or simply be a documentation of his or her study participation. The latter information can be as general as a review of the study procedures, conclusions, and a summary of what such procedures will provide for the researchers. If there is additional, clinically relevant information yet to be obtained, plans for getting this information to the subject should be arranged.

When a study is randomized and blinded, its original design may indicate how the subjects will be informed about their group assignment. It is likely that even if such information did become available to investigators when a subject completed randomized procedures, the information will not be distributed at least until all randomized subjects have completed their participation in the randomized, blinded components of the study. Premature "unblinding" can interfere with the validity of data analysis and should be avoided. If some subjects learn of their randomization status before all subjects have completed study procedures, the prospect for inadvertent unblinding is increased because of interactions among subjects and their families.

C. Provision of Information Long After Study Completion

Clinically relevant information frequently comes to the attention of an investigator long after a subject's individual study participation is over or even after the study has been terminated completely. For many studies, data are analyzed only after all subjects have completed study procedures. A subject in such a study should be informed during the consent process that if any clinical information relevant to him or her is obtained, the researchers will provide the information only after the completion of data collection and analysis. The subject can be requested to provide a phone number and address to the research team and to update these as necessary for a specified time to enable the team to communicate any potentially relevant information after the analysis. During this process, researchers can discuss with the prospective subject whether personal contact after study completion will require any special arrangements for maintenance of privacy. If so, mechanisms can be devised and documented in the research record for that subject to ensure that privacy and confidentiality will not be inadvertently breached.

It is possible that long after the study is completed and perhaps even long after it is published, new information is discovered, perhaps through reanalysis of old data or as a result of new data that provide important new insights into old findings. What is an investigator's obligation to a subject under these circumstances? There is no clear answer to this question, in part because there may be no consensus about what information is clinically relevant to the participant. Team members will have a general consensus about a specific piece of information. For example, if a lung mass were found in a subject undergoing routine chest X-rays for study purposes, such information will need to be given to the subject promptly. But, as discussed more fully in the next two sections of this chapter, other kinds of information that may be uncovered during a clinical research study will cause disagreement among researchers and research ethicists as to whether it should be provided to the subject, the subject's surrogate, and/or the subject's community physician. If such unveiling of questionably meaningful information can be anticipated to occur during the course of a study, we recommend that the consent process recognize the possibility and give the prospective subject the choice of whether to be contacted by the investigator long after study participation is completed. If contact is requested, the record will indicate whether special care to protect the subject's privacy and confidentiality in the contact process is needed.

Consider the study of persons with heart valve replacements. As part of the study, blood and tissue was taken and stored. The study was finished, and papers were written and published over 10 years ago. New techniques for analyzing the samples, however, have emerged that may shed some light on genetic propensity for valve deterioration. A new researcher who wants to run these studies has joined the team. The original consent process allowed for this situation in that it included discussion of the possibility of studying the samples in the future for diseases related to the condition of the patients in the original study. Those who consented had their blood drawn and stored. These samples are used by the new researcher. In the course of this new study, data are incidentally discovered that show evidence of predispositional genes for a neurological condition completely unrelated to the subjects' valve problem. Further, the new findings are about predispositional genetic mutations, so having the gene variant does not mean that the individual will develop the neurological disorder, only that the person is at increased risk. To make matters more complicated, there is only one treatment for the neurological disorder, and it is not well tolerated. The disorder also has a highly variable course across patients. What should the researcher do with this information?

If a subject wishes to obtain any news of potential interest well after study termination, the effort required of an investigator to deliver that information is the second part of the ethical problem. Again, there is no consensus. We recommend that the researcher make a good faith effort to contact the subject; once the researcher has tried to contact the subject, the researcher can view his or her obligation as being met. A good faith effort includes a letter sent to the subject's most recent address on record that explains to the subject the importance of contacting the researcher. If there is no response, additional measures will depend on the clinical relevancy, certainty, and urgency of the information that the investigator believes it important to convey. We suggest that this determination be made not by the investigator alone. Rather, this process is best accomplished in consultation with an IRB that can help design any further steps (if any are considered prudent) and that will assist in implementing a means of contact that protects the subject's privacy and confidentiality.

D. Counseling Subjects

The type of information that could be generated during a study should determine whether counseling of subjects should be a part of the study design. For example, if infection with HIV is an exclusion criterion and the prospective subject will be tested to determine his or her study eligibility, counseling the individual about HIV and the implications of having or not having the test should be part of the study's initial informed consent process. If the counseling is adequate, a prospective subject will be able to understand the implications of the test and of receiving a positive HIV test result, including the necessity of reporting and the need to obtain referral for follow-up care. The individual can weigh those implications against interest in study participation. If the individual goes on to have the HIV test as part of study screening and receives a positive HIV test result, the counseling needed to meet standards of appropriate clinical practice must also be part of the protocol's screening processes. Other protocols require provision for other kinds of counseling. Investigations of genetic mutations that predispose carriers to serious diseases definitely require a substantive counseling component.

When designing a study, the first question is whether special counseling is needed. If so, the next question is who will provide the counseling. Physician/investigators often believe incorrectly that they are sufficiently knowledgeable and skilled to provide the counseling. The decision may be influenced also by financial constraints and/or the sources of counseling that are available. In many cases, it is important not to underestimate either the need for counseling or the skills needed to provide it. For genetics studies, counselors who specialize in this field are often the only professionals with adequate training, knowledge, and experience. Unfortunately, the numbers of genetics counselors available are insufficient to meet the demand resulting from the explosive expansion of clinical research in this area. A genetics study requires on-site genetics counselors as well as provision for referrals, remote consultations, investigator training sessions, and other ancillary services to ensure appropriate counseling for subjects. The addition of counseling to a protocol may pose additional considerations for how information generated during the study will be kept confidential (Berry, 2003; Chen, 2001).

IV. WITHHOLDING PERSONAL INFORMATION FROM A STUDY SUBJECT

Some information may be best withheld from research subjects. This view is very controversial. Certain investigators and clinical research ethicists believe, on the basis of rights of autonomy, that any information collected about a subject as part of a research study should be shared with the subject if requested. We believe that withholding information from subjects should be done only infrequently and only with the approval of the IRB and/or IEC. We also believe, however, that some information need not be provided to subjects. These informational categories include data that are scientifically uninterpretable and information that can reasonably be expected to produce severe harm, such as evidence of nonpaternity. There may be research settings, however, where even the prudent withholding of research-generated information is not allowed. For example, at the time of this book's publication, legal interpretation is that research information produced by federal government-employed researchers, such as those within the NIH's Intramural Research Program, cannot withhold any information generated about a research subject that is requested by a research subject because of the requirements of the Federal Privacy Act.

A. Withholding Meaningfully Uninterpretable Clinical Research Information

Unless researchers plan to provide subjects with all research-generated information, including raw data, which is unheard of, decision about what information to provide is a matter of judgment. As discussed in the previous sections of this chapter, some clinically relevant information, by general agreement, should be provided to subjects expeditiously. Beyond the most obvious, however, there are no clear guidelines. Some investigators, subjects, and ethicists believe that information about genetic predisposition to disease ought definitely to be provided. Others argue against disclosing disease predisposition, especially when minors and/or late onset disorders for which there is no treatment or medical prevention are involved. Many of the arguments concerning these issues hinge on concerns about potential psychological harms to subjects and/or families related to genetic information that has a high degree of uncertainty. For example, a child who has a BRCA1 mutation will not necessarily grow up to develop breast cancer. Even in subjects with Huntington's disease, where evidence of the mutation predicts with certainty its development, the age of onset and clinical course are uncertain.

Uncertainty becomes unmanageable when even the scientific meaning of research findings is uninterpretable. Most would agree that, when a scientific area of study or field is at an early stage of development, clinical research goals are to make observations upon which more definitive studies can be based. Virtually any, save the most basic, molecular interpretation of findings is premature. Provision of this kind of information to subjects is simply not useful. This belief is based on the ethical notion that **provision of information, in and of itself, is a morally neutral act. Provision of information is beneficial only when it serves some useful end; in other words, providing information without understanding its implications may be harmful.** The primary obligation of clinical researchers is to conduct scientifically sound research in a manner that protects the rights and welfare of research participants. When the implications and potential risks of information are unknown, we believe that protection of a subject's welfare takes precedence over autonomy rights to have access to scientifically uninterpretable data.

A strong counterargument claims that only the subjects themselves can reasonably be expected to be interested enough to follow the development of the science long enough to link their own early stage data with scientific progress evolving over years or decades.

Consider a subject afflicted with a genetic disorder for which there is no treatment, no cure, and virtually no understanding of etiology and pathophysiology. Imagine, also, that the results for many of the molecular studies performed on the subject's blood samples during the study will be and can be expected to remain uninterpretable for many years. Nonetheless, the subject, who not only suffers but whose family suffered for generations from the disease and can be expected to continue to suffer through future generations, wants copies of all data generated about himself or herself from the study. This research participant argues that because the subject and his or her family will maintain interest for a very long time, they ought to be able to hold their presently uninterpretable data until future studies provide insights that allow for interpretation. Certainly, this is a difficult request to turn down. This request is compelling from a clinical perspective for the researcher; it is also an accurate reflection of who would be most interested in and willing to follow the research over a period of years and decades. What should a researcher do?

We suggest that when a researcher's subject wishes to access and hold onto data that will not be interpretable for a number of years, this researcher might want to consult the IRB and/or IEC of the institution for consideration in a manner analogous to a compassionate use request. Doing so, however, does not negate the default position that protection from potential risks comes first in an early phase study with data that are clinically uninterpretable. If disclosure of clinically meaningless information might ultimately contribute to stigma and discrimination, withholding of scientifically uninterpretable data is the ethically preferable option. This position is strengthened by the reasonable probability that by the time there are scientifically interpretable data having clinical relevance for individuals, testing will be developed so that data collected in the preliminary studies can easily, and perhaps more accurately, be resampled for validity.

B. Withholding Highly Volatile and Possibly Destructive Information

We recommend that data that can be predicted with a reasonable degree of certainty to lead to serious harm for the subject, especially violence, be withheld. Such kinds of information include evidence of nonpaternity, misattributed maternity, and incest. The arguments for and against withholding information offered in the previous sections are essentially applicable here as well. **The morally relevant difference is that although there may be important and useful applications of such harmful information in decisions regarding the medical care and/or future reproductive choices of subjects, the same information can be obtained outside the research setting.** Therefore, although this information may be of current relevance and/or interest to a research subject or the parent(s) of a research subject, because this kind of information can be obtained outside the research setting, it should not be divulged within the research setting except under the most constrained of circumstances. When such rare circumstances emerge, provision of this kind of highly volatile information should be provided only with guidance from the IRB.

Nothing in the canons of clinical research ethics suggests that investigators provide, in the name of autonomy rights, information that is incidental to the information sought in a study where the incidental information can reasonably be anticipated to cause grievous harm. Instead, clinical research ethics and regulations governing clinical research call for minimization of risks to human subjects. **Researchers are obligated to protect subjects, especially from risks that can be anticipated.** The threat of emotional damage or family violence, as in matters like nonpaternity and incest, suggest that investigators should not provide such information found incidentally during a study.

To protect subject privacy, however, when such information (often held for years as family secrets) might be obtained, it is important that persons who hold that information in secret know ahead of time that such information may emerge during the research study.

A family with a rare genetic disease may hear of a research project that would be relevant to their disease. If family members decide to go through the informed consent process, researchers interviewing them can inform them of the type of troublesome information, such as nonpaternity, that might be generated from such a study. Here, it is not sufficient simply to inform the prospective subject. Researchers can inform subjects in such a way that allows a family member who does not want to participate, because participation might result in discovery of the "family secret," to decline participation with protection of his or her privacy and confidentiality.

Creating a process to accomplish the disclosure or withholding of potentially harmful kinds of private information will require thoughtful creativity by both investigators and IRBs and/or IECs. The potential for family violence that breach of privacy and/or confidentiality poses, however, demands that this issue be well considered and planned for each protocol before a problem occurs.

When such matters are the core questions to be investigated, how this information will be collected, stored, and conveyed or not conveyed to subjects are considerations central to the study design and approval process. In such studies, strategies for protecting privacy and confidentiality are among the central ethical concerns of the protocol.

V. PROVISION OF INFORMATION AT STUDY CONCLUSION

Investigators should provide an extensive summary to each subject after a study is completed. A common complaint of study subjects is that they contribute their time, effort, and bodies and never hear about the study after it is finished. This lack of feedback contributes to human research subjects feeling like guinea pigs. This summary of information can take on two forms. One form is a **summary report of the subject's personal participation.** This is essentially a lay rewriting of any medical information that is provided to the subject and that is to be given to his or her community physician or that goes directly, with the participant's permission, to the subject's community treating clinician. This kind of study summary, at least the technical version, is common practice and ordinarily required for sound discharge of a volunteer patient from a clinical study. It is the translation of the technical transfer report that is a novel suggestion here.

The second form of summary that is recommended is one that is rarely provided. This is a **summary of the study findings written in lay**

language that is sent to all study participants. Investigators ought to make a greater effort to share the findings of their studies with the individuals who served as partners in the production of those findings. One important means of doing so is to send summaries of study findings to all participants after the data are analyzed and published. This lay summary might include reference to, or a copy of, any professional publications that resulted from the study. This is another way in which researchers respect the dignity of their subjects and maximize benefits of clinical research participation.

The ethical controversy is not whether subjects should receive such information, but what measures researchers need to take to protect the privacy and confidentiality of subjects when reporting findings, either in summary form to subjects or in publications. When providing data in summary form to subjects and/or in a publication, a writer can quite easily mask personal identity when the study is large and/or deals with commonly occurring conditions or diseases. This masking may not be easy for a study involving a rare disease or a small cohort of subjects. In studies of genetic diseases, whether pedigrees can be altered and how subjects can be protected from identification by their own family members and/or communities are topics of hot debate in the field of scientific publishing.

VI. RELEASE OF RESEARCH INFORMATION TO OTHERS

Protecting privacy and confidentiality of research subjects is all about keeping identifiable research information private. **The expectation, in ethics and regulation, is that information collected and/or generated within the clinical research setting will stay with the researchers unless the subject gives expressed specific, written consent for its transfer.** Ordinarily, permission will specify to whom and under what circumstances the information can be conveyed. It is important to remember, however, that there can be no iron-clad guarantee of absolute protection of privacy and confidentiality. For many studies, research records may be accessible to a variety of individuals and organizations, and there is always the theoretical possibility of an accidental breach.

Historically, it has been common for researchers to share data among themselves. This may mean sharing clinical research data between one research institution and another or among otherwise unrelated research groups within the same institution. If there is a possibility of such sharing of personally identifiable research data, prior written consent of the subjects should be obtained.

Situations may exist in which there is no transfer of information from the researcher to a third party, yet subjects feel forced to offer information, either on insurance and/or employment applications. For example, if an individual is seeking insurance or a job, applications may ask if the individual has ever participated in a genetics research study. Subjects should not be encouraged to lie on such forms. Rather, an ethically acceptable informed consent process will ensure that potential subjects understand the implications and risks of the information to be collected and developed during the course of a study and that privacy and confidentiality cannot be guaranteed. With this information and understanding, an individual can make his or her own decision about whether to participate in the study.

VII. CERTIFICATE OF CONFIDENTIALITY

A **Certificate of Confidentiality** is a novel mechanism to improve protection of the confidentiality of research records from legal and/or administrative disclosure. A Certificate of Confidentiality is a documented agreement on the part of the DHHS that researchers conducting a particular study will not be required to divulge any personally identifying information about the study's subjects in any administrative or judicial court proceedings other than those already required by law, such as in child abuse cases. If a study that collects highly sensitive information, such as on spousal abuse and/or illegal activities, requires data to be collected and stored, along with signed informed consent documents, it may be a good idea to obtain a Certificate of Confidentiality. The Certificate of Confidentiality was originally developed by the DHHS to protect subjects in studies investigating illegal drug use and mental illness. HIV research started using the certificate, and it is now applied to studies of genetic and other diseases and conditions.

The Certificate of Confidentiality is a subject protection mechanism that is implemented through the investigator. The Certificate of Confidentiality has already withstood court challenges and is a protection expected to be more widely known and used in the future. It is important to remember, however, that Certificates of Confidentiality protect study data only from involuntary disclosure by the researcher(s) in court or administrative hearing situations. It does not protect the data from being disclosed by the research participant nor does it exempt researchers from having to disclose research data in cases where such disclosure is already legally required, such as in child abuse cases.

VIII. WRITING THE PROTOCOL SECTION ON PRIVACY AND CONFIDENTIALITY

Writing the protocol section on privacy and confidentiality requires the investigator to have considered how best to employ strategies

and mechanisms to protect individual- or group-identifying information generated and stored. When few or no data are generated in written form and data collected are of a sensitive nature, careful consideration of what individual-identifying information needs to be collected and/or stored is important. When scientifically acceptable, it is important to consider avoiding collection of personally identifiable information. When data must be collected in identifiable form, the researcher would be wise to be aware of conditions under which the identifiers can later be eliminated or stripped. When personally identifiable information must remain with research data, the investigator should explain in this section how such data will be managed, coded, and stored.

IX. WRITING PRIVACY AND CONFIDENTIALITY STATEMENTS IN CONSENT FORMS

Inclusion of a statement about privacy and confidentiality in a consent form is required. The U.S. regulations require that, where appropriate, adequate provision be made for protecting the privacy of subjects and maintaining the confidentiality of data. **Informed consent documents should contain a statement of how privacy and confidentiality will be accomplished.** If identification of subjects is a risk, the researcher states how subjects will be shielded from recognition. If data are to be coded, the researcher explains where the list connecting the coded numbers to subject names will be kept and who will have access to the list. The researcher also indicates which groups, such as sponsors, the FDA, and insurers, will have access to research records and can include a statement such as "Privacy and confidentiality will be protected vigorously to the extent permissible by law. We cannot, however, guarantee privacy or confidentiality." It is important that subjects understand that privacy and confidentiality are difficult to maintain completely and that accidental breaches do occur. There should also be a statement to inform subjects that maintaining privacy and confidentiality does not protect them from divulging information themselves if they are asked about the research on insurance and/or employment forms. Finally, it is likely that a HIPAA disclosure and/or release form will be required as part of an investigator's institutional policies. This form will most probably be standardized text supplied to investigators through their IRB administrators.

10

●●●●●●●●●

THE "ETHICS" SECTION

●●●●●●●●●●●●●●●●●

I. THE DIFFERENCE BETWEEN AN ETHICS SECTION AND A COMPLIANCE WITH ETHICS REGULATIONS SECTION

Many protocols have a section entitled Ethics or Ethical Considerations. For the most part, however, these sections focus on regulatory compliance and not substantive ethics. Commonly included in these sections are the consent and assent documents, a statement that the protocol adheres to the principles of the Declaration of Helsinki (which it often does not), a statement that the protocol follows good clinical practice (GCP) guidelines and, where appropriate, the ICH guidelines. Such sections should be renamed to reflect more accurately their focus on regulatory compliance. They are necessary, and they address ethical issues, but they do so within the context of regulatory compliance, which is quite different from a section that addresses the specific ethical issues relevant to the particular protocol. In addition to the standard focus on regulatory compliance, there should be an expanded discussion of ethical issues and a means for differentiating those that require protocol-specific analysis from ethically driven compliance issues generically required of all human subjects protocols.

The ethics section that we recommend is additional; this section is a true ethics section that is best placed at the end of the design portion of the protocol. Placement of this new section in the design portion of the protocol ensures that there is a presentation of the full range of substantive ethical concerns related to each protocol and that these are specified and explained.

Such a new ethics section will distinguish the protocol from one that merely indicates compliance with the ethics regulations from one that demonstrates a meaningful level of ethical sensitivity on the part of the investigator and/or sponsor. This is not to suggest that simply writing the section will ensure that the study will be conducted properly. Rather, it will assist investigators in making a good faith effort to identify the full range of ethical concerns raised by the protocol. Further, by making the substantive, protocol-specific issues explicit, it will assist review groups in focusing on the ethically important issues it is their job to consider. Too many IRBs and IECs waste precious time reviewing the consent forms. The effort that most review bodies invest in overhauling consent forms could be accomplished by well-trained research review administrators. The critical task that can be performed only by the IRB and/or IEC is to probe the ethical implications of the study itself. Having a well-articulated, highly focused section illuminating the substantive ethical issues integral to the particular study advances the prospect that the design will be ethically sound and that appropriate subject protections will be built into the protocol. The following questions will assist investigators in deciding what needs to be in this new ethics section:

- Is this a study that needs to be done?
- Is the information to be gained of importance sufficient to place human subjects at risk of even a mere inconvenience?
- Are there any subject characteristics that might make subjects vulnerable to manipulation?
- What aspects of the protocol present concern for subject safety?
- Are there any aspects of the protocol that diverge from accepted standards-of-medical practice?
- If so, what are they and in what ways do they diverge?
- What risks of harm are created for subjects by the divergence?
- What is the ethical justification for the divergence and the risks posed?
- What are the benefits of the study?
- Might the benefits pose an undue inducement to study participation or a reluctance to withdraw?
- Does the protocol call for additional subject protections?
- If additional subject protections are to be used, what should these additional protections be and why?

Assuring the reader that regulatory compliance will be followed does not answer these questions. Only a vigorous defense of the specific study components (e.g., inclusion or exclusion criteria, randomization with or without a placebo arm, payments to subjects or to parents of minor subjects, mechanisms to protect subjects from dangerous premature withdrawal) leads to vigorous discussion by the review body. Only through such vigorous discussion can the review body fully exercise its responsibility for study approval and oversight. A study can comply fully with regulatory requirements yet have ethical issues integral to the study be insufficiently considered and/or discussed. For example, studies involving placebo arms are permitted, in principle, by regulation and by the Declaration of Helsinki and CIOMS. In many studies, the default bias of the FDA is that a placebo arm is necessary for adequate statistical analysis. But it is the responsibility of investigators and review bodies to decide whether a placebo arm is ethically acceptable in each specific study. There are many examples far more subtle.

> Consider investigational development of pain medications to be taken on an as-needed basis. In the face of regulatory body preference for fixed dose designs, when might it be acceptable to require a fixed-dose design to test for safety that results in overdosing subjects?

Meeting regulatory requirements and adhering to the Declaration of Helsinki can never get investigators and review bodies to the level of specificity of study design demanded by the ethical analysis of the design issues of a particular study. Therefore, we recommend that each clinical research protocol include a section that focuses both investigators and review bodies on the particular ethical issues embedded in the particular study under consideration.

II. AN EXISTING MODEL OF A SUBSTANTIVE ETHICS SECTION

Since 1997, the NIH Clinical Center has had a policy requiring all intramural program protocols to include a substantive ethics section. This policy requires that all intramural research program protocols include the rationale for subject selection based on a review of gender, ethnic, and race categories at risk for the disease/condition. Inclusion of any special classes (i.e., pregnant women) of subjects must be justified. A discussion of strategies and procedures for recruitment (including advertising, if applicable) and justification for any exclusion are also required. The NIH policy requires; that this section include an evaluation of benefits; and risks/discomforts; physical, psychological, social, legal, or other vulnerabilities; and an assessment of their likelihood. Protections of privacy and confidentiality are to be specified. This policy requirement represents an important advance in explicitly addressing ethical issues on a per-protocol basis. NIH grantees have comparable requirements.

In addition to specific issues that such a section needs to cover, flexibility needs to be built into the ethics section so that investigators do not fall into the habit of only considering the specified items, dulling the moral imagination needed to pick up subtle ethical issues embedded in different studies. Instead, it may be better to leave open the ethical issues to be covered, forcing study sponsors and investigators to analyze each protocol individually.

III. WRITING A SUBSTANTIVE ETHICS SECTION

The new, substantive ethics section may best be situated at the end of the design portion of the protocol. **The investigator should fully articulate the ethical issues presented by the protocol and justify the proposed study design.** That means that the person or persons writing the protocol need to understand the difference between ethical considerations and regulatory and/or compliance issues. One of the best ways to learn how to articulate the ethical underpinnings of a study is to ask, for each section of the protocol, questions that focus on the principles and theories discussed in Chapter 2. That is, for each major section of the protocol, ask the following:

- What ethical principles does this study section raise? The following are examples:
  - Is there anything in this section that presents concerns about a subject's ability to make his or her own decisions? If so, what might either assist the person in doing so and/or protect the person who cannot?
  - Are there ways that the study can be altered to reduce risks further? What are we calling a study benefit? Might that be controversial? Might that be coercive?
  - What justice concerns are raised by this study's design? What are the socioeconomic conditions in the country or community of the trial? What are the socioeconomic statuses of proposed subjects?

- If we do X, what might be the short-term/long-term potential positive/ negative consequences? The following are examples:
  - Is there anything in this study design that diverges from standards of practice for the subject's disease or condition? If so, in what ways? Might the divergence produce short-term or long-term problems for symptoms or disease course?

o   If there is little experience with the agent or device in humans, or in humans with the condition or disease under study, how well do the animal and/or computer models predict the behavior in the proposed subject population?

o   Related to each study section, what are the investigator's obligations to subjects?

o   Is there any way, either medically or nonmedically, that the proposed subjects for this study might be considered vulnerable, or possibly become vulnerable and/or decisionally impaired during study participation?

o   Can all the proposed subjects provide their own ethically and legally valid consent?

o   If not, what protections might be helpful/required?

o   Given other ethically complex aspects of study design, what other and/or different kinds of additional protections or ways of minimizing risk and maximizing benefit can/might/should be built into the protocol?

Identifying the ethical issues embedded in a protocol and then deciding how best to address them is complex and difficult. That is why the primary goal of this book is to impress upon clinical researchers that the science and ethics of a clinical study cannot be separated. If we have made this point clearly it will be obvious that identifying, articulating, and addressing the ethical aspects of a clinical trial require the same effort and collaborative process that has long been applied to the seemingly purely scientific aspects of designing a clinical trial. Consideration of the ethical issues and how and where they are integrated into other aspects of the protocol requires a process of collaborative discussion with clinical researchers and clinical research ethicists. Such discussions are most successful in coming to ethically appropriate and scientifically valid solutions when researchers and research ethicists discuss specific protocols together and start their discussions early in the design process.

The following section presents specific language, with blanks to be filled in and expanded to address the full range of substantive ethical issues considered for a proposed protocol.

The primary ethical issue(s) raised by the scientific design of this protocol is/are...

(Issues that should be inserted here include randomization and blinding, placebo control or issues related to the statistical validity of the study, characteristics of the study population suggesting degree of vulnerability, and/or potential problems with capacity of

subject to give valid consent. When ethical concerns are additive, such as in studies involving psychiatrically ill minors or frail, elderly subjects with life-threatening conditions that also produce mental status declines, addressing the additive nature of the issues is a central ethical requirement.)

Although these aspects of the study mean that this protocol is ethically complex, the scientific information to be gained is important because...

(Inserted here should be the justification for why this study will be useful. The researchers are advised to be conservative, focusing on why knowledge to be gained is needed. Is the information to be gained novel or confirmatory? Does the information to be gained address a compelling, unmet need?)

The risks to subjects and/or their community are...

(Here, the investigator needs to think broadly, elucidating the full range of potential risks and/or harms.)

It would be impossible, however, to obtain this information without this design....

(i.e., including placebo arms, randomization, minors, a multicenter trial in undeveloped countries, adults with questionable decision-making capacity)

because...

(It should be explained here why a less ethically complicated and/or ethically problematic design would not allow accomplishment of the scientific ends of the protocol.)

Therefore, we believe that to manage appropriately the ethical complexities inherent in this study, it is necessary to put the following additional protections of human subjects/study population(s) in place. They are...

(Additional protections may include medically responsible non-research-affiliated clinicians, consent monitors, research durable powers-of-attorney, assessments to provide ethically and legally valid consent on an intermittent basis throughout study participation not merely for initial consent, special strategies for follow-up and for ensuring safe and orderly premature termination of study or of participation of a subject in the study, provisions for continued drug provision after study conclusion.)

By instituting these additional protections, the risks have been appropriately minimized, and a reasonable and an ethically acceptable balance between risks and benefits has been established.

By including in the design portion of the protocol this kind of substantive ethics section, consideration by investigators and review bodies of the ethical aspects of the protocol will exceed regulatory compliance, addressing more fully the substantive ethical questions raised by each protocol. Through the writing and review of such a section, analysis of ethical issues during the design phase of the protocol will be more thorough and investigators and review bodies will be more conscious of sponsor's and investigator's justifications for each protocol. By becoming more explicit about the ethical issues embedded in a study, the proposed justifications, and what, if any, additional protections sponsors and investigators have proposed to be built into the study design, discussions by review bodies will be more focused on whether the review bodies agree that the study is ethically justifiable and that the protocol appropriately protects the rights and welfare of the particular subjects proposed for inclusion. In addition, anecdotal evidence indicates that protocols containing such sections enjoy streamlined IRB and IEC review and encourage smoother communications among IRB and IEC bodies, investigators, and study sponsors.

section

III

....

PROCEDURES, METHODS, STATISTICS, DATA MANAGEMENT, AND RECORD KEEPING

....

11

· · · · · · · · · ·

PROCEDURES AND METHODS

· · · · · · · · · · · · · · · · ·

The study procedures and methodology section describes the manipulations that will be carried out, in what sequence, and by whom. This section must be explicit and complete with a specification of how measurements will be taken and how data will be analyzed; an explanation of whether subjects will be randomized or blinded; and, if interventions will be performed on subjects, a clarification on how they will be performed, how often, and by whom.

For example, in a genetic study, what kind(s) of sample(s) will be taken? Who will do the procedures? In a surgical device trial, who will perform the surgery and what qualifications of experience and background will be required of the surgeon(s)? Regardless of the subject of a study, descriptions of data to be collected and the means of collection are required.

Researchers also realize that depending on the length and scope of the study, some measurements may be taken at different time intervals or frequencies than others. How this will be done must be fully recorded in this section of the protocol. In addition, it is often useful to present this information not only in narrative form in this section but also in the form of flow charts or diagrams, included in appendices and/or consent documents that are attached to the protocol.

Procedures should be established and described in the protocol to meet the criteria for reducing bias and protecting subject safety. For example, blinding and randomization reduce bias. Explicit and easy-to-follow procedures for breaking the code for a blinded study in an emergency contribute to subject safety.

I. RANDOMIZATION

Randomization is a process of selecting groups for comparison of the efficacy of one intervention over another; subjects are allocated to the various arms via a random selection process, as already explained in Chapter 4. If a study involves randomization (which will have been justified in the study design section), the procedures and methodology section explains how subjects will be randomized. Will randomization be affected by simply assigning each subject to the various study arms as they enter, or will there be a computerized assignment process? Researchers specify who will have access to the randomization assignment during the trial and explain how the information that determines where a subject will be placed is protected from unauthorized access.

If the randomization strategy is straightforward, explaining how subjects will be assigned is sufficient for this section of the protocol. But if the study calls for a more complex design, such as a crossover or random assignment after a run-in and/or a washout period, explanation will be required for ensuring subject safety.

Related most closely to the reporting of randomized trials, investigators of a randomized trial can familiarize themselves with the CONSORT statement (CONSORT, 2004) in the design phase of the protocol. The CONSORT statement is an important research tool that uses an evidence-based approach to improve the quality of reports of randomized trials. Used widely throughout the world, the CONSORT statement's information and its accompanying checklist and flow diagram can help investigators during study design to enhance comparability of data across related randomized trials and strengthen the ability of others to evaluate data validity. Doing so advances the ethical requirement to maximize study benefits. Designing studies so data can be compared across multiple different trials increases data utility.

II. BLINDING

Many studies are **double-blinded**, meaning that neither the subject nor the investigator knows to which study arm the subject has been assigned. If a study is blinded, how the blind will be created and maintained will have to be fully described. The protocol will need to provide enough information to convince reviewers that the group preparing the study medications, including placebos, is competent and trained to do so. Researchers may consider the following list of questions when writing this section of the protocol:

- How, precisely, will one arm's intervention be made to look like the other arm's intervention?
- Who will prepare the blinded agents?
- What will the procedures be for breaking the blind, if necessary, for medically indicated reasons?
- When will the blind be broken for data analysis?
- If some measurements are to be taken without being blinded, which ones are going to be explained and what strategies will be applied to reduce bias in analysis of the unblinded measurements?
- What will be done to reduce the risk of blinds being broken by subjects communicating among themselves?

III. DRUG TESTING

If the protocol is testing a new agent with the expectation of developing a marketable drug by a U.S. sponsor, at the very least the procedures will be governed by FDA regulations, GCP guidelines, and the applicable ICH guidelines. It is likely that the drug trial will require multiple IRB and IEC approvals and involve many different countries and/or multiple study sites within various countries. Most pharmaceutical companies have their own protocols that describe study procedures in exhaustive detail. This information needs to be comprehensive to educate nonresearch personnel, such as unit nurses, residents, and fellows, in the administration of study agents and procedures.

A. Drug Information

The section on drug information describes the physical properties of the agents, formulations, and strengths. This includes the colors, sizes, shapes, smell, taste, viscosity, and other such information concerning the tablets, capsules, solutions, powders, or other compositional attributes. If the study involves a placebo, the placebo's physical properties and attributes should be described as well. Information is included that demonstrates that the processing of the active and placebo agents, such as the manufacturing and packaging, is safe and meets appropriate safety and purity standards. Although for studies sponsored by drug or device companies many of these details will be in the investigator's brochure that accompanies the protocol, the investigator's brochure is rarely provided to all IRB and IEC members. Enough detail should be included in the protocol to ensure that IRB and IEC members can satisfy themselves about safety issues related to these aspects of study design.

This section includes a description of agent packaging, such as bottles, blister packs, vials, or tubes. Any special aspects of the packaging needed for proper administration, such as packaging information about dose adjustments, can be highlighted. What need not be included is the type of information that could change during the course of a study, such as information about the number of pills per blister packet. Child-resistant packaging should be the default and so stated. If alternative packaging, such as blister packs, is to be used, this should be made clear in the protocol.

Labeling information goes in this section as well, including information about how labels will be made to ensure proper randomization or to protect blinding. Not to be included, however, are the protocol elements of a label that are standardized in regulation or are already covered by ICH guidelines, such as drug strength, sponsor/institution name, or protocol number. Rather, boilerplate language such as the following may be sufficient: "Labeling information meets applicable regulatory requirements. Specifics are available upon request or in Investigator's Brochure."

What is important to include in detail is the information needed for safe preparation and handling, such as for reconstitution procedures, temperatures to maintain agent viability, intravenous or oral suspension preparations, and other such information. The level of detail will be site/protocol-specific for preparation and handling requirements. Processes and directions for any special handling and/or storage requirements should be described if transport after preparation will be required. Any equipment needed for preparation, handling, administration, and/or storage (e.g., syringes, blood sampling tubes, scales, and any other special equipment) should be listed. It is important to describe who will be providing supplies and equipment, how these supplies will be conveyed to the site, and whether strict accounting will be required.

Accountability for drug supply, including sponsor and investigator responsibilities for maintaining drug accountability and drug record keeping, should be stated. Researchers should also explain the procedures for tracking study drug intake by subjects, when this is relevant. For example, in some out-patient studies, strategies for protocol compliance will need to be well-developed and clearly explained in the protocol and consent and/or subject or surrogate information materials. This issue may be critical to ensure both subject safety and scientific validity of study findings.

B. Dosing and Administration

Dosing and administration information needs to be fully specified. The level of detail needed has implications for subject safety and

for ensuring data quality. Selecting study dose or doses has important ethical implications that go well beyond safety concerns. Depending on whether the study is a phase I, II, or III trial, determining the dose has implications not only for subject risk but will also impact potential for subject benefit. The study may be a single bolus administration, or the study may test dose ranges and/or a number of different doses. Often, the choice of a starting dose for an initial study of a new drug is based on a variety of factors. These include comparison of the drug's potency and activity with that of known standards with a similar mechanism of action. Increasingly controversial is the historically common practice of obtaining values for the initial study from the LD50 (i.e., the dose that kills 50% of test animals, which is the median lethal dose). These tests have come under increasing attack and are expected to be used less frequently in the future. This evolving concern for the kinds of animal data to be obtained prior to initiating human studies is reflected in the change of the most recent Declaration of Helsinki (2000) (Appendix, No. 13). In this revision, the traditionally firm requirement for gathering animal data prior to initiation of clinical trials has been limited. The new language no longer makes such data an absolute requirement for moving to human trials. Rather, the new declaration (2000) calls for animal studies to precede human trials only to the degree absolutely needed.

The initial studies will also seek to establish pharmacokinetic and pharmacodynamic data. All of this information will be pooled to determine a conservative dose that is expected to represent the threshold of the dose–response relationship in humans. A fraction of this low dose is usually selected as the starting dose in the early phase II trials.

This dose determination process is obscure to the general, non-research public and to the majority of research subjects. If, however, patients volunteer for research seeking direct medical benefit, the potential for benefit in a trial with a starting dose at a weak level for the early entry subjects is virtually nothing. This fact of the clinical research process should be explained to participants. Although one suspects that even if this were fully explained to subjects, the psychological mechanisms underlying the therapeutic misconception would block appreciation of the implications of dose escalation for potential direct benefit, such a possibility does not relieve the investigator from making a good faith effort to provide an explanation.

This problem has generated some discussion but little change in practice. Conversations have started at professional clinical research meetings of the need to develop novel clinical research designs allowing individual subjects to pick their risk level and decide at which dosing cohort they would want to be entered, but these discussions have not yet resulted in concrete protocol strategies. A novel study design that is being seen more often is a rapid cohort escalation approach. This design allows for moving fewer persons more quickly through early stages of a study so that doses of an experimental agent that are anticipated to be too low to have any meaningful expectation of direct medical benefit will be completed as expeditiously as is reasonably safe. What is considered reasonably safe by some, however, is considered too risky by others, and this design continues to be controversial. Discussions have also centered on whether it is ethically appropriate to provide subjects ongoing information of efficacy and/or safety data accrual well ahead of meeting study end points (Veatch, 2002). This is an area of study design that can be expected to garner increasing attention in the future.

As demands increase for maximizing subject benefit and autonomous choice in risk taking, these ethical considerations will influence the degree of sponsor and investigator justification for dose levels, ranges, and regimens required in the future by review bodies. Investigators can use this section, in which the objective dosing information is presented, to include justification for the proposed dosing strategies. The objective information and justification cover the proposed strategy for dosing frequency, dose escalation, titration, tapering, and termination. Where graded toxicities have been established to guide this process, they can be included here. Strategy justification includes not only a consideration of the risk/benefit analysis for subjects but also an explanation of how the selected dosing strategy has a reasonable probability of answering the questions posed in the study.

Also described in this section are procedures for dose modifications, especially those that will and will not bring a subject to off-study criteria. Routes and methods of administration should be fully explained. Justification for routes and/or methods of administration being selected for ease of scientific analysis should be made when methods less burdensome on and/or disruptive of subjects' daily lives are available. This applies also to descriptions of timing of dosing in relation to meals, fluid intake, concomitant medications, strenuous physical activity and exercise, bed rest, as well as other study procedures. Procedures related to the subject and to record keeping in the event of a missed or partial dosing should be included.

For drug studies involving patient volunteers, it is critically important to have a clear and detailed explanation of processes for rescue intervention. This will include a full list of rescue medications, differentiating those that can be used without the subject's removal from study from those that meet off-study criteria. If there is any reasonable expectation of efficacy differences across these two groups, an explanation and justification will be required.

Here also the protocol will explain the criteria and how they will be met for needing rescue medications and/or removing a subject from study. Criteria and evaluation of subject distress and/or symptomatology, resulting in administration of rescue medication and/or study termination, is a highly contentious area of human subjects research ethics. Much of the publicity about unethical clinical research stems from the concerns of the psychiatric research volunteer advocacy community. Among the many charges by psychiatric research volunteer advocates of unethical conduct in clinical research is that psychiatric research subjects experience psychic harm and distress too long and at unacceptable levels before initiation of rescue interventions. This issue gets entangled in the placebo ethics debates (Carpenter *et al.*, 2003; Lewis *et al.*, 2002; Weijer, 2002) and counter claims, particularly by the FDA (Temple, 2002; Temple and Meyer, 2003), that assert the ethical need is great to ensure that ineffective medications do not get approved. According to the FDA position, the threshold for rescue and termination (i.e., prevention of harm beyond which society cannot ethically ask any research volunteer to tolerate) should be set at the level of irreversible harm or death. The contentiousness concerns whether the FDA risk threshold is set too high. Although it is unlikely that the questions about appropriate placebo use will be settled any time soon, they illustrate the importance of clarifying such issues as rescue criteria in a protocol. Highlighting the issue as a substantive ethical issue raised by relevant psychiatric studies in the ethics section of the protocol, and including a vigorous justification in the protocol for how a particular study proposes to handle this ethical complexity in study design, will assist in finding the ethically acceptable balance on a per-protocol basis.

C. Compliance

Procedures to measure subject compliance with experimental regimens and/or exclusionary events, such as pregnancy and/or illicit drug use, should be described in this section. Compliance strategies to ensure adherence to study regimens might include instruction cards, food diaries, calibrated syringes or other measurement instruments, pill counts, tube weights, blood, urine, or other body concentrations of study agents. Special documentation processes may exist for recording adherence or problems adhering to study regimens.

Measuring and recording adherence to other kinds of study requirements, such as avoidance of illicit drugs, may require regular administration of toxicology screens and thus may generate clinical research information with legal ramifications for subjects. If this or other kinds of sensitive information is being collected to ensure protocol adherence, such as HIV testing, intermittent drug testing, or testing for alcohol consumption, a description of special protocol protections, such as the Certificate of Confidentiality, related to obtaining, storing, protecting, and discarding such information should also be described here.

D. Concomitant Therapies

Decisions about allowable concomitant therapies are based on many of the same considerations noted in the previous paragraphs. The listing of what will be permitted, during the study and at screening, should be described here. Drugs and therapies should be listed that will make a prospective subject ineligible or cause an ongoing subject to meet off-study criteria. Drugs and nonmedication therapies, such as radiation therapy, should be described.

After an individual is enrolled in a study, whatever therapy a subject requires for short-term management of symptoms or other medical problems that surface during a trial should be provided at least long enough to ensure stabilization and appropriate referral and transfer. This is ordinarily considered standard practice. It often aggravates IRBs and IECs, however, that the way this is worded appears to put scientific need before clinical protection. That is, it is common to see protocols state, "Prohibited/disallowed medications are..." followed by a list of what medications will result in subject removal from study. To avoid this confusion, we recommend wording such as: "Subjects will be provided any medical intervention necessary to address their short-term clinical needs. These will be maintained while the subject's clinical condition is being stabilized. Care will be continued until the subject can be safely transferred to appropriate clinical care. The following list of medications, if administered, will result in the subject being removed from study." This kind of statement will make clear which medications will result in meeting off-study criteria without suggesting that any needed intervention will be withheld.

It is important to justify why particular therapies are permitted (i.e., will not confound data analyses) and why others are not. Further, the subject should be given the time frame during which the subject will be monitored for events (e.g., administration of off-study medications, exclusionary illnesses) that will render that subject off-study.

E. Open-Label Extensions

Open-label extensions are becoming a common feature of drug trials. An **open-label extension** meets the needs of subjects who are benefiting from trial participation and allows sponsors to continue collecting data. This is a design innovation that typifies the spirit of ethics evolution. An ethical consensus appears to be developing that finds that it is an unacceptable harm to subjects to remove from them a benefit, if they are obtaining benefit, because a study has met its statistical and other scientific end points. That is, it is no longer ethically acceptable to use subjects for the study period without regard to ensuring continuation of a benefit generated within the research context. In an expected-direct-benefit study, consideration is given to ensuring that subjects who are determined to be benefiting from an experimental agent or device do not have that benefit terminated too abruptly. An open-label extension may be a useful way to continue to allow subjects to receive the experimental intervention, at least for some transitional period of time. This permits continued benefit for the subjects until they can be safely transferred to receiving an equivalently efficacious agent or until the agent under study becomes commercially and practicably available. In the case of a placebo controlled study, crossover designs are often preferred so that all subjects have an opportunity to benefit from the experimental agent or device. Then, after the crossover periods have been completed, persons who are or were benefiting can go directly into an open-label extension study.

Open-label extensions are also being added to no-direct-benefit studies to encourage potential subjects to participate in no-direct-benefit procedures. Some might find this approach a reasonable trade-off; others consider this design coercive.

> Consider a study of pharmacokinetics (PK) in pediatrics. Drug A is approved for lethal heart arrhythmias in adults and in children as young as 3 years of age. The drug is widely used in infants and toddlers under 3 years of age and the sponsor's national regulatory body wants PK and safety data in this younger age group. The drug sponsor designs a short PK trial with a long-term (1 year), open-label extension trial. Study subjects will be children in the age group of interest with intermittent lethal arrhythmias.

Procedures of an open-label extension will be quite different from the procedures and processes of the trial to which it is attached. All the relevant details for the performance of the open-label trial can be in this section, with the subject-pertinent details in the consent as well. Also, the justifications for the open-label trial will need to be as fully explained as the justifications for the original trial, including discussion of any ethical concerns the open-label extension trial poses, such as those related to lack of medical infrastructure at the study site and unknown risks of extended use—raising concerns about the adequacy of subject monitoring and required refrigeration of experimental agents.

IV. SURGICAL TRIALS

Surgical trials present many considerations similar to those of medical trials, but they are distinct in important procedural and

methodological ways. To begin with, the history of surgical research has developed much differently and has been controversial in different ways from medical trials. The evolution of surgical improvement has been a history of nonvalidated interventions. While this may be said of medical interventions, the creation and growth of research regulation since the mid 20th century for new drug development has been far more restrictive and vigilantly applied than oversight of surgical developments. There is disagreement in the surgical research community about when a minor modification of surgical technique becomes a research project requiring formalized submission to and approval by an IRB or IEC. One guideline is "that any modification that places patients at an increased risk during or after surgery should be submitted to an Ethics Committee/IRB" (Spilker, 2000, p. 327). This guideline may be inadequate, however, since risk assessment is too subjective to ensure that those surgical interventions needing scrutiny and oversight of IRB and/or IEC review and approval will get them. Rather, the approach taken by the U.S. federal regulations in its definition of research as "a systematic investigation, including research development, testing and evaluation, designed to develop or contribute to generalizable knowledge" (45 CFR 46, 46.102) can be applied. This definition is grounded in virtue ethics in that it is an intentions-based definition. Making the determination of whether a surgical intervention is research requiring IRB and/or IEC approval on the basis of the intent of the surgeon(s), rather than on risk assessment, increases the likelihood that technical interventions that are truly research-driven will be handled as such.

The designs used in medical research to reduce bias, such as randomization and blinding, are either more difficult or more controversial when applied to surgical research. Unlike the progression of experience with a medical treatment, where *ad hoc* patients receive a novel prescription or other intervention, a new surgical technique will be ready for testing when some surgeons have used it enough to perfect their own techniques. At this point, it will be ethically difficult for those surgeons to randomize patient volunteers to a previously used technique that they no longer employ. Although this condition theoretically represents the same clinical equipoise that provides the ethical justification for a medical treatment study, the complication of surgical skill adds a new dimension. Surgery requires a different kind of technical skill than prescribing and administering drugs. While the skills needed to prescribe and administer drugs tend to stay stable over time, this is not the case in surgery. Surgical techniques change over time as does the technical skill of a particular surgeon. Performing more surgeries increases surgical skill so that there may be substantial differences for the same surgeon in patient outcomes over time. There is great variability in skill level among surgeons as well. These idiosyncrasies make the procedural and methodological issues of surgical research quite different from drug development research.

Perhaps the most ethically important implication of this difference will be the training built into a surgical protocol. This section of a surgical protocol will need to provide exhaustive detail about who will be performing the surgical procedures, what their training will be, who will be providing the training, and how long the training period will last.

If the study is to be randomized and/or blinded, the particular design will have implications for training as well. Implications are addressed in these questions:

- If the randomization strategy is to assign different surgeries to different surgeons, how will training be made equal across surgeons?
- Will surgeons of equal experience be involved in the protocol, or will there be a mix of senior and junior surgeons?
- If the blinding strategy is to have one or more surgeons perform the procedure and have a different surgeon evaluate the outcome, what will be the required skill level for the surgeon or surgeons making the evaluations?
- Will the surgeons making the evaluations be trained similarly to the surgeons actually performing the study procedures?
- If surgeons are not trained equally, what is the justification to ensure that the evaluating surgeons are capable of making adequate evaluations?

Surgical outcome is also influenced by the hospital in which the surgery is performed. If the surgical procedure under study is going to be performed at multiple hospitals, this section will need to describe what strategies will be applied to take these environmental and staffing patterns as well as skill level differences and differences in team configurations into account.

Sham surgical (surgical placebo arm) designs may be the least biased, but they will be the most ethically controversial (Jones *et al.*, 2003). Placebo effects have been demonstrated in placebo controlled surgical trials, with estimations comparable to the placebo effects in many medical trials (Beecher, 1961). But there is also the feeling that risks of a surgical placebo arm, commonly termed **sham surgery**, pose greater risks to subjects than the typical placebo arm in a medicine trial. When a sham surgical arm is proposed, which would have been justified in the ethics section of the protocol, the researcher will have to include a detailed discussion of how the sham will be performed, specifying clearly what will be left out of the sham surgery arm compared to what will be performed in the experimental arm(s). For an example of a sham surgery trial, see the Case of Brain Tissue Transplantation in Parkinson's Disease Studies in Chapter 15.

V. DEVICE TESTING

Device testing presents ethical and methodological issues more similar to those of surgical trials than to drug trials. As with surgical trials, device trials commonly involve a surgical procedure or device involved in a surgical or other kind of invasive procedure. This means training requirements for study personnel can be expected to be more complicated and extensive than for personnel in a drug trial.

Although device development is less regulated than drug development, the 1976 passage of the Medical Device Amendments to the U.S. Federal Food, Drug, and Cosmetic (FDC) Act brought device development into the modern era of medical research regulation. The relevant statutes, found primarily in Sections 501 to 520 of the act, were promulgated to elevate safety and efficacy standards for the medical device industry. Divided into Class I, II, and III devices, **Class I** presents the least risk, and the devices in this class are governed by the standards that apply to all medical devices prior to the 1976 Amendments. Class I devices are not designed to support or sustain human life or prevent impairment. **Class II** devices pose some risk and are subject to controls that continue to evolve. Class I and II devices are marketable on the basis of performance standards. **Class III** devices require premarket approval. Class III devices include those that are life supporting or sustaining, have substantial activity in preventing health impairment, or have the potential to cause injury or illness. More difficult to classify are the combination devices (i.e., those devices that include medication). A common example is an antibacterial wound dressing. A more modern example involves implantable cardiac devices with antibacterial coating.

For device trials, the researcher might start by describing the users of the device. The instructional and training descriptions that were delineated in the previous paragraphs for surgical trials apply equally to device trials. Device trials are often conducted in two main parts: **the pilot in which the design and materials are tested for feasibility** and **the clinical part in which the device is tested in conditions of its anticipated use**. This section also covers the procedures and methods that will be conducted during both the pilot and primary parts of the protocol.

Much of the weakness in the device literature relates to the frequency with which devices are introduced into clinical use without well-controlled trials. Whether the proposed study has a control will have to be justified in the design section of the protocol. Whatever the design features of the study are, there will need to be a description of how that design will be implemented. Any additional tests, such as those for stability and biocompatibility, will have to be listed and described in this section as well.

VI. ASSESSMENTS

In designing the methods for any proposed study, it is important to avoid the common trap of overassessing, overmeasuring, and over-recording. The scientist has a natural tendency to want to characterize his or her study population more fully than may be needed to answer the scientific questions of the study; to assess, measure, and record such a voluminous amount of data makes the possibility of finishing the study in the allotted time with the allotted resources unattainable. Rather, this is the section in which the writer wants to be concise. For each iteration of protocol drafts, the researcher can exclude items that are not essential to testing the hypothesis or answering the study question(s). The word *essential* is not elastic. It is important to judiciously limit assessments, measurements, and recordings to the scientifically and ethically permissible minimum. The challenge is to focus on the data as narrowly as possible to ensure optimal precision and practicality. Although a useful safety strategy is "the less done to subjects, the less their risk," finding the optimal amount and kinds of data to collect is the goal. Even the lowest risk study is unethical if the expectation of obtaining useful data is not realistic. When studies present more than minimal risk, the risks posed demand that data be mined to the greatest degree possible to maximize the production of useful knowledge. These seemingly contradictory ethical norms calling for doing as little to subjects as is reasonable (i.e., putting subjects through as few procedures as possible to minimize risk) while gaining the most utility from data obtained requires that investigators wisely plan the kinds and amount of data to be collected.

A. The Subject's Standard Physical and Patient History

Whether the study is to test a drug, surgical technique, or device, the initial study procedures will often include **performing a standard medical history and physical. The primary ethical issues raised by obtaining these baseline measurements in the clinical research context are the ways their purpose is differentiated from the purpose of a standard history and physical in clinical care.** Although the procedures and processes involved may be virtually identical, the reasons for performing them are greatly different. This difference presents ethical concerns in the research setting that do not exist, at least not to the same degree, in the clinical arena.

The first of these differences involves the kind of information obtained. In the clinical setting, learning about such potentially sensitive behaviors as drug and alcohol consumption and sexual habits may have important implications for diagnosis and treatment decisions. This is not the case in clinical research. No matter how much investigators and subjects hope that a particular subject will benefit from the study, research is never individualized treatment. Acknowledging this difference illuminates how, for example, in a procedure as routine as obtaining information from a history and physical, the distinction between the goals of clinical care and clinical research demands different approaches to protection and disclosure.

Therefore, this section of the protocol describes exactly **what will be done with information obtained from the history and physical**. Presumably, a subject will need to meet certain physiological parameters, already specified in the inclusion and exclusion criteria. What if a drug screen is positive? If the result leads to a study exclusion, what will be done with the subject's records? Now the investigator has created a legal risk for someone who will not be in the study. If the study was an expected-direct-benefit study, the subject is now denied the opportunity for research benefit and is merely left with increased risk.

> The implications of subjects being excluded from a study because of a preliminary patient history or screening result are illuminated by the case of HIV testing. Because many protocols exclude HIV-positive individuals, many studies test for the condition. If testing comes back positive, what kind of counseling will be provided? HIV is still stigmatizing. How will the HIV test result be protected, given the individual's need for adequate referral?

A second kind of problem related to information obtained from a research history and physical has to do with individuals other than the subject. **In a clinical history and physical, it is common to obtain information about others to which the patient is related either genetically or socially.** Some studies, such as those researching mental health, drug/alcohol abuse, or family violence, specifically investigate psychiatric and behavioral histories about a subject and his or her genetic kin and social contacts. Again, in the clinical setting, this information is obtained for the sole purpose of helping a patient get well. In research, the information is being obtained for the benefit of others. What level of protection and/or limitations should be placed on the particular kinds of information obtained in the research setting about others who are connected to the subject? Although there is no clear answer to this question, the issue has already been raised in the courts (Botkin, 2001). Any potentially sensitive information about individuals other than the subject obtained during the study should be clarified in this section, including details on the specific information obtained and the strategies for protecting the privacy and confidentiality of these individuals as well as the information.

Another part of a standard history and physical that increases research risk to subjects in a way that differs ethically from the risk posed by clinical care is **radiation exposure**. Many standard physical exams include a chest X-ray. Although a chest X-ray may be considered minimal radiation exposure, any exposure is worse than none. Hence, it is important that a history of the prospective subject's past radiation exposure be taken and this section of the protocol can mention and describe the radiation history.

B. Sexual Maturity in Minors

Another part of a standard history and physical, when examining minors, is an evaluation of sexual maturity. Evaluating sexual maturity can be embarrassing to children, especially for adolescents. If such a test is to be part of a study, this needs to be explicitly mentioned in this section of the protocol and included in the assent part of the protocol and/or the assent document as well as the parental permission form.

C. Capacity to Provide Ethically and Legally Valid Consent

It is so important to obtain the knowing, informed, voluntary consent of subjects to participate in research. The history of human subjects research is blemished by involvement of persons who have not been capable of making an informed decision on whether to participate in a study. Thus, the ethics of assessing capacity to provide ethically and legally valid consent is evolving. Capacity assessment is fully discussed in Chapter 5 and Chapter 8.

VII. Laboratory Studies

The laboratory studies included in the protocol should be listed in the procedures and methods section. **Laboratory tests, both standard and experimental, may be conducted as part of the clinical research**

protocol. The investigator lists the laboratory tests and gives their justification. Because both standard clinical and experimental laboratory tests may be used, the IRB and/or IEC should be made aware of the validity of the testing procedures and whether they are being used for medically indicated reasons or for research purposes. If the tests are being subjected to statistical analysis as part of the primary or secondary end points of the trial, the researcher should provide that information in this section. A literature review may be helpful in assessing the validity of experimental tests.

VIII. OBSERVATIONAL METHODOLOGIES

To this point, the study designs discussed have lent themselves to quantitative research methodologies. This is not to suggest, however, that more qualitative approaches, such as observational methods frequently applied to social science studies, are not of equal value. **Observational studies and other qualitative methods of research are critically important and of equal value to all other methods that produce valid findings.**

Observational methods are useful in biomedical research just as they are in social science research, but as for any other methods, they must be appropriately applied. The excuse for the U.S. Public Health Service's Tuskegee Syphilis Study (Jonsen *et al.*, 1998) was that there was no treatment for syphilis and so it was necessary to observe the disease course to learn more about the condition. This was simply a lie. Although the treatment available at the time was nonvalidated and eventually proven ineffective and probably harmful, there were standard-of-care interventions available at the time the infamous study was initiated. The original injustice was compounded when effective treatment, penicillin, was introduced into clinical care but was withheld from subjects. The justification, again, was the scientific need to learn more about the disease by continuing to observe its course.

When there is truly no treatment for a condition, however, observational studies may be ethically appropriate. This point reiterates our position that before there can be studies with a reasonable expectation of direct medical benefit to study participants, there must often be research from which no direct benefit can be expected. Before interventions for disease can be developed and tested, identification and elucidation of the mechanisms underlying the disease process are usually needed. This is a distinction between hypothesis-testing and hypothesis-generating research. When behavioral evaluations are to be the core of studying a question and/or hypothesis, the only means of collecting data may be through observation of the behaviors, themselves, often under field conditions.

To determine if a biomedical study might benefit from including observational data collection strategies, it is important that investigators consult professionals skilled in qualitative research methodologies. Often, studies planned with quantitative methods could maximize benefit by adding specific qualitative methods to the study. Because few biomedical researchers are well trained in such methods, there may be an unwarranted bias against qualitative methodologies, and opportunities for developing data to the greatest degree possible are missed.

IX. VIDEO AND/OR AUDIO TAPING

Although the addition of observational methodologies to more quantitative biomedical studies can help encourage maximum use of all data collected, the use of video or audiotapes poses risk to subjects of breach of privacy and confidentiality. **Even if identified by code, research subjects are usually quite recognizable in a video or audiotape. When these forms of data collection are to be used, special protections will need to be in place to protect subject identity.** These protections include obtaining the subject's specific consent for these data collection methods, procedures for protecting identity such as taping subjects without showing their face, and consideration of destroying these data earlier than might be the case for written research records.

X. QUALITY-OF-LIFE MEASUREMENTS

Collection of **quality-of-life information** is being added to a wide range of protocols. Quality-of-life (QOL) information covers a wide spectrum of data related to subject well-being. Some QOL surveys examine how subjects function throughout their daily activities related only to what the subject is experiencing in the research setting. Other QOL surveys investigate the well-being of subjects across many sectors of a subject's personal and public activities. Discussion continues about whether QOL data are sufficiently objective to be scientifically meaningful. Nonetheless, a growing number of instruments to assess quality of life have been tested for reliability and validity and are being included in medical protocols. Because QOL information is growing in importance, such data collection could be a useful adjunct to the primary data set of the study. Consider the following situation.

An oncology research group is planning its next study of an experimental agent for prostate cancer. The experimental drug has gone through its phases I and II trials and the group is now planning the phase III trials. It is anticipated that, if approved, the agent will be used in early-stage prostate cancer in patients who have had their tumor surgically removed and in whom the tumor has not spread outside the prostate. For this group of patients, there is a dizzying array of postsurgery possibilities, including hormonal treatment and/or radiation. Some physicians believe that a watch and wait approach is also reasonable. Because of this variability, designing a randomized, double-blinded, placebo-controlled trial is acceptable. The group is considering a large, complex, 6-arm trial. Arm A is the experimental agent at the maximum tolerated dose from the phase I data that showed efficacy at the phase II stage. Arm B is a lower dose that also showed efficacy in the phase II trials. Arm C is an approved hormonal treatment. Arm D is radiation alone. Arm E is radiation plus the hormonal treatment in Arm C. Arm F is watch and wait. With 6 arms, this phase III trial is going to be multisite and multinational, and attempts will be made to enroll several thousand subjects. Given the complexity and large subject enrollment numbers projected for this trial, the group agrees that this is an ideal study in which to add a QOL data collection component. The various postsurgical treatments for prostate cancer differ widely, particularly in terms of side effects that have substantial QOL impacts. The utility of any new treatment for prostate cancer will be maximized if it not only produces efficacy advances but also has a more favorable side-effect profile than existing treatments. Adding a QOL component, such as a survey and a few QOL questions during follow-up visits, can produce additional information that may help determine optimal dosing characteristics if the drug is approved, such as time of day and intervals.

XI. Follow-up Procedures

Many clinical research studies include collection of follow-up data that can be an integral part of the study. Follow-up procedures can involve a single phone call to determine whether a subject has contacted the person/facility to whom he or she had been referred at study conclusion. The follow-up may also be annual visits to the research site for repetition of all study procedures. Whatever the form of a follow-up, it needs to be detailed in the protocol.

The form of follow-up should meet the criteria established for subject safety and scientific validity of the findings. For example, patient volunteers may have medical needs that continue beyond the end of a clinical research study. The extent of follow-up will be dictated by how serious and acute these needs are. Novel follow-up strategies have been designed to include family members to ensure that subjects whose safety is at risk are protected (Schooler and Baker, 1999).

An example of such a study is one in which persons with schizophrenia participate in an out-patient study of a novel agent versus a standard-of-practice, approved drug to reduce the negative symptoms of schizophrenia. The study is designed to run for 6 months. At the end of the 6-month study period, subjects are weaned off their study medications and transitioned back to the care of their community treating physicians. There is one follow-up visit post–active study termination. This follow-up visit calls for the subject to return to the out-patient study clinic for an interview to evaluate how he or she has done since ending active study drug administration, to learn if the subject has stayed on his or her community-administered medications, and to record the names of those medications. Many persons with schizophrenia relapse because they fail to take their medications, and they may be lost to follow-up for this reason. Knowing this, the original study built into the protocol and the consent process agreement on the part of the subject permission to contact a family member to attempt to find the subject if he or she does not return for this follow-up visit. This assists the researchers in obtaining the data the protocol includes and it allows the researchers to assist patients and families in postprotocol treatment needs.

XII. Adverse Reactions and Adverse Events

Requirements for reporting adverse reactions and adverse events in clinical research are well established although their occurrence, and the extent of their recording, became a public issue after the death of Jesse Gelsinger at the University of Pennsylvania in 1999 (Committee on Assessing the System for Protecting Human Research Participants, 2003; Committee on Assessing the System for Protecting Human Research Subjects, 2001; Lemmens and Freedman, 2000). Gelsinger's death in the University of Pennsylvania gene therapy study; subsequent media attention; and public outcry about adverse reactions and adverse events, their attribution, and reporting resulted in a flurry of responses. Institutions developed enforcement policies to ensure that when adverse events occur, they are reported fully and promptly. Now that reporting of adverse events has been improved, the need to improve the interpretation and attribution, specifically of adverse reactions, has become more obvious. Because of the bias of investigators to hope that their experimental interventions will be helpful and not hurtful, there continues to be an inclination to attribute adverse reactions to causes other than the experimental intervention. Often the attribution bias is to assume that an adverse reaction is not attributable to the experimental intervention unless there is good evidence to suggest that the adverse reaction is related to the study. Instead, it is important that there be a high level of suspicion that the adverse reaction is in some way connected to the study. This ensures that possible problems with the experimental agent are investigated as vigorously as is reasonably possible.

A. Definitions, Classifications, and Attribution

An adverse reaction is most broadly understood to be an undesirable response to medication. Adverse reactions are not invariably bad. Adverse reactions may indicate that the experimental agent can produce a physiologic change in the subject, provide information useful for dose adjustment, and serve as a clue to previously unsuspected activity. A benefit of the last option is notably demonstrated by the success of Viagra, a drug whose development had nothing to do with sexual performance but for which an adverse reaction led to a new use for the agent. Regardless of how useful the information generated from adverse reactions might be, however, they ordinarily represent a previously unrecognized side effect. Adverse reactions are ordinarily attributable to the experimental agent, such as infection in a subject in a study of a novel immunosuppressive agent. Adverse events often are not attributable to the experimental agent, such as the death of a research subject by being a passenger in a fatal car crash. Some adverse reactions are anticipated, and others are not; some adverse events are serious, while others are not. Some adverse reactions are systematized through the use of adverse reaction dictionaries, which are compilations of anticipated adverse reactions, while others are defined in the context of a particular study. When the latter method is used, definitions should be included in the protocol before initiation of the study, in so far as possible.

B. Reporting

However adverse reactions are defined, determined, and, attributed, they, along with any other adverse event(s), must be reported properly and in a timely manner. Some adverse reactions must be reported to the FDA, to other regulatory bodies, to study sponsors, and to the IRB and IEC, each within its own specified time limit. Requirements for reporting of some adverse events are determined by institutional policy only, based on such criteria as whether the adverse event or reaction was anticipated and/or severe. **The problem with the severity criteria, however, is that definition of severity is often vague, and its determination may be left to the investigator.** Attribution is often complicated by the possibility that adverse reactions mimic or exacerbate symptomatology that is consistent with disease progression.

By leaving to an investigator's discretion the decision of whether an adverse reaction or event meets a vague or hard-to-define threshold, there is the risk that the investigator may consciously or unconsciously unduly influence attribution and reporting patterns to minimize the causal connection with the experimental agent. We recommend, therefore, that protocols and or IRBs/IECs include a pharmacist and an information specialist so that maximal use can be made of the extensive literature on drugs and devices.

12

··········

STATISTICS, DATA COLLECTION AND MANAGEMENT, AND RECORD KEEPING

··················

The statistics and data collection, data management, and record keeping section of the study protocol describes how the data will be collected, recorded, and maintained. Applications of appropriate statistical strategies to data analysis and proper data collection and management procedures have important ethical implications. These include ensuring that subjects do not take on risk without a reasonable expectation of benefit to medical progress. Well-designed and implemented data management and record keeping procedures protect subjects from breaches of privacy and confidentiality.

I. STATISTICS

To make certain a protocol's statistical analysis strategy is appropriate and that it includes optimal analysis design to achieve scientific validity, investigators are encouraged to consult a biostatistician early in the design process. Once the investigator has begun to shape the study question and/or hypothesis, he or she can consult and collaborate with a qualified statistician who is experienced in the design of the proposed study. Consultation and ongoing guidance on the variables to monitor and/or manipulate data collection strategies and methods for data analysis are essential during all stages of the study. For large, complex, and/or multisite studies, statisticians will be performing the data analyses, perhaps even in blinded fashion, after all the data have been collected. Statisticians should be considered as full members of the research team and viewed as integral to the design process and perform-ance of most studies.

A. Qualitative and/or Quantitative Data

While the study is being designed, the primary methods of evaluation need to be identified. Is the study going to be qualitative, quantitative, or both? **A bias exists toward quantitative statistics and hypothesis-testing studies. But quantitative and qualitative methods are important for progress in medicine.** There are areas of medical research without enough knowledge to devise hypotheses to test. In such cases, well-devel-oped study questions can lead to innovative hypothesis-generating research as important to medical research as more fully formed hypothe-sis-testing studies. When the knowledge base is premature and calls for hypothesis-generating research, quantitative methods may still be appro-priately applied. The reverse may also be true depending on the study question. Mature, hypothesis-testing research may call for application of qualitative methods of data collection and analysis. The examples dis-cussed in Chapter 11 concerning the growing attention to quality-of-life data illustrate this point.

The body of literature about quality-of-life issues is quite large, with much of it reporting on measurements that apply qualitative data strate-gies. **These quality-of-life data are considered a double-edged sword. Qualitative methods produce literature rich in what is sub-jectively important to a wide range of patients of different ages, disease processes, and social circumstances. This "qualitativeness" and subjectivity, however, result in many discounting their ability to provide meaningful and useful insights.** If the data are to be used for regulatory drug approval depending on the ends of the study, the strategies applied to data collection and analysis will influence the appli-cation of the data and thus have implications for the risk/benefit balance of the study.

Investigators will want to seek out a biostatistician and/or research methodologist who has experience in testing the kinds of hypothesis under examination in the study. Researchers may need to consult more than one methodologist. The probability of need for multiple statisticians and/or methodology consultants increases markedly if using both qualitative and quantitative analysis strategies. This level of design and analysis strategy, however, may be critical to the ethical requirement for maximizing benefit from research participation in relation to research risk.

Research in the area of spousal violence is needed. A heated controversy exists about how to effectively treat victims and perpetrators. Are perpetrators simply "bad people" who should be punished and sent to jail? Or might these perpetrators have a disordered physiology that medical intervention could correct or ameliorate? Should victims and perpetrators be separated? When the pair want to stay together and work out their problems, is couples therapy useful or potentially dangerous? These are complex issues that have grave implications for victims, perpetrators, and society. Much more data are needed to be able to shape hypothesis-testing questions. One can imagine study designs that might combine biologically driven questions solved with quantitative methods and behavioral and psychologically driven questions best pursued with qualitative methodologies. This combination adds methodological and ethical complexity.

B. Sample Size and Power Calculations

Sample size and power calculations must be fully justified and explicit in this section of the protocol. Involving more research participants than required to answer a question or test a hypothesis unnecessarily puts extra individuals at risk. **Underpowering** a study means there is less expectation of answering the study question or adequately testing the study hypothesis, which puts all participants at risk for no benefit to anyone (Halpern *et al.*, 2002). Both situations are unacceptable. What is needed, ethically, is to find Aristotle's golden mean—the number of subjects that is not too many, not too few, but just the right number to meet safely the scientific ends of the study.

The protocol needs to include a clear justification for why the proposed statistical approach has been selected, including the mathematical justification. Having the formulas in the protocol means the statisticians on, or adjunctive to, the IRB, IEC, and other review committees can quickly make their own evaluations. Including the formula is, however, not sufficient. Along with formulas, the text needs to provide sound justification for subject number and the effect size that is being sought.

The ethical aspects of this issue concerning the use of statistical approaches are beginning to surface most notably in the area of cancer research. To date, the trend has been to have larger and larger trials with small effect sizes. There has been, however, an interesting challenge raised to this approach, suggesting a total reorientation of the statistical goals of late phase oncology trials (Horrobin, 2003). Given a presumption that subjects enter oncology trials in the hope of gaining a personal direct benefit, it has been suggested that rather than continue to run large trials powered for small effect sizes, oncology trials—or trials in any disease that has a high probability of patient mortality within a 2 to 5 year period—should change orientation toward initiating small trials that look for large effect sizes. Although such a shift is unlikely because of the major systems alterations demanded by such an approach, it is a provocative thought that deserves consideration.

C. Variables and End Points

The number and type of variables and/or end points will be a balance between the minimum burdens on subjects and the scientific optimum. For example, by adding an extra measurement that does not increase risk (e.g., an additional set of laboratory values with already acquired blood) and increases the quality of the data, the risk/benefit balance is tipped in favor of running the extra tests. If, however, obtaining one more set of laboratory values is intended to make data graphs more elegant, and the additional measurements require a research-only needle stick, the balance tips against getting those values.

In deciding whether the study is best designed to be cross-sectional or longitudinal, the same ethical considerations apply. **Although data may be more generalizable with a longitudinal design rather than with a cross-sectional design, longitudinal studies present their own difficulties.** When a longitudinal study is planned, what if the methods of data collection and evaluation used during the study's early years become obsolete as the study matures? Will numbers of subjects involved have to be increased? Will data from the initial subjects be wasted? The variables and study end points should be selected to maximize the knowledge gained and minimize burden or risk to subjects.

In phase II and III drug or device trials, the ideal is to identify efficacy end points that demonstrate biologically measurable improvement. Sometimes, however, efficacy will not be directly measurable for safety reasons, and surrogate markers will have to suffice. The problem with surrogate markers is they are often more susceptible to interpretative challenge than directly measurable biologic end points. Therefore, this section should include an explicit discussion of why the particular end points have been chosen, including a presentation of what the perfect end points might be as well as why, if applicable, these end points cannot be used.

D. Pharmacokinetics and Pharmacodynamics

Pharmacokinetics is the study of the absorption, distribution, metabolism, and elimination of a drug. The goal of a pharmacokinetic study is to characterize the effect of these bodily functions on drug action. This information is critical in developing appropriate dosing range and schedules as the experimental agent moves into later phases of development and study. Pharmacokinetic data are among the first collected in humans. Some individuals advocate obtaining pharmacokinetics data in as many populations as possible. Ordinarily, the first human pharmacokinetic trials are in healthy volunteers, often in a single-dose administration of the experimental agent.

This practice has evolved for safety and scientific reasons. Regulatory bodies require this practice as it is necessary for continued characterization of the experimental compound. It is unclear, however, how much clinically useful information this data collection method provides. How long a drug stays in a healthy body and is used by the tissues of a healthy body is often quite different from these parameters in a sick body. Although prudence, regulation, and scientific need dictate that the majority of experimental agents be tested in healthy humans before patient populations, the transitional stage may create false expectations. Thus, the critical ethical considerations of pharmacokinetic studies rely on the quality of conclusions being conveyed to future subjects and review bodies as well as the protection of the healthy normal subjects in these early investigations. For example, many phase I trials are single-bolus administrations, and the phase II trials involve multiple dosing. Thus, there may be no human experience in the patient populations involved or in the dosing regimens applied at the phase II level. Phase I pharmacokinetic trials are usually only designed to statistically evaluate toxicity and safety measures. They will often look for activity, and once detected, the expected-direct-benefit potential of the experimental agent is emphasized. It would be more efficient if any trial in a new population, with a new dosing schedule or route of administration, was labeled as a phase I trial. Given that the present conventions are unlikely to change, it is important that the lack of experience with the agent in a population, with a particular dose or dose range, schedule, or route of administration, be specified in the protocol and consent process. The protocol should include a specification of the numbers of humans previously tested with the agent, an explanation that the previous tests were for pharmacokinetics, and details on the population previously tested (e.g., healthy volunteers or patient volunteers with conditions different than those in the present study).

Pharmacodynamics is the study of how medications affect the body (i.e., the biological and clinical effects of an administered drug). Many start the evaluation of pharmacodynamics concurrently with early trials of pharmacokinetics. The pharmacodynamics of an agent, however, are central to study questions throughout all phases of clinical trials.

E. Placebos

Ethical considerations of placebos have surfaced intermittently throughout this book. Here, the relevant aspect of the ethical complexities presented by placebos is the problem of data interpretation resulting from high placebo responses. **Because placebo responses are high, especially in certain kinds of clinical trials (e.g., drug development in psychiatry), regulatory agencies have a pronounced bias in favor of placebo use.** Sponsors want to continue to use placebos because of their claim that to show differences between experimental drug and approved interventions will require such large study numbers that the research becomes impossible or prohibitively expensive.

Research consistently demonstrates that some persons in a placebo arm of virtually any kind of trial, be it drug, device, or nonmedical intervention, respond to placebo. The range of placebo response varies widely depending on the experimental intervention and the way the response is measured, with responses commonly 35–65%. **Briefly, the central ethical concern about placebos is that situations will arise in which it will be unethical to have a study arm that withholds standard medical intervention.** Most fully articulated in the Declaration of Helsinki and the CIOMS guidelines, the ethical claim is that clinical research subjects ought not be placed at risk of harm by being deprived of potentially efficacious intervention. That is, many believe that a placebo arm provides no prospect for benefit, but that any study arm providing either approved existing intervention or an experimental arm is potentially of benefit. This claim is grounded in the notion of **equipoise**: the only ethically justifiable basis for randomization is the belief that one arm has the potential to be as beneficial as any other study arm. On the face of it, this logic would preclude use of placebos altogether. But the reality of a placebo response makes for a more complex ethical analysis.

It is common for a study with three arms to present results of 34% response in the approved drug arm, 33% in the experimental agent arm, and 30% in the placebo arm. On the face of it, this looks like a bad outcome.

Actually, it may be sufficient for drug approval and represent an important advance in treatment of the condition under study. Coming in at 1% less response than the approved agent may not be statistically significant, and if the approved agent came into practical use without sufficient testing, the 34% response may not be fully interpretable. Because of the placebo use, at least it is clear that the agent is better than nothing. Given the serious ethical problem of having so many nonvalidated standard-of-practice drugs, devices, and procedures, many of which once tested are shown to be useless or harmful, assuring others that a drug is better than nothing is a critical threshold to surpass.

As with virtually all ethical judgments, broad claims, such as not placing research subjects at risk of harm by being deprived of potentially efficacious intervention, require additional specification to be credible. In the case of placebos, the most frequent specification is the same as in most other aspects of the clinical research process. Reduction of risk to zero means no clinical research, so the relevant question is how much risk is too much? In the case of placebos, how much risk is tolerable when withholding an approved or experimental intervention?

The answers to these questions and the arguments that surround them are very complex and often defy logic. Consider first the experimental arm. This discussion has already pointed out that what are commonly referred to as phase II expected-direct-benefit trials may expose patient volunteers to experimental agents that have never been administered to patients previously in some dose ranges and routes of administration. Common sense and previous clinical research experience suggests that there is no reasonably accurate way to predict whether the experimental agent will work at all, work well, or be harmful in this setting.

The experimental arm in such a trial is virtually identical in its withholding of approved intervention as is the placebo arm. Further, the experimental arm is equally or more likely to produce harm than is the placebo arm. Thus, we do not accept the claim that withholding potentially beneficial intervention from a patient is substantially different in the experimental arm than it is in the placebo arm, at least not in early human experience with the experimental agent. The claim we accept, however, is that **once an experimental agent has been demonstrated to be potentially beneficial, the concern about inclusion of a placebo arm increases with the severity of the condition.**

Discussions of problems with placebos often use the examples of cancer trials and studies of cold medicines to set the boundaries for discussion. For the most part, placebos are not used in oncology trials. Even if a study could employ a crossover design, by the time the placebo group crossed over, disease progression might be beyond remedy. On the other hand, most would

Continued

> agree that placebos in the development of common cold medicines are acceptable. Subjecting individuals to cold symptoms is of less consequence than risking approval of a cold remedy that does not work. The placebo battle is being fought on the middle ground.

One of the arguments in favor of including a placebo is the following: without a placebo arm, the study will require so many subjects that enrollment requirements would be unobtainable and/or the study prohibitively expensive. When applying conventional statistical strategies, these arguments appear sustainable. There may be sufficiently rigorous novel statistical strategies, however, that mitigate the numerical problem. Although these strategies are published, they have yet to catch the attention of research sponsors (Finkelstein *et al.*, 1996a, 1996b). As newer statistical approaches develop, the concerns about subject numbers as an argument for study designs that omit placebo controls may decline. Also, it is worth noting here that although the FDA appears to have a strong bias in favor of placebo use, FDA regulations for drug studies with a new drug or device application (NDA) only require two well-controlled studies.

F. Modeling

Modeling is a computer strategy that can be used to justify the involvement of humans in research. Like the novel statistical strategies for avoiding placebo arms, modeling processes are relatively new to the clinical research arena and techniques are not yet widely employed within the clinical research community. **In modeling, computer models are built as early data emerge. They develop statistical projections of the probability of experimental compounds having unacceptable side effect profiles and/or efficacy potential to stop or warrant continued human trials, respectively.**

When modeling can bolster assumptions that an intervention will ultimately be approvable, its use should be explained in the protocol as additional justification for involving human subjects. When modeling can predict that lack of efficacy or unacceptable side effects will cause termination of a study program, terminating the study sooner rather than later may be optimal, reducing the number of individuals exposed to research risk. Therefore, use of computer modeling is encouraged to the degree it can be integrated into the planning process of clinical trials.

II. DATA COLLECTION AND MANAGEMENT

The section on data collection and management should include explicit procedures for developing and collecting data; methods for coding, recording, storing, and protecting the data; and instructions given to research subjects and study personnel to ensure that study procedures are followed. Although the design of these procedures may evolve through the course of the protocol development and the review process, the information in this section should be as complete as possible at the time the protocol is submitted for review. This information should be so concise that anyone reading the protocol can understand what data are to be collected and how they will be handled by the various categories of personnel involved in data collection and management for the study. The level of detail is critically important to subject safety.

A. Instructions for Subjects, Investigators, and Other Study Personnel

Development of instructions for research participants and study personnel can begin as soon as the general design and proposed subject population are determined. Too often, preparation of the written instructions for subjects is done at the last minute. When such instructions are mere afterthoughts, they turn out poorly written and confusing. Important points are often left out. To avoid this problem, instruction sheets can be written and attached to the protocol. Although they may be attached as an appendix, including them in the section with all other collection forms may be better placement to ensure thorough review. That they are reviewed thoroughly will be important to ensure their content is complete and readable by subjects, research surrogates, and research personnel as applicable.

Instruction sheets for subjects will repeat some of the information found in the consent documents but not much. Where there are repetitions, the repeated information will be provided in abbreviated form. For example, it may be useful to start the information sheet with a condensed version of the purpose of the study. Other information regularly included in research participant instruction sheets are names and phone numbers of contact persons in case a subject experiences a problem; information about device use or malfunction, dosing, contraindications, self-administered rating scales, and keeping of diaries; instructions on what information to bring to clinic, laboratory, or study visits; and timing and scheduling for clinic, laboratory, or study visits.

Instructions for study personnel call for detail. These instructions include those for investigators if the protocol is being prepared by a sponsor. The instructions for study personnel may include processes for scheduling subject visits; instructions on obtaining, coding, and storing biologic samples; and information on how to complete, code, and store data collection forms. For complex studies, especially for multicenter and multinational trials, these instructions and forms will need to be incorporated into manuals for study procedures.

Many of the forms will be required by the regulations of the jurisdictions in which the studies are conducted. A study can only come to its optimal conclusion through strict processes for ensuring that study procedures are followed by study personnel for collecting, coding, and storing data. One of the first decisions to make about the design and management of **study report forms** (sometimes referred to as **case report forms**) is how they will be categorized:

- Will all forms for a particular subject be kept together by date of activity such as for a clinic visit?
- Or will all clinic reports be bundled together and all report forms related to subject scans and X-rays be bundled together?
- Where will the code linking subject number to personally identifying information, such as name, address, and/or social security number, be kept?
- Will a code be stored in a locked cabinet? If so, who will have the key or access to the key or combination lock formula?

Each data collection form should be standardized to the greatest degree possible. That is, collection and/or coding of a particular piece of information should be done the same way and recorded in the same place each time and across forms. Data collection forms will need to be signed and dated by an investigator.

B. Data Entry

Data entry processes have become increasingly complex as research has become increasingly complex, computerized, and conducted at multiple sites. For multisite and multinational studies, much of the data entry will be remote. Some researchers will input some data on site and electronically transport these to a remote center, but then they will ship data report forms for remote entry of other data. Even in studies that are designed and implemented in one location, data entry can involve multiple processes across several study team members and various institutional departments. To ensure that data entry is accurate, it is important to have sufficient and explicit procedures in the protocol and/or appendix. Whether remote or on-site, data entry procedures need to be worked out and explained in the protocol in sufficient detail for reviewers to determine whether quality control and confidentiality protections are adequate.

C. Clinical Research Coordinators and Contract Research Organizations

The individuals responsible for overseeing day-to-day operations of the trial will have a substantial impact on ensuring that the study procedures, data collection and management, as well as subject safety and protection are maintained. Ordinarily, a **principal investigator** (PI), often a physician or a medical scientist with a Ph.D. degree, will assign to a clinical **research coordinator** (RC) the responsibility of overseeing the daily performance of a study. The RC, often a nurse, will be responsible for a vast array of research activities, often everything up to the signing and dating of documents by the investigator. We recommend that if a study team includes an RC, this person's curriculum vitae or some documentation of this individual's qualifications should be included with the protocol submission packet to the IRB and IEC. Because RCs are often involved in recruitment, consent processes, and study performance oversight, it is essential that they have the skills, training, and experience to perform their jobs in a way that ensures subject safety.

For large studies, especially pharmaceutical industry drug or device studies, **study monitors** will be included in the protocol. Study monitors span a wide range of disciplines and educational backgrounds, from physicians to persons with a college degree in a nonscience area. Monitors can be identified during the design of the study. Roles and responsibilities can be shaped during the design phase of protocol development and finalized prior to study initiation.

Who the monitor(s) may be will be influenced by who is conducting the trial, such as whether the study is being managed by a medical contract organization. Although some study monitors are independent consultants, most are employees of the sponsor or of the contractor hired to manage and oversee the performance of a trial. Referred to as CROs or SMOs, contract research organizations or site management organizations, these study contract organizations provide sponsors with a range of services to ensure that the study is conducted properly and in accordance with the protocol approved by the IRB and/or IEC.

The goal of having an RC, a study monitor, and/or a CRO involved in the day-to-day performance and oversight of a study is to ensure subject safety and the integrity of the data collected. As a study becomes more complex, with studies involving multiple sites and/or conducted in several countries, the monitoring processes for the study become more complex. Decisions about oversight and monitoring personnel can be started during the design phase and made explicit in the protocol submitted for IRB and IEC approval.

D. Academic and Pharmaceutical Industry Collaborations

Much of the increased complexity of clinical trials relates to the shift in the funding source of clinical research. When clinical research was beginning to flourish after World War II, the majority of funding for clinical trials came from the public sector. The majority of investigators were in academic institutions. Since the last several decades of the 20th century, these sources of funding have been changing. **The private sector provides an ever-increasing amount of clinical research funding. Investigators are increasingly recruited from the ranks of community private practice.** These shifts are in large part a function of money. Public support of academic institutions has diminished rapidly over the last several decades. Academic institutions have turned to lucrative collaborations with the private sector to keep their research portfolios and large segments of their academic departments afloat (Eichenwald and Kolata, 1999; Lind, 1996; Press and Washburn, 2000). The more recent phenomenon of community physicians adding participation in pharmaceutical industry research to their clinical practice activities parallels the rise of managed care and declines in personal income and other less tangible rewards of the practice of clinical medicine.

When universities benefit from the influx of private money, independence in organizational oversight may suffer. Conflicts of interest proliferate. For community physicians who move into the clinical research arena, conflicts of interest exist, and there are even fewer oversight mechanisms governing investigators often with less training and certainly with fewer colleagues from whom to learn (Williams, 2004). Thus, although the swift invasion of private research support into academic and community settings holds out the promise of quickening the pace of medical progress, it also sets the stage for new problems that require thoughtful attention. At the protocol design and approval level, the most effective means for protecting research participants from potential harms from these arrangements is to make the arrangements explicit in the protocols. Reviewers may then make sound judgments about whether the pressures are countered by adequate subject protections. Such protections include disclosing conflicts of interest in informed consent processes and documents. At the institutional level, protections include policies and procedures to reduce the impact of conflicts of interest or to avoid them altogether. Where such policies do not exist, it will be up to the IRB and/or IEC to evaluate the impact of such collaborative arrangements and ensure that adequate subject protections are built into the protocol.

III. RECORD KEEPING

One of the most important protections for subjects is proper and adequate record keeping. By keeping appropriate, adequate, and accurate records, anyone with approved access will be able to make a reasonable assessment of how well the performance of a study complies with the approved procedures. Design of good record keeping practices is essential and should be made explicit in the protocol.

Study data should be kept on data report forms developed as part of the design process. Strategies for storing and keeping the consent, assent, and permission forms up-to-date will be somewhat different. Many institutions are moving to a system of stamping dates on these types of documents. The reasoning behind this new process is to ensure that these documents are updated and current, consistent with at least annual reviews required of each protocol. It also means that IRBs and IECs are more likely to review these documents once more at the time that the protocols are reviewed again. The process for ensuring that consent, assent, and permission documents are up-to-date should be instituted during the design stage of a protocol. When these documents are amended, whether there is a date stamp requirement at the site, researchers need to make certain that a method exists for keeping them current and available. Whatever the chosen method is for documentation management, guidelines concerning this management should be part of the instruction provided to study personnel.

Examples of bad record keeping litter the field of research. In the Jesse Gelsinger case (see Chapter 15), one of the problems uncovered during the investigation of Jesse's death was that there were deficiencies in research record keeping. Deficiencies in record keeping may be a portent for all sorts of other problems. Poor record keeping may signal a general lack of attention to study details or it may signal merely a mismatch between PI and study monitor. In a situation wherein a study is being conducted by a well-known, perhaps egotistical, senior academic investigator and being monitored by a junior person without an advanced degree, the study monitor may have a difficult time impressing on the PI the need to attend to details the monitor sees as critical to record keeping, but the PI sees only as a paperwork nuisance.

Continued

One way to increase the probability of good research record keeping is for the oversight bodies to do a sample record check prior to a protocol's annual review. Some IRBs include this process as part of their standard annual reviews. Such an IRB process might be that the IRB chairperson assigns a primary reviewer to each protocol up for its annual review. The primary reviewer has the responsibility for not only reviewing the protocol, but also for going to the protocol implementation site and reviewing the records or some sample of the records, to assure that all documentation is as it is supposed to be by the protocol requirement. Then, for any protocol having deficiencies, the PI will be required to appear at the IRB to explain what corrective actions have been instituted. Such a process often has salutary effects. The PI learns that it is not only the study monitor who is insisting on proper record keeping. Word gets out around the institution that the PI had a protocol problem, and this increases institutional awareness of any problem that might turn out to be widespread, rather than protocol-specific. Such an experience, for the conscientious investigator, is ordinarily enough to ensure improved practice.

section

IV

· · · · · · · · · ·

SPECIAL ISSUES

· · · · · · · · · · · · · · · · ·

USE OF HUMAN BIOLOGICAL MATERIALS

· · · · · · · · · · · · · · · ·

Human biological samples have long been a rich source of research material. **Materials for biological research come from a variety of sources, including cells collected during research, biopsy specimens obtained for clinical diagnostic purposes, and tissues removed during surgery or at death. A wealth of technologies has emerged to optimize use of such specimens for medical progress. These new technologies create ethical questions.** Technological advances that allow such specimens to be used in ways not contemplated at the time of harvest and storage require scholarly attention to the ethical implications of applying new research methodologies.

One of the reports of the National Bioethics Advisory Commission (NBAC, 1999) highlights the ethical complexities in this area of clinical research. Because new technologies for sample analyses are rapidly becoming available and because of the diversity of regulatory responses to this expanding area of clinical research, ethical and legal issues can be expected to be unsettled for some time.

I. ANONYMOUS, ANONYMIZED, CODED, AND IDENTIFIABLE SPECIMENS

Categorization and labeling of biological samples pose a challenge. **Important, and often subtle, inconsistencies exist in nomenclature**

and designation of categories. For example, the NBAC report (1999) defines the categories of human biological materials as follows:

1. Repository Collections
   a. Unidentified specimens: Specimens for which identifiable personal information was not collected or, if collected, was not maintained and cannot be retrieved by the repository.
   b. Identified specimens: Specimens linked to personal information that identifies the person from whom the specimen was obtained by name, patient number, or location in a pedigree (i.e., his or her relationship to a family member whose identity is known).
2. Research Samples Supplied
   a. Unidentified samples: Sometimes termed **anonymous**, these samples are supplied to investigators by repositories from a collection of unidentified human biological specimens.
   b. Unlinked samples: Sometimes termed **anonymized**, these samples lack identifiers or codes that can link a particular sample to an identified specimen or human being.
   c. Coded samples: Sometimes termed **linked** or **identifiable**, these samples are supplied to investigators by repositories from identified specimens with a code rather than obviously identifiable information, such as a name or Social Security number.
   d. Identifiable samples: These samples are supplied by repositories from identified specimens with a personal identifier (such as a name or patient number), which allows the researcher to link the biological information derived from the research directly to the individual from whom the material was obtained.

Rather than simply adopting the NBAC's categorization system, some in the U.S. pharmaceutical industry have their own nomenclature. In this language, terms such as **double-coded** or **de-identified** samples are used, and substantive difference in definitions regarding anonymized samples were introduced. In the pharmaceutical industry version, double-coded or de-identified samples are labeled with a second coded number. The link between the first code and this second code is recorded. Anonymization is accomplished when the link between the two codes is destroyed. The intent is that the double-coded or de-identified samples cannot be linked back to their personally identified source. The fact is, however, that regardless of intent, this **relinking** is technologically possible.

Legal definitions differ among countries and in the United States about what information identifies a sample. That is, the U.S. HIPAA regulations clarify information covered such as what information characterizes personalized, identifiable information. As just noted, different professional groups have different definitions. **Because of this variability, one of the most important pieces of information in a human biological materials protocol is the definition of category or categories of samples to be used and/or generated.** Samples of several different categories may be included in a single protocol. Each needs to be clearly labeled and defined.

Each category presents its own specific ethical questions to be addressed clearly in the protocol. The following list includes some of the questions that are relevant to a protocol in which biological samples are collected and/or generated:

- Is the study generating new samples, does the study material already exist, or will both new samples and previously obtained data be used?
- If the study uses preexisting samples, how were they obtained, and were the donors informed of their intended use?
- Whether preexisting or obtained for the study, will the samples be taken anonymously or with identifiers?
- If samples originate with identifiers, will they later be coded or anonymized?
- In either circumstance, when, in what sequence, and how will the coding and/or anonymization be effected?
- Are the anonymized samples anonymous, or could they, theoretically, be relinked to their source?
- How will the donor's privacy and confidentiality be protected?
- Are there risks to relatives from breach of confidentiality regarding identification of a subject's sample?

II. ANTICIPATED PRESENT AND FUTURE USE(S) OF TISSUE

Which questions apply to which samples is, in large part, determined by the use of the sample described in the protocol and whether there are plans for additional future uses of the sample. Although the possibilities for future use are often difficult or impossible to predict, even if only a theoretical possibility, a description of possible future applications needs to be considered in the protocol.

A. What Is Known and What Is or Can Be Anticipated

The precision of description of studies to be performed on a biological sample has been increasing. In the mid-1980s, a protocol might have stated simply that laboratory tests will be performed. Today, it would be considered unwise for an IRB and IEC to accept such vague language. At a minimum, an IRB and IEC can be expected to require language that limits laboratory tests on human biological samples to those relevant to the disease under study. If the sample will be used for genetic or DNA testing, the minimum additional specifications should indicate whether any family linkage analysis will be included and/or whether the testing will provide diagnostic and/or prognostic information. The goal is to provide the reviewers with enough information to make a reasonably accurate prediction of risk so that they can decide whether the protections proposed are sufficient. Although this process might seem constraining, nothing prevents an investigator from submitting to the IRB and/or IEC a protocol amendment to allow sample analysis not specified in the approved protocol. If the additional tests do not increase previously approved risk, the amendment can be expedited.

It is conceivable that tests will be anticipated but not requested at the time the study is designed. For example, the scientific community may anticipate a new analysis technology that will become operational in 2 to 3 years, but it is impossible to describe such tests adequately at the time of protocol preparation. The techniques are simply not advanced enough to permit satisfactory explanation to the IRB and/or IEC although the investigator anticipates their applicability to samples being used and/or generated in the proposed study.

Discussion of the anticipated testing, however, can be in the protocol. In a section that might be entitled Future Studies, the investigator can describe what is known about the upcoming technology. When it is time to conduct the studies, they should be approved in an amendment to the protocol. If at the time of submission of the original protocol to the IRB and/or IEC the researchers can indeed anticipate that future tests with the new technology are expected not to increase risk, it can be so stated. It is prudent to include this information, also, in the consent form. That is, it is wise to inform the subject in the consent document that the investigators may want to contact him or her in the future to ask permission to perform tests that are not yet available.

The situation is much more difficult when scientists can envision tests to be run on samples, but the technology to run such tests is not quite operational. These are the tests that are already imagined but cannot yet be done with the existing or developing tools. Even these vaguely anticipatable tests can be considered during the planning phases for the study. In so doing, it is worth trying to collect these vague possibilities into requests for permission for future studies.

Finally, with technological progress moving at such a dizzying pace, it is expected that methods for testing will evolve in the future that will encourage testing of stored samples in ways that cannot yet be contemplated.

This prospect, too, ought to be planned for and explained to research participants.

B. Storage Procedures

It is important to the approval of a protocol that will use and/or generate human biological samples to be as precise as possible in explaining how the samples will be stored and maintained. Concerns about privacy and confidentiality are particularly great when it comes to the storage of identifiable DNA samples or materials from which identifiable DNA can be extracted. Although review of the ethical discussion about whether or not genetic information is qualitatively different from other medical information is beyond the scope of this book, that a number of people believe that such a difference exists and that this difference is morally relevant makes it advisable to apply a heightened attention to the protection of privacy and confidentiality of such materials.

Although genetic information is generally thought to result from use of DNA, it is now increasingly obvious that genetic information can be obtained by protein analysis or proteomics. Thus, serum analysis may lead to information related to genetics or a disease. It is important in the consent process to try to anticipate the use of such materials and to help a prospective research subject understand the multiple ways in which genetic information can be generated. Similarly, a blood specimen can be used to generate cell lines that can be perpetuated, used for decades, and shared with investigators around the world. Investigators need to anticipate these possibilities and to explain their use in the protocol and consent processes or documents.

Sources of stored human biological materials include large tissue banks, repositories and core facilities, pathology specimens, specimens in newborn screening laboratories, forensic DNA banks, umbilical cord and other blood banks, organ banks, and specimens kept as part of longitudinal research studies. These samples/organs are kept with or without identifiers. For studies that generate new samples, the investigator needs to decide whether they will be taken and stored with identifiers or with a code and whether they will be (if ever) stripped of identifiers before or sometime after storage.

There are advantages and disadvantages to storing samples with personal identifiers or a linkable code and to storing them anonymously (or in "anonymized" fashion). Storing identifiable samples allows clinical researchers to relate the findings of sample studies to whatever clinical information was collected or might be added to the record of a particular patient or research subject.

For the subject, this direct connection to the source allows voluntary withdrawal from the study. What withdrawal means operationally, however, will need to be made explicit in the protocol. The researcher will want to consider distinctions that need to be specified in the protocol and consent process. The following questions are those that an investigator might consider when determining how to deal with voluntary withdrawal:

- If a subject withdraws and no further experiments will be done on the individual's sample(s), will that subject's stored samples be destroyed?
- Will there be an attempt to remove that subject's data from the records?
- If samples from minors are included in a study, how will the subjects be afforded the opportunity to withdraw?
- What kinds of records need to be kept so that a minor subject who has reached the age of 18 or 21 can withdraw from a study?

Under some circumstances, storing samples that are identifiable can increase the potential for direct medical benefit to a subject. For example, the subject can expect to benefit when clinically relevant information is found that could be of importance to his or her health. Maintaining identifiers and linking sample data back to individuals also has a potential for harm. For example, the data could result in future job or insurance discrimination for the subject. For the investigator, the benefit of storing samples with identifiers allows the possibility of linking a sample to other information about the subject, perhaps providing novel scientific insights or suggesting questions that lead to new clinical research. Additional layers of regulation intended to protect the privacy and confidentiality of the subject and the information as they pertain to different levels of consent place an additional burden on the investigator.

These potential benefits and burdens for both subject and investigator apply to samples with personal identifiers (such as name or Social Security number). As long as it is possible to connect a sample with an individual, protections to ensure subject privacy and confidentiality, as well as plans for the appropriate return to the subject of clinically relevant information, are needed. The same responsibilities exist whether a sample is immediately identifiable or is coded. This difference can confuse investigators and IRBs or IECs. Often, reviewers and investigators think that as long as the investigator obtains the sample in coded fashion and has no intention of linking the sample back to the source, there are no risks to subjects. But this assumption of limited risk is only as sound as the procedures used to ensure that no relinking will be made. It is more likely that if a sample can be linked back to the source and if the sample is stored long enough, some new technology or novel research question will stimulate an investigator to want to use the stored sample in a way that will lead a clinical researcher to identify the sample so more clinical information about the subject can be obtained. Therefore, if samples, whether generated in a study or obtained from a stored supply, are to be used in a coded fashion, there must be explicit discussion in the protocol of procedures implemented to preserve privacy and confidentiality. Who will keep the list linking code to personal identifiers? What provisions will maintain confidentiality of the link during the study or at any other time during the existence of the sample?

Many of the concerns related to privacy, confidentiality, storage, and record keeping can be avoided if samples are obtained or stored anonymously. If there is no way to identify the donor source of a sample, there is no risk of harm to any individual subject. Although the study of truly anonymous samples does not remove potential risks to social groups (discussed in Chapter 5 and Chapter 6), it does, at least, reduce individual risk. Generating and storing samples in an anonymous fashion provide the researcher with greater freedom to use the samples repeatedly. Federal regulation in the United States even allows researchers to take samples from identified specimens without need to seek consent from the source if they are to be used anonymously. After the samples are made anonymous (or they are "anonymized"), they can be held indefinitely and used for studies without further review. As new technologies become available, samples can be used and reused without review or approval, beyond that required by the researcher's institutional policy. The cost of this freedom for investigation, however, is loss of the potential value of related clinical data.

A compromise is to use a sample, either with personal identifiers or a linkable code, for the duration and purposes of the study being proposed, followed by anonymization of samples at a specified time. This allows the researchers to maximize scientific use of available information about a subject, albeit not indefinitely. It also provides a period during which withdrawal of a subject (or on behalf of a minor child) is possible. Setting an explicit time for removing identifiers defines the point when the samples will be beyond the possibility of linkage to any particular subject and subjects are beyond the possibility of withdrawal.

C. Sharing Samples with Other Investigators

The time-honored tradition of sharing biological samples with other researchers is becoming increasingly complex. **The free and open sharing of materials among researchers has been a hallmark of the scientific**

enterprise. The practice of sharing samples is part of the tradition of openness in science, the need for studies to be replicated, and the progression of scientific knowledge from earlier findings. **Increasing concerns about breaches of privacy and confidentiality and increasing levels of secrecy related to the commercialization of scientific knowledge, however, have led to a creeping restrictiveness in the sharing of human biological materials.** At the very least, most institutions and businesses have explicit policies governing the transfer of materials. Some transfer of materials across state or national boundaries is governed by state or international laws. In addition to legal and regulatory concerns, ethical questions center on issues of prior consent and the degree that a sample can be identified:

- Was the subject's consent obtained?
- Is the subject's consent needed? If so, how might another consent process take place, and can the consent be practicably obtained?
- If a researcher has samples with identifiers, might it be ethically permissible to share them with identifiers retained?
- If sharing the samples is not currently possible, might it be ethically permissible to share them after the identifiers are stripped?

The many possible ways and reasons for sharing samples need to be considered and planned in the original protocol design. Forethought can reduce problems if sharing is later requested.

III. TISSUE SAMPLES FROM THOSE WHO ARE DECEASED

A consideration that is currently absent from regulatory oversight is the use of tissue from deceased individuals in clinical research (although DHHS regulations do address the issue related to tissue from a dead fetus, as discussed in Chapter 5). **DHHS regulations define a research subject as a living individual. In general, it has been assumed that those who have died no longer have interests that need to be protected.** Thus, regulations focus on protection of living research subjects, excluding from oversight research involving tissue from those who are deceased. This assumption, however, is false. **With the advent of genetics research, it is quite possible that information obtained from tissue from deceased persons can represent a harm for living relatives.** It is possible, also, that an individual who specifically declined use of his or her tissue while alive could have his or her wish disregarded with impunity after death. Each of these possibilities requires thoughtful attention during protocol development (Annas, 2005; DeRenzo *et al.*, 1997).

The spirit of the regulations and the canons of clinical research ethics are to protect human subjects from potential harms posed by the proposed research. The regulations are silent, however, concerning research oversight of studies using samples from the dead which can present risks to living individuals. For example, genetic studies using specimens from deceased persons may lead to information important to living relatives. These relatives, perhaps unknowingly, may become research subjects. It is prudent that appropriate protections for relevant studies be considered and implemented.

Consider the following possibility. The IRB at Western Plains State University has a problem. The IRB chairperson and university dean of research have just learned that one of the university's most well-respected investigators, Dr. Dillion, has been named in a local newspaper article that is unfavorable to the university and to Dr. Dillion's research. It turns out that Professor Dillion has been collecting blood and tissue samples from sets of deceased twins in which one twin had autism. He has been creating this database for 20 years and because the samples have come from persons after death, there has been no oversight of the research. In fact, the IRB chairperson and the dean only vaguely know about the database. It turns out that although Dr. Dillion has stored the samples without identifiers, he has kept the samples coded. That means he could link the samples back to the deceased twin. The numbers of twins who meet these criteria are relatively small and most know of each other's families through a national patient advocate group for twins with autism. Since Professor Dillion started collecting these samples, certain genetic markers have been identified that appear to predispose offspring of the healthy twin with blue eyes to autism. Dr. Dillion has never contacted any family members of the deceased twin. The newspaper story is about several of these offspring who have learned of Dr. Dillion's database, understand the reproductive implications, and are upset by Dr. Dillion having the data. Some persons interviewed in the article objected on the basis that if Dr. Dillion has information that might be useful to reproductive decisions of potentially affected or carrier offspring, he should contact them and give them the information so they can make more informed reproductive decisions. Others objected to the data being identifiable because they are concerned that such information, if linked to living family members, could result in employability or insurability risks. Others interviewed for the article objected because they felt that information, even in the form of a blood sample, should not be provided to researchers without permission of the deceased person's heirs. When the article appeared, the university was caught by surprise. Dr. Dillion has broken no university, state, or federal regulations. Because, however, the university did not have any policy on collection of data from dead persons and the IRB had never had any involvement in oversight of the database, it reflected adversely on the school's reputation for the thoughtful conduct and oversight of its human subjects research portfolio in general.

IV. WRITING THE PROTOCOL SECTIONS ON THE USE AND STORAGE OF HUMAN BIOLOGICAL MATERIALS

The consent form sections on use and storage of human biological materials are expanding in size and scope. Only a few years ago, it was common that the only risks cited for such studies were the discomforts of a finger stick or a punch biopsy. Today, clinical researchers have a greater appreciation of the potential risks and benefits of research involving human biological materials. A consent form for a study of biological materials includes the same sections as any other consent form. If the material to be tested will be for genetic testing, the consent document will need to explain this point fully in clear language that is easily understood by a reader. For example, the purpose section might read something like the following text that is directly addressed to the subject.

What Is the Purpose of This Study?

The purpose of this study is to learn more about the genetics of heart disease. To do this, we will examine the genetic material taken from your blood. Your blood cells contain a molecule called deoxyribonucleic acid, or DNA for short. This DNA is in your blood cells and all other cells in your body. Your DNA that you receive from your parents has a code used in genes that translates into your eye color, blood type, hair color, and other characteristics that combine to make up your body. DNA determines or works in combination with the environment around us to shape how our bodies look and how they work. This means that our DNA plays important roles in how our hearts work or how our hearts get sick. By studying the DNA of persons with heart disease now, we expect that some day in the future, we will learn how to prevent, more effectively treat, and perhaps cure heart disease. We will also be growing cells from your tissue to establish lines of the cells that can live for long periods of time, allowing us to investigate your disease more fully. The parts of the cell may also be studied to understand your disease more fully.

What Will We Be Investigating in This Study?

In this study, we will be examining the genes for . . . We already believe that genes . . ., . . ., and . . . may play a role in the kind of heart disease you have. We will also be looking at other genes to learn if they might, also, be related to . . .

What Are We Asking You to Do?

We are asking you to do three things:

1. We are asking that you consent to give us a small amount of your blood for testing of genes . . ., . . ., and . . .
2. We are asking that you consent to let us use your blood to test for other genes that might be related to your heart disease.
3. We are asking that you allow us to store your blood so that we can test it in the future for genes that might be related to your heart disease but are at present not recognized. If you agree to allow us to store your sample for future studies that we cannot now specify, all identifiers will be removed from your sample before long-term storage. We are asking that you permit us to grow cells from your blood for future use.

You may agree to one, two, all, or none of these requests. Declining to agree to one, some, or all will not cause you to lose any benefits to which you are already entitled.

If you agree to one, two, or all of our requests and then change your mind during the study, you can withdraw your permission at any time without penalty. What it will mean to withdraw is that . . .

A. Storing the Samples

In addition to the examples provided in the text on the previous pages, the investigator will need to add a section on how the team will store the samples. Storage methods and means of identifying the biological samples will be determined by the needs of the study and the kinds of materials to be stored. Here, the investigator needs to explain whether the samples will be taken and/or generated with identifiers. If identifiers will be used, will they ever be removed? If they are to be removed, when, how, and by whom will they be removed? Often, the explanation that is in the protocol can be used in the consent document after translation into language understandable by an 8th grader.

Whether the material to be stored is specifically genetic, risks and discomforts are of two different kinds. They are the risks of the procedures used to obtain the samples and the risks of breach of confidentiality for the information generated from the research. First is the discomfort and/or risks occasioned by procurement of the material. Simply drawing blood causes minimal discomfort, but obtaining tissue or organs during major surgery may be associated with substantial risk and/or discomfort. The risks of procurement, however, might still be minor if the research activities do not add significantly to risk or discomfort inherent in the clinically indicated procedure(s) from which the samples will be produced. If samples are to be stored with identifiers, however, it is prudent to categorize the study at a greater-than-minimal risk level because the real risk of genetic research is most often not encountered in obtaining the sample but from information potentially derived from study of the sample. It is important that investigators become comfortable and skilled at thinking through the full range of these nonmedical potential risks.

All of these points need to be understood by the potential subject. The following text can be used as a guideline for information to be included in a consent document. Note that one or multiple topics can be presented depending on the study risks; these examples in the following paragraphs are options that could be included as explanations.

What Are the Risks, Discomforts, and Benefits of Participating in This Study?

A. Minor Medical Risks

Discomfort associated with participation in this study comes from the blood drawing, punch biopsy, surgical procedure, and other such procedures to obtain the sample and is expected to be minimal. The needle stick needed to obtain the blood sample may cause bruising at the needle site, fainting, and, in rare cases, infection. These events are easily treated and reversible.

B. Major Medical and Nonmedical Risks

Although you will be undergoing a major operation, that operation is part of your standard clinical care. Your care provider or surgeon will explain what will be involved in this surgery and a separate consent form will be used for those procedures. Here, our research team is asking that a little bit of . . . (e.g., tissue) from your . . . (e.g., lung) that is being removed and discarded during your surgery be given to us for our research.

The real risk of participation in this clinical research study relates to the possibility of misuse of personal information (or information that can be linked to a particular group of persons) discovered during our research tests. If you agree to participate in this study, your blood, tissue, or organ will be studied in a way that will produce information that can be connected to you personally (or to the group of persons whom you represent). This is assuming that the material will be taken and stored, at least for some specified time period, with personal or group identifiers.

C. Risks of Revealing Genetic or Personal Information

Misuse of genetic information, although rare, has caused problems for subjects related to their employment and their life and health insurance. There is also a risk that participation in this genetics study could cause you to feel psychological distress or to experience tension with family members or others in your social, racial, tribal (or other types of delineators) group.

Although there can be no absolute guarantees, every reasonable effort will be made to keep your personally identifiable information secret so there will be no misuse. Although the information is kept secret, if you are asked whether you have ever been tested for a genetic disorder, answering "yes" to the question could cause you problems.

If you agree to participate in the study, no risk to you, personally, can be anticipated from your participation because your blood sample will not be individually identifiable. It is possible, however, that the findings of the research could result in (additional) stigma or discrimination for the group of persons represented in this research.

D. Benefits

You will receive no medical benefit from taking part in this genetics research study. It is anticipated, however, that information gained through this research will, in the future, help people who have the same or a similar illness. Reimbursement of expenses or any additional payment that may be provided is not considered to be a benefit.

14

·· · · · · · · ·

SPECIAL ISSUES RAISED BY EVOLVING AREAS OF CLINICAL RESEARCH

·· · · · · · · · · · · · · · ·

Each study presents its own set of ethical considerations. **Certain kinds of ethical issues are inherent in particular areas of clinical research, regardless of specific ethical questions associated with a specific study.** In this chapter, some of the most common special areas of clinical research are presented, highlighting the ethical issues most frequently associated with each.

I. GENETICS RESEARCH

Genetics is the fastest growing area of clinical research. The pharmaceutical industry is eager to attach pharmacogenomics components to a vast number of their more traditional clinical trials. The mushrooming biotechnology industry is virtually synonymous with genetics research. Academic research is not far behind, either through collaborations with the pharmaceutical and biotech industries or through its own publicly and/or privately funded research. Much of the genetics research fervor arises from public efforts engendered by the Human Genome Project, organized through the National Human Genome Research Institute (NHGRI) at the National

Institutes of Health (NIH). More and more frequently, clinical research today includes a genetics component because the value of relating human physiology and disease to inborn genetic determinants is increasingly recognized.

Given this ubiquity, it is crucial that investigators, institutional review boards (IRBs), and institutional ethics committees (IECs) recognize and are sensitive to the ethical issues most frequently encountered in human genetics research to determine how they can be addressed most appropriately and effectively in protocols and consent documents. (A voluminous amount of rich literature exists on ethical issues in genetics research. For the junior investigator, a useful starting point is the seminal work produced by the Institute of Medicine reviewed in Andrews *et al.*, 1994.)

A. Risks to Subjects

The substantive risks to subjects reside not in obtaining the genetic material for study but in the information generated from the study. When the information suggests potential or existing health problems, to whom that information is given (whether intentionally or accidentally, with permission or not) can have negative implications for a subject's job status and insurability. Discovery of genetics information may affect family dynamics, and it may put other family members at unknown risk. It is crucial that these risks be explicit in the consent section of the protocol and in the consent form. There is evidence that jobs as well as life and health insurance have been jeopardized, albeit rarely, by information generated in a study, and potential subjects need to appreciate these risks.

Information that predicts the risk of disease may affect a research participant's or his or her family members' psychological status. For example, a study of Huntington's chorea, a disease that in an individual progresses to involuntary movement disorders and dementia, may involve testing of multiple family members. Some who are at risk will be positive for the genetic abnormality, while others will not. Both results have the potential for psychological impact. Individuals who are positive will have to adjust to the expectation of developing Huntington's disease if they live long enough. Those who are negative for the abnormality may suffer what is referred to as "survivor's guilt." To assist subjects through these often difficult transitions, pre-test counseling and post-test counseling as well as both traditional nondirective genetics counseling and psychotherapeutically focused counseling may need to be included in a genetics protocol. Although genetics counselors are scarce, their lack of availability cannot excuse inadequate counseling when it is needed for study subjects.

Genetics information may carry with it the key to uncovering more serious family secrets, such as discovering nonpaternity, as already mentioned in Chapter 9. Views differ on how to convey to subjects the possibility of generating this information as part of the research process. It is generally agreed, however, that if misattributed parental status is revealed, the information ought not be provided to the subjects. That does not mean that on rare occasions, when the information is important for clinical care or future reproductive planning, this information must never be conveyed. It just means that the default position is not to convey such information. If an investigator believes that it is important to inform the subject, the investigator should consult with the IRB and/or IEC and other relevant institutional personnel about whether, and if so, how such information is best disclosed.

It has been proposed that such personal information need not be explicitly mentioned in consents as long as the protocol provides a method for nondisclosure. This is a weak ethical argument seemingly grounded in beneficence. The stronger argument, consistent with the principles of respect for persons and nonmaleficence, is that this risk must be described in the consent process and documents. Divulging such a secret can be psychologically destructive and lead to family dissolution and/or violence. Because misattributed paternity is quite common among the population, its discovery in a genetics study is surely not improbable. Potential subjects should know that such information could be generated during the study, and there needs to be a plan to enable a potential subject who is concerned with such information to decline study participation without alerting others to the reason. This may have implications for arranging to have consent discussions with the prospective subject in an area separate from other family members and suggesting more than one possible reason that a prospective subject may be ineligible.

The paternity issue can become quite contentious when minors are involved in a study. Paternity of offspring is often contested by spouses or unmarried partners. In a divorce and/or custody dispute, it is not unusual for the father or putative father to demand evidence for or against paternity from the investigator through access to the minor child's records. Parents have been assumed to have the right of access to the research records of their minor children. If nonpaternity has been determined, how it will be recorded in the child's records is an important issue. Planning for such an event is recommended, including a refusal on the part of the researcher to provide any information about nonpaternity. This information can be obtained outside the clinical research setting and researchers are not obligated to share such information. Some genetics researchers have taken the extra step of having their research covered by a Certificate of Confidentiality (see Chapter 9) to ensure that research records cannot be obtained by warring parties in divorce or custody proceedings.

B. Subject and Family Member Conflicts

Information gained during a study may compromise relationships of a subject with other family members. For example, even in genetics studies that do not involve family linkage analysis, information gained about a subject may have implications for other family members. A study subject may find out something about himself or herself that others think should be shared with other family members. This can be a privacy question for the subject who does not want to share personal genetics information, which might have health implications for others in the family.

Another frequent scenario is a genetics study involving a family with certain members who do not wish to participate. This situation can produce family discord as some family members attempt to persuade others either to or not to participate in a family genetics study. Although investigators cannot take responsibility for what family members do or say to each other, the well-planned protocol may be able to avert such family discord. Perhaps not all family members need to be involved to achieve the scientific ends of the study. To the degree that this is true, it should be clarified in the consent documents. Family members who are to be involved in the recruitment process will need to be educated about refraining from pressuring other family members. Voluntary participation is the hallmark of ethical research, regardless of who does the recruiting. Plans for education of family members should be explicit in the recruitment section of the protocol. Investigators are advised to have an established mechanism to enable any person who feels coerced by other family members but who does not want to be a study subject to decline gracefully, with appropriate cover provided by the protocol. This can be as simple as the use of an exclusion criterion that gives the investigator the option of excluding a prospective subject if, in the opinion of the investigator, it would not be in the person's best interest. It can then be said honestly by both parties that the family member did not meet study eligibility criteria.

C. Risks to Communities

Even when genetics research presents no risk to a particular subject or family member, the research may present a risk to a group. Chapter 5 cited the example of the stigma attributed to Ashkenazi Jewish women that ultimately resulted from anonymous genetic research. This case, like many in genetics, resulted not only from a bit of serendipity but also from the way in which genetics research progresses. To find genetic variability that is clinically meaningful is difficult under the best circumstances. The best prospects for doing so occur when defined populations with as little genetic variability as possible can be studied. Such a population is a gold mine for genetics research. Because such populations are scarce, the risk of stigmatization is high when the population is intensively studied. Published reports of newly discovered genes tend to involve particular populations first (Arcos-Burgos and Muenke, 2002; Biesecker, 2002); only afterward is the gene pursued in more heterogeneous populations. **Therefore, when investigators plan studies of particular populations, especially those in which conditions such as alcoholism, cancer, or psychiatric illness have already been identified, ways to minimize or avoid additional negative effects of the research findings on the population need to be considered.** Although the shape of the protective mechanisms is a matter of judgment (Weijer *et al.*, 2003), mention of the possibility of community harm should be included in the consent process and documents, even if there is no apparent risk to an individual because the data are anonymous. If the group can be identified, there is the possibility for group harm. With a prospect of harm to certain groups of people, some individuals may not want to participate so that they, themselves, can avoid contributing to the risk.

D. Genetics Studies or Genetics Study Add-ons?

Is the genetic study independent, or is it a part of another broader protocol? The question to be asked or the hypothesis to be tested determines the optimal design of a genetics study. Sometimes adding a genetics component to a larger study makes the ethical considerations more complex. The PI of the primary study might have his or her own biases for or against genetics studies, which could influence recruitment for the genetics component. Adding a genetics component to a larger study, however, may be an effective way to recruit sufficient subjects into the genetics component. Although it could make the informed consent process longer, more cumbersome, and more difficult, integrating the two might make collection of samples much quicker and more efficient by integrating sample collection into other study procedures. This is a design issue that needs to be carefully thought through in collaboration with the investigators responsible for the related nongenetic primary research study. Through such discussion, mutual interests might be identified that would facilitate scientific progress as well as improve procedures for obtaining, maintaining, protecting, and analyzing samples for a genetics study. Such decisions have implications, also, for whether to include genetics study considerations in the consent and assent documents of the primary protocol or to append separate genetics research consent documents to the primary protocol. This question may be decided differently depending on whether the genetics research primarily involves genotyping, phenotyping, or gene expression studies.

For example, Better Health Drug Company (BHDC) has made the scientific and commercial decision to add a genetics component to the majority of its drug development studies. This is in part because national regulatory agencies are beginning to ask for such data and partly because such data are needed to make the promise of personalized medicine a reality. Personalized medicine is expected to result from advances in pharmacogenetics and pharmacogenomics, which will lead to the creation of drugs targeted to patient groups and/or individuals with genetic characteristics that predict increased efficacy and reduced harmful side effects. The BHDC therapeutic division for gastrointestinal (GI) diseases and obesity is now working out procedures for complying with the new company initiative. First in the GI group's development pipeline is a trial of a new drug to be given to obese patients, post-gastric-bypass surgery, that is hoped to both suppress appetite and reduce anxiety. The design of the genetics add-on component is that blood that is left over from a clinically required postoperation blood draw, which would otherwise be discarded, will be turned over to the company's Pharmacogenomics Research Group (PRG). The PRG will then store it for its own studies. The PRG group's standard protocol and consent language has already gone through internal company review and review by the company's outside panel of pharmacogenetics/pharmacogenomics medical research consultants. The generic protocol and consent is approved for inclusion or attachment to any company protocol the PRG group deems appropriate. The GI group is now debating whether to incorporate the company-approved protocol and consent language into the primary protocol or to make it a separate add-on. Those in favor of incorporating the genetics add-on language into the primary protocol and consent think it will increase recruitment into the genetics component, which they support strongly. Others on the GI team are worried about those community investigators and members of the public who are particularly wary of genetics research, especially when a private, for-profit pharmaceutical company will be doing the research with samples it both controls and will be storing for long periods of time, if not indefinitely. These GI team members think by integrating the genetics add-on study into the main protocol they will jeopardize accrual to the primary study. It would be better, they argue, to make it a separate add-on, so those investigators and potential subjects who don't want to participate can decline more easily, even though it will be made clear that the add-on is optional regardless of where the information is provided. Making the add-on separate, these team members continue, makes reading the information for the primary protocol less cumbersome and thus, less likely to scare off potential subjects. They argue vigorously for separating the add-on from the main study.

E. Use and Storage of Genetic Samples

Ethical issues related to the use and storage of identified, coded, anonymized, and anonymous samples were addressed in Chapter 13. Protocols need to thoroughly explain where such genetic material samples are being used and stored specifically for DNA analysis. Regardless of whether genetic information is qualitatively different from other kinds of medical information, many in the field believe that it is. Investigators must take special care to protect DNA samples in ways often not required in studies with no genetics component.

Consider the following difference. Dr. Jenkins is a psychology professor at Sunset College. Her area of expertise is cognitive performance under stress and she has been conducting both animal and human studies in the area for many years. The majority of her human subjects studies are pencil and paper tests that include the stressor of background noises of different kinds. Sometimes the background noise is pleasant, such a soothing music. Other studies involve more distressing noises such as noise of highway traffic, sometimes including a car crash. Usually, the pencil and paper tests are anonymous, but they do include a detailed demographic section so information can be stratified according to age, gender, and other variables of interest. Dr. Jenkins has been conducting one longitudinal study, however, for the past 17 years. In it she gives the same set of tests under the same set of background noise conditions to a cohort of subjects. These data are kept with personal identifiers. Because Dr. Jenkins has been conducting much research over the last 20 years, her office is full of file cabinets. The ones in which she keeps anonymous data are unlocked. The identifiable data she keeps in a locked cabinet. The IRB has always considered this sufficiently protective.

Dr. Pearson, a faculty member in the same department, conducts genetic research. He is looking for genetics connections between genotype and persons of different personality types. Some studies divide persons into extroversion/introversion groups. Other studies differentiate these two groups further. Once a subject has tested into the extroversion or introversion group, the subject is tested into such types as uninhibited/shy, respectively. Dr. Pearson has been doing this research for many years. He has always kept his personality inventory data with identifiers because some of his subjects continue to serve in studies year after year. Now that Dr. Pearson is taking blood and/or saliva samples to do genetic testing and is combining the genetic information with the personality data, his IRB is questioning whether or not his data storage procedures are adequately protective. The genetic material is coded and Dr. Pearson keeps only one list linking the code to the name of the subject. This list is kept in a locked drawer in his office. But now that there is identifiable genetic material that can not only be linked to the coded genetic samples, but also to the subjects' personality data, the IRB thinks Dr. Pearson needs to come up with a more protective strategy for all of the data.

F. Minors: Participation in Genetics Research

The participation of minors in genetics research poses several interesting and important ethical concerns that should be addressed in relevant protocol preparation. The complexities of devising and implementing mechanisms for handling stored samples from minors were addressed in Chapter 13. Simply deciding whether a minor ought to be a part of a particular study can produce much discussion and disagreement. For example, genetic studies that include minors will often involve testing for a particular disease. There is, however, much controversy about when and for what kinds of genetic diseases minors should be tested. Many professionals in the pediatric genetics counseling and research communities believe that minors should not be tested for any genetic condition with a late onset of disease, especially those for which there is presently no treatment or cure. This view is not always shared by parents of minors in families with a history of specific genetic conditions or by the advocacy groups that speak for such parents and families. A reason given for not testing minors for late onset disorders is that such knowledge can result in what is often termed **closed futures**. This term refers to the denial of opportunities to subjects with genes for a late onset disease, resulting in a sort of defeatist approach for the minor subject's future. Alternatively, the information might cause a child to be nurtured in aberrant ways as a result of having this kind of knowledge about his or her future. The principle of autonomy asks researchers to assist persons in being as self-determining as possible in the face of potentially life-changing information. If knowledge of the genetic information is of no immediate benefit to the minor child, respect for his or her developing autonomy suggests that testing wait until the child can consent or decline independently. At the very least, these concerns suggest that if a minor child is included in a genetics protocol, he or she should have the opportunity to dissent privately from his or her parents. Also requiring consideration in the design phase is how minors will be given the opportunity to withdraw stored samples when they reach the age of maturity.

G. Variability in Ethical Standards, Vocabulary, and Regulations

One of the most frustrating problems for genetics researchers is the considerable variability in ethical standards, vocabularies, and regulations among states and countries. This variability requires that each protocol present the ethical arguments that support the study and refute convincingly all the expected arguments against it. The reasons for doing the study will be in the rationale section, with argumentation in the ethics section of the protocol. Clarification and definitions will be in the procedures section, and the regulatory compliance section of the protocol can identify the regulations and international guidance documents that govern the conduct and oversight of the protocol.

Consider the following problem. The prospect of race-based therapeutics is rapidly becoming a reality. Now that studies have shown that African-American subjects with class III or IV heart failure with dilated ventricles benefit from being given isosorbine dinitrate plus hydralazine over placebo (Taylor *et al.*, 2004), a biotechnology company working with university investigators across the country and in different parts of the world wants to move this work forward. The idea is to genotype African Americans with any heart disease. Objections within the company to this approach include concerns about discrimination. The company librarian is asked to do a search of state and federal legislation and legislation in several European countries to look for mention of genetic discrimination. The librarian comes back to the group frustrated and explains that this is going to be a very difficult search to run because genetics and genetic discrimination is defined differently across the states and by foreign legislative bodies. Ultimately, the biotech group decides to limit the genotyping to only two U.S. states and two foreign countries in which the librarian can find state and national legislation that defines terms like *genetic information* and *genetic condition* comparably and has similar kinds of legislative protections against housing and/or employment discrimination based on utilization of genetic information.

II. PSYCHIATRIC RESEARCH

Psychiatric research has been a magnet for controversy regarding research ethics since the mid-20th century. The first presidential ethics commission, The National Commission for the Protection of Human Subjects of Biomedical and Behavioral Research, produced *The Belmont Report* and a series of authoritative reports now embodied in the federal regulations that govern research on human subjects in the United States. The commission also produced recommendations about studies of people with mental illness that were not implemented at that time (The National Commission for the Protection of Human Subjects of Biomedical and Behavioral Research, 1978). Another presidential ethics commission, the National Bioethics Advisory Commission (NBAC), submitted its report and recommendations 20 years later for the ethical conduct of research involving these psychiatrically ill subjects (National Bioethics Advisory Commission, 1998). The many complex ethical issues central to studies involving subjects with a psychiatric impairment already mentioned throughout this book ought to be considered by investigators when designing a protocol concerning these subjects.

A. Capacity to Give Consent

One of the most difficult and important ethical issues in research involving psychiatric patients relates to the subject's altered mental status and poor judgment that are a part of the disease process and relates to the effects of these conditions on decision making. As a result of severe stroke or coma, a subject's clear lack of capacity requires that a surrogate make the decisions. In the case of severe stroke or coma, there is no disagreement about whether or not the individual is decisionally capable. The individual's lack of decisional capacity is obvious. That is not the case for psychiatric illness. Psychiatric symptoms wax and wane over the course of an individual's disease. The impact of psychiatric illness on decision-making capacity is variable across subjects who all share the same diagnosis and at different times within the same individual.

Research involving subjects with other kinds of mental disturbance, such as late life dementia, also presents different problems from those presented by psychiatrically ill persons. For example, the family histories of individuals with a psychiatric illness can be expected to be strained in different ways from families with elders who became demented later in life. That is not to say that families of psychiatrically ill persons do not care about their psychiatrically sick family members. It does, however, acknowledge that the symptoms of psychiatric illness have a high probability of disrupting family relationships and separating family members throughout the subject's life. **Thus, in psychiatric research, there is a high probability that the ability of subjects to provide informed consent may be diminished and that ethical issues involving surrogate decision making may be complex.**

Some in the research field take the position that if subjects cannot provide their own informed consent, they should be excluded from a study. Others believe that psychiatrically impaired research subjects, if decisionally capable of providing consent but who might be anticipated to lose it during the study, ought to be involved in research only if they are willing and able to assign a research surrogate prior to study entry. There are those in the research community, however, who believe that both approaches raise concerns for increased stigmatization and pose therapeutic problems on the basis that such protective mechanisms may exacerbate feelings of powerlessness and paranoia in an individual with psychiatric disease. Whether an autonomy-driven approach or a more protective, beneficence-driven approach is proposed will depend on the ethical perspective of the investigators and review bodies responsible for the trial. Either approach will present its own set of ethical complexities, and whichever approach is taken will need to be justified in the body of the protocol, particularly in the Ethics Section (Chapter 10).

Controversy also surrounds the dispute about how capacitated a psychiatrically ill individual has to be to provide ethically and legally valid consent. The ethical and legal notion of consent is that it is decision specific. Assessment of a subject's ability to provide ethically and legally valid consent needs to be built into any protocol where subjects can be expected to have questionable capacity. Although processes for such assessment are becoming increasingly refined, they are and can be expected to continue to be a subjective determination, as discussed in Chapter 5.

Protocols involving psychiatrically ill subjects will need to address the capacity issue with better specificity. Discussion of how capacity is to be assessed should be built into the protocol. Such protections may include consent monitors, non-research-affiliated physician advocates, and non-research-affiliated individuals performing the capacity assessments.

Other protections include the increased demand for more patient advocates joining IRBs and IECs. Progress on meeting this demand has been slow but mounting, with programs to train and place patient advocates on IRBs and to create institutional policies and practices for including greater numbers of patient advocates and/or former research subjects in the review bodies. It may be wise, also, for investigators to more fully use psychiatric patient advocates in the design and development of protocols.

B. Risk of Placebo Arms

Capacity issues in adults are not the only seemingly intractable ethical questions raised by psychiatric research. The literature representing what has been dubbed "the placebo wars" focuses on concerns for the well-being of psychiatric research subjects. Mentioned previously in Chapter 6, part of the ethical concerns about the use of placebos comes down to the seemingly unanswerable question: how much risk is too much risk? When translated into the language of psychiatric research, the question includes whether the harm of psychological pain is equivalent to harm of physical pain. Part of this question is empirically answerable in that future data may reveal whether or what kinds of mental illness have ill effects on somatic health or psychic health. Questions about the potential for psychological pain and suffering need to be considered where relevant. The investigator's justification for particular answers in the protocol and a well-described set of protections for questionably capacitated subjects should be expected to minimize the risk of such harm.

C. Minors: Participation in Psychiatric Research

When pediatric subjects are involved in a study, the level of ethical complexity increases. Adding minors to any protocol, as discussed in Chapter 5, adds a whole new set of questions. These include the growing autonomy rights of adolescents, possible differences in parental authority regarding research and clinical care decisions, and the vulnerability of young children or anyone legally incapable of giving informed consent. Involving psychiatrically ill minors in research raises additional specific questions. One of the most complicated is the following: **to what degree should mental conditions in children be addressed through medical intervention?** Data about mental illness in younger and younger children are being obtained. Mental diseases not previously recognized in children are increasingly well documented, yet concern about the effects of any pharmacologic intervention on development, especially neuroleptic intervention on brain development, remains.

Another concern in involving these subjects is the appropriateness of surrogate (i.e., parental) decision making. While the care and attention devoted by parents to their mentally impaired children are ordinarily presumed to be in the best interest of the child, there may be lingering suspicions about the quality of care that parents may be providing. Mentally ill children are an enormous burden on their families. This does not mean that children with other diseases may not also be an enormous family burden. There is, however, an intuitive difference between behavioral and physical disorders that may result in **strains on families of children with behavioral disorders differing from those on families of children with somatic diseases.** In addition, some children with mental illness may have parents with similar, or comparable but different, emotional problems that do not render them unacceptable parents legally, although ethically they might be considered less than optimal decision makers for their children. These differences create concerns about the motivations of parents who enroll their children in psychiatric research, especially research that has little or no expectation of direct medical benefit. These issues need to be presented squarely in a protocol for the reviewers to consider. Justifications for conducting the study need to be thorough. Concerns about the appropriateness of administering psychotropic drugs to children mandate a particularly high level of justification for such studies. Rescue end points will need to be specific. When subjects will be paid, serious thought is required to decide the specifics of compensation (e.g., what kind, how much, and to whom, such as to the parents, child, or both). This area of research can be expected to expand rapidly over the next several years as a result of the interest of treating physicians, the pharmaceutical industry, and the U.S. FDA in increasing the inclusion of minors in research.

III. RECRUITMENT AND RETENTION OF WOMEN AND MINORITY POPULATIONS

During the second half of the 20th century the traditional perspective that research is an activity from which vulnerable persons must be protected and/or excluded changed to one in which all persons, particularly women and persons from minority populations, should have access. This philosophical change was given practical shape by the NIH Revitalization Act of 1993, which required established guidelines for inclusion of women and minorities in clinical research. The guidelines call for all NIH-funded clinical trials, especially at the phase III level, to collect sufficient data to elicit information about subjects of both genders and diverse racial and ethnic groups. The influence this guidance has had on changes in clinical research populations is immeasurable. Prior to 1993, it was common for women to be excluded from clinical trials, even of medical interventions that, if approved, would be taken by women as well as men. There was a general lack of appreciation of the possibility that differences in female and male chemistry and physiology might result in substantial differences in the ways therapeutic interventions affected each gender. Couple this lack of attention to differences in treatment impact with the variability in women's bodies resulting from menstrual cycles—it was just considered easier to study men. As data mounted that significant differences in drug metabolism and outcome existed between the sexes, however, data also accumulated pointing to differences in health patterns across racial and ethnic groups. These scientific awakenings were taking place within a social context of attention to injustices towards women and minority populations in other sectors of society. The resulting 1993 act literally changed the face of clinical research, regardless of funding source. Progress has been swift in some ways and in other ways it has been slower. Today, women, even women of reproductive potential, are regularly included in clinical trials. The shift from excluding women completely to only excluding women of childbearing potential to including all but pregnant women (see discussion in Chapter 5 and in the next section of this chapter) has been accomplished quite completely. For studies in which a fetus would need to be protected from an experimental agent, protocols and consent documents include clear and explicit language on requirements for birth control. Also, an increased equalitarianism has surfaced when scientifically appropriate. When relevant, birth control is required for both female and male study participants. This attention to gender issues in reproduction can be seen in other ways as well, such as discussions of egg and sperm banking in relevant protocols.

The swift shift to a reasonable and fair balance of the benefits and burdens of research participation that can be seen between males and females, however, has not been achieved as successfully concerning inclusion and retention of minority populations. Recruitment and retention of minority populations in research continues to exist at lower levels than would be hoped for on the basis of fair access. There appear to be multiple reasons for the reduced numbers of minority subjects. Fear and mistrust on the part of minority communities of the majority-dominated research community account for much of the problem. Few discussions of problems in recruiting minorities escape reference to the lingering effects of the Tuskegee Syphilis Study (see Chapter 15). It is unlikely, however, that mistrust is the only cause of low minority recruitment. Researchers are working to learn better techniques for community outreach. The 1993 act specifically requires the creation of outreach programs to recruit the populations covered by the act, and as researchers gain knowledge of which outreach strategies work best (Arean *et al.*, 2003; Meinert *et al.*, 2003) it can be anticipated that the numbers of minority subjects will increase.

IV. INVOLVEMENT OF PREGNANT WOMEN OR FETUSES

As was noted in Chapter 5, the ethical involvement of pregnant women or fetuses in research is a controversial topic in the research and political arenas. The DHHS regulations described in 45 CFR 46 (Appendix, No. 15) that relate to involvement of pregnant women or fetuses were revised in November of 2001. The revised regulations explicitly state the circumstances under which Common Rule agency-funded research may involve pregnant women, fetuses, and neonates; and after delivery, the placenta, the dead fetus, or fetal material. In the case of pregnant women, a fetus, or a neonate, research can only be performed when risk has been minimized and there is an expectation of direct medical benefit to the subject. In the case of the neonate, the anticipatable benefit must be the enhanced prospect of survival to viability. In all cases, the potential benefit must be obtainable only through the research proposed. For research after delivery involving the placenta, the dead fetus, or fetal material, the research must adhere to any applicable federal, state, or local laws. In addition, if information associated with the material is recorded so that living individuals are identifiable, these individuals are considered research subjects, and all pertinent regulations apply. Research of this kind presents substantial religious, cultural, philosophical, and political controversy and can be expected to continue to do so for the foreseeable future.

V. EMERGENCY MEDICINE RESEARCH

Research in emergency medicine is an area of study that has acquired its own set of regulations over the last decade. This expansion of regulations resulted from the identification of an improper practice for obtaining consent that was endemic throughout the emergency medicine research community. In many emergency medicine studies, the consent mechanism judged to be outside the bounds of ethical justification and regulatory compliance was referred to as **deferred consent**. The practice was that investigators enrolled individuals into emergency medicine studies who were unable to provide their own consent and had no one to consent for them. Later, when the subject was able to consent and/or an appropriate surrogate was available, consent for the completed procedures plus permission to continue were sought.

When the federal government realized that this was a widespread practice in emergency medicine research, guidance letters were mailed to thousands of investigators to inform them that deferred consent is not acceptable. Consent must be prospective and continuing until terminated. It can never be retrospective. Needless to say, this "cease and desist" directive brought emergency medicine research to a virtual halt. Although the U.S. FDA regulations were a bit more liberal than those of the U.S. DHHS, it became immediately apparent that for emergency medicine research to progress, regulatory relief and clarification were required.

Regulatory relief came in the year 2000 in the form of FDA guidance and regulatory clarification. Perhaps the most interesting, ethically complex, and innovative aspect of this regulatory guidance is the requirement for community involvement in the development of an emergency medicine study. The terminology in the regulations is **community consultation**. Any emergency medicine research protocol that requires an exception from the standard requirements for informed consent must obtain it from the IRB. The IRB must document the PI's consultation with representatives of the community or communities in which the study will take place and from which the study subjects can be expected to come. The guidance document has detailed information about what will not be accepted as meeting the community consultation requirements. Final determination of what meets the standards for community consultation and public disclosure is left to the discretion of the investigator and the review bodies. This is an ethically difficult issue because there has been much disagreement in the ethics literature about just what constitutes a community representative. There is, as of yet, no consensus on who might be the appropriate community representative for any particular group, community, or population. Effective implementation of this new federal regulation will be a challenge for investigators and IRBs or IECs; data of the impact on research of the new regulations is just beginning to appear in the literature (McClure *et al.*, 2003; Shah, 2003).

The guidance includes several other requirements that are not specified for other kinds of research: the study must hold out the possibility of direct benefit to the subjects, and a licensed physician must concur in IRB approval. Previously existing regulations had already required an IRB to add consultants for review of any protocol for which it does not have the requisite expertise. The regulations for emergency medicine research now require all such protocols to include a physician not affiliated with the research who will concur with the IRB that the regulations have been met at the initial and continuing reviews of the protocol.

Another important and novel regulation governing emergency medicine research is the requirement for public disclosure at completion of the study. It is stipulated that at the end or termination of an emergency medicine study, a public report of sufficient information, including demographic characteristics of the study population, identifies the lay and research communities that were involved. Disclosure is intended to provide a timely and comprehensive summary of results in formats appropriate for publication in both scientific and lay media. Like the requirement for community consultation, the new regulations provide a reasonable level of detail to allow investigators, IRBs, and IECs to carefully evaluate whether a particular protocol meets the proposed regulations and appropriate ethical standards.

VI. COMMUNITY-BASED RESEARCH

The requirement for community involvement discussed in the preceding section reflects just one aspect of the discussion on ethical considerations regarding research and its effects on community or communities. Growing concern about how a community or communities ought to be involved, treated, and protected in the research setting has led to the reasonably new research area of community-based research. **Community-based research is community-driven, community-organized, community-focused, and community-managed.** Unlike traditional research that is investigator- or sponsor-initiated and focuses on their interests, even in the studies that ask questions about particular communities, community-based or participatory research (PR) reverses this process. **Community-based or participatory research addresses concrete problems and issues of interest to the community that are generated from within the community through equal partnerships with researchers and, thus, present unique ethical challenges to the conduct of trials** (Marshall and Rotimi, 2001).

Much of this research is ethnographic or applies other qualitative methodologies. It frequently focuses on services and educational aspects of community activities and addresses problem areas that communities, themselves, have an interest in studying. The focus is often on research that can be used to influence public policy. Research agenda priorities are commonly set by the urgency of the community's need to address a particular aspect of its services.

For researchers embarking on community-based research, the design phase can be expected to be much longer than for traditional studies. A lot of work will be required to familiarize the researcher with the community in which he or she chooses to work. A special characteristic of this kind of research is the locus of control (e.g., the community as sponsor), which involves a lengthy process of community organization and agenda creation. The role of each partner in the collaboration needs to be clarified and agreed upon before a protocol is drafted. Funding mechanisms can be cumbersome and also need to be well defined early in the design process.

VII. QUALITY IMPROVEMENT AND QUALITY ASSURANCE RESEARCH

Research for quality assurance (QA) has been around for a long time. The questions being raised about how much oversight QA research ought to receive and how QA is the same or different from quality improvement (QI) research are new (Bellin and Dubler, 2001; Casarett *et al.*, 2000). **Quality assurance research** has never been considered academic research in the scholarly sense. It is conducted in hospitals and other health care delivery organizations to ensure that the quality of care provided is adequate. Historically, QA research was most frequently of the retrospective chart review variety or involved anonymous patient satisfaction surveys. With the economic implications of diagnostic related groups (DRGs) and other cost-cutting innovations of the past 30 years for hospital care, QA projects evolved into **quality improvement research** projects. QIs are now the byword of evaluating and continually upgrading standards in health care organizations. As the need for increasingly sophisticated methods of assessing and improving quality grew, the kinds of studies conducted to produce information about QA and QI have become more sophisticated. This has translated into many QA and QI projects that increasingly resemble academic-level, quantitative research. The more such methodologies have evolved, the more attention has been brought to placing QA and QI projects under some sort of oversight system.

For those interested in performing QA and QI projects, it is important to understand that there have been a few attempts in the literature (ibid) to assist investigators and IRBs or IECs in deciding whether QA or QI research should receive IRB/IEC oversight and whether it requires a subject's consent. Consent issues in this area of research promise to present ethical challenges to the investigator and the review bodies that will ultimately take responsibility for oversight of this area of research. Some of these issues are presented in these questions:

- If QA and QI projects are required as part of a hospital's ongoing accreditation processes, can patients simply decline to give consent?
- Will written consent be required?
- Might some less obtrusive means for honoring dignity rights, such as information sheets, be sufficient for deciding that all patients must be willing to participate in projects designed to increase the quality of care for all patients?

These and other ethical issues related to QA and QI research are only just beginning to be discussed in the 21st century. This is an area of research and research oversight that is in flux and can be expected to receive increasing ethical, procedural, and regulatory attention over the next decade.

VIII. TRANSLATIONAL RESEARCH

Translational research is the "buzz word" for research that moves between the laboratory bench and the patient's bedside at an ever quickening pace. **Translational research** is designed to move basic research findings into therapeutics and to accelerate the flow of insights from clinicians that are shaped into questions answered at the bench. Investigators can expect to see funding for translational research growing at a dizzying pace over the next several decades. One of the primary ethical concerns of this research relates to the types of contractual agreements that are attached to many of the studies and the concerns the agreements raise for continued free exchange of scientific information. That is, translational research is characterized by the kinds of public/private collaborations that produce serious conflicts of interest for investigators and institutions. Another ethical concern raised by the push for translational research is that there will be a reduction in funding for undirected basic research. Because so much of medical and scientific progress results from serendipitous findings, directing scientific inquiry towards therapeutics may have an effect opposite to that which the proponents of translational research seek. By attempting to move basic research too quickly into areas that have a specific therapeutic focus, the natural meandering of scientific interest will be constrained, and the possibility that scientific surprises can emerge will ultimately be reduced. A final and related concern is that the push of translational research will result in moving science so quickly from the bench to the bedside that subjects will be harmed in ways that might have been avoided, had the process been slower. A glaring example of how this problem might evolve is discussed in the presentation of the research focused on brain tissue transplants in Parkinson's Disease in Chapter 15.

IX. Epidemiological Research

The ethics of epidemiological research are evolving. **Epidemiological research is research designed to study processes, characteristics, or other facets of particular populations or phenomenon**. Epidemiological studies are among the oldest and most common human subjects research studies. Historically, this area of research has attracted little attention or controversy. The ways in which epidemiological studies are carried out, however, especially restrictions on researcher access to study populations, have tightened markedly (Coughlin and Beauchamp, 1996; Horner, 1998). The kinds of databases that researchers automatically have access to without a requirement for study-specific consents from subjects have declined. The days are over when researchers would obtain the names, addresses, and other contact information of family members from a proband (primary research subject) and contact these family members directly. In light of the QA and QI issues just discussed, the sun may be setting on days when it was possible to simply access patient charts without institutional review and oversight. IRBs and IECs now commonly require that investigators provide probands and/or database registry administrators with researcher contact information and request that the proband and database registry administrator do the contacting. With the advent of HIPAA, epidemiological research is likely to become increasingly complicated.

For example, Dr. Samuels is a community geriatrician who regularly admits her patients to the Downtown Teaching Hospital. She has been sensing that an increasing number of her patients have been having infectious complications after cardiac surgery. She wants to conduct a study of the hospital's infection rates in cardiac surgery patients over the age of 65. She approaches the physician in charge of resident research projects, Dr. Yee, and suggests the project. Although interested and expecting that the project is doable, Dr. Yee is unsure how to manage the transfer of hospital information about patients other than those under Dr. Samuels' direct care. Dr. Yee tells Dr. Samuels that he will contact the hospital's HIPAA compliance officer and get back to her.

X. SURGICAL RESEARCH

Norms and practices for clinical research involving surgical interventions are also changing. Most IRBs and IECs review fewer surgical protocols than they do drug or biologics protocols. This is in large part because of the differences between regulatory processes for the approval of pharmaceuticals and those for devices. In sum, the U.S. regulatory apparatus for the approval of drugs is voluminous compared to the regulatory apparatus for the approval of medical devices. The extent of the regulatory apparatus for surgical interventions can be expected to change in the near future, with surgical innovation coming to rest on a research foundation that looks more like its pharmaceutical cousin in both understanding and application of norms of clinical research ethics and the imposition of more regulatory requirements (Horng, 2003). Nonetheless, blurred lines between what some might consider research and what others define as innovative surgery can be expected to continue. That is because surgical procedures, *per se*, are not regulated and regulatory bodies are appropriately hesitant to appear to be seeking authority to regulate medical practice.

A group of orthopedic surgeons at a community teaching hospital come back from a surgical conference having learned about a new technique for repairing complicated ankle breaks. They want to apply the new procedure, but some are not convinced that it will be better than presently used techniques. Because surgical procedures themselves are not regulated, some of the surgeons just want to invite the surgeon who presented the information at the meeting to their hospital to train them so they can start using the new technique. Others want to set up a formal test of the procedure so that, once all the surgeons have been trained, as eligible patients are identified, they are invited to participate in a randomized trial of the old technique versus the new. The chief of surgery asks that his group think it over and to come back for a meeting the following week prepared to defend one option or the other.

XI. Biologics

Although vaccine research has been conducted for at least the last two centuries, research with biologics is expanding quite rapidly. **Whereas traditional drugs have been developed from nonliving chemicals, biologics are derived from living sources such as viruses, animals, and people.** Many traditional drugs are administered by mouth; most biologics if administered orally would be destroyed by the digestive system, so they are most often administered through injection. Traditional drugs have the potential for altering immune system response, while biologics hone in on specific cells, often intending to produce an immune response. These differences in source and mechanism have implications for the ethical considerations necessary during the design process. For example, if there is even the theoretical possibility that a subject could shed either administered virus or a new virus produced by the combining of the administered virus with virus harbored in the host, what provisions will be made for containing the subject? How long might such a subject need to be quarantined? If quarantine is needed, what social amenities (e.g., free telephone access) might need to be provided? In designing protocols with biologics, there may be ways the biological agent presents risks and/or benefits similar to or different from traditional drugs. Investigators, sponsors, and review boards will want to think about these differences and/or similarities carefully in the study design and review process. Consider the following example.

> A group of researchers have been working with a pharmaceutical company on a biologic intervention for liver cancer and the agent is now ready for its move from the bench to its first in-human trial. Because the biologic is not expected to have any serious side effects—one of the advantages over standard chemotherapeutic agents—the company wants to get PK data in healthy humans before conducting tests in patient volunteers. The company's clinical research and development (R&D) team leader convenes a meeting of scientists and clinical research ethicists to consider whether the risks of this biologic are different than a standard chemotherapy agent, and if so, how such a difference(s) might affect the risks to healthy human research volunteers.

XII. Prisoners

DHHS regulations at 45 CFR 46, Subpart C, lay out constraints on research involving prisoners (Appendix, No.15). For research governed by the DHHS regulations, Subpart C applies when any subject is or becomes a prisoner. This last point may not be well-appreciated by researchers and review bodies. It seems that some have not understood this aspect of the regulations, rather interpreting the regulations only to apply to those incarcerated at the time of study entry. A prisoner is defined as any individual involuntarily confined or detained in a penal institution. The term covers those sentenced to such an institution under criminal or civil statute and individuals detained in other facilities by virtue of statutes or commitment procedures that provide alternatives to criminal prosecution, such as institutions housing individuals deemed too psychiatrically impaired to stand trial. The term also covers individuals detained pending arraignment, trial, or sentencing. When a study includes a subject(s) who meets the definition of prisoner, special composition of the IRB is required. With the exception of prisoners, IRB members must not have association with the prison(s) involved. Also, at least one member of the IRB (or one of the reviewing IRBs) must be a prisoner or a prisoner representative with appropriate background and experience to serve in that capacity. There are additional conditions that must be met for research involving prisoners related to avoidance of undue influences on prisoner informed consent, fairness of subject selection, subject selection immunity from arbitrary intervention by prison authorities or other prisoners, parole board actions concerning study participation, and specific details about poststudy follow-up care. These constraints and the additional logistical complexities they bring to research involving prisoners have resulted in little prisoner research since the regulations were created. Today, an appreciation for the need for information related to health and other medical issues pertinent to prisoner status has led to these regulations being reviewed by various groups. It is anticipated that there may be changes to these regulations in the future.

XIII. CLINICAL RESEARCH AND BIOTERRORISM

Since the terrible attacks on the World Trade Center and the Pentagon on September 11, 2001, the United States and the rest of the world have been irreversibly changed. Fear and concern about more terrorist attacks have become commonplace. Talk of terrorism has become the stuff of everyday conversations. For Americans, whatever sense of isolation we may have felt from the horror of terrorism that others around the world have experienced for generations is gone. A sad recognition for the need for clinical research into protection from terrorist attacks has set in, and much attention has focused on bioterrorism. This realization has been accompanied by attention to the ethical considerations raised by this new menace in our midst (Moreno, 2003). Old concerns about the ethical conduct of military research (Moreno, 2001) have resurfaced. New concerns have emerged about how such research will be conducted in other public and private sectors (DeRenzo, 2003; Fleischman and Wood, 2003; Meslin, 2003). Many hospitals, public health authorities, and state and local governments are developing plans for bioterrorism response requiring studies to predict how well such plans might work. This is an area of clinical research that can only be expected to expand in the immediate future and the years ahead. It may be prudent for researchers, research sponsors, and research review bodies to begin thinking about the ethical issues related to such clinical research. One of the concerns about bringing such protocols forward is that there will be an urgency attached to them that might reduce the time for design and review needed to assure that these scientifically and ethically complex protocols receive the required degree of thoughtful preparation.

CASE HISTORIES: LEARNING FROM EXPERIENCE

· · · · · · · · · · · · · · · · ·

The case method has long been used for teaching medicine and law and is equally effective in teaching research ethics. That is, **research ethics case histories** are an excellent source of instructive insights and are an important means of illuminating ethical issues that call for thoughtful analysis. This final chapter presents, with commentary, several cases that may be useful in the mentoring of junior clinical investigators; we hope that these cases are of interest to our readers. The first three cases are landmarks in the evolution of clinical research ethics, and the last three are contemporary cases that may become central to the continuing evolution of clinical research ethics. The first three are important because they initiated the development of regulations that continue to guide the performance of human subjects research. The last three were selected because they illustrate how thinking about ethical problems continues to evolve. All address common problems in clinical research: difficulties in appropriately balancing risks and benefits, protecting the vulnerable from exploitation, and obtaining truly informed consent.

To some, the recurrence of the same problems may seem a disheartening commentary on the improvement in ethical standards for clinical research, but the cases do reveal significant evolution. Over time, the ethical flaws in many of the most notable cases have become increasingly subtle. Although U.S. regulations have not been substantively altered since they were promulgated over 20 years ago, their interpretation continues to change as the public and the scientific communities have become more sensitive to the ways in which ethical lapses can occur in the clinical research setting. This enlightenment and the public and professional debates responsible for it continue to refine the definition of the boundaries of acceptable ethical conduct in human research. Thus, although the nature of the core problems is the same, the more specific ways in which they manifest indicate that clinical research involving human subjects continues to benefit from higher ethical standards.

I. Classical Cases in Clinical Research Ethics

A. *The Tuskegee Syphilis Study*

The Tuskegee Syphilis Study (Reverby, 2000) was intended to document the natural history of syphilis in Black males from Macon County, Georgia, and it was active from 1932 to 1972. This study represents one of the most infamous violations of clinical research ethics in U.S. history. The multiple, egregious breaches of research ethics included misrepresentation of study procedures, which were of no expected direct medical benefit to subjects, as special treatments; the failure to provide life-saving treatment to subjects when it became available; and the unmistakable fingerprints of racism. Here, we omit discussion of the ways in which some subjects were provided standard care and others were not as well as the intentional denial of beneficial treatment when it became available. Rather, we focus on the specific decision not to disclose information discovered during the experiment that would likely have made subjects unwilling to remain in the study.

During World War II, penicillin was discovered to be effective against syphilis; researchers prevented the men of the Tuskegee Syphilis Study from finding out about this remarkable new treatment. An argument in favor of this outrageous behavior offered by the U.S. Public Health Service investigators was that continuing the study was more important than informing the subjects. Informing them may have made them drop out of the study, which might have resulted in its termination prior to its meeting its scientific end points. This woefully flawed argument points most directly toward two ethically complex and related issues in research: informed consent and risk/benefit analysis.

> *Today, we recognize that no data are important enough to supersede the principles of respecting the research participants enough to allow them to make their own informed decisions about research participation. The accumulation of data is also not more important than a subject's well-being and preventing subjects from being placed at risk of grave harm.*

- But when does information become important enough that informing certain subjects becomes the priority?
- How should the information be provided?
- In addition, the intractable questions remain: how much risk and how much harm are too much? How much information is enough?

Determining the answers to these questions has been, is, and will continue to be at the heart of the difficult task of determining whether a study is ethically acceptable.

Informed consent presumes that adults capable of decision making and those who speak on behalf of children or adults unable to speak for themselves will make sound judgments, provided they have sufficient information and adequate understanding and are not subject to undue influence or coercion. These requirements for informed consent do not end with the process that takes place before entry into a study, regardless of how well it is accomplished. Throughout the study, the investigator(s) must continue to provide subjects or their surrogates with timely information that can reasonably be expected to influence their willingness to continue participation. In the Tuskegee Syphilis Study, the Macon County men were never told that a new drug had become available to treat syphilis.

Sometimes, it is difficult to decide whether information that emerges during a study is important enough to transmit to subjects or their surrogates. In the case of the Macon County subjects, there is no disagreement. Information that a new drug is available to cure a fatal or debilitating disease must be provided to subjects promptly. But less obvious cases illuminate the other ethical problem raised by the flawed argument of withholding the information in the Tuskegee study. **Conducting ethically sound human subjects research requires repeatedly weighing the value of accruing new knowledge for benefit of future persons and the protection of the rights and welfare of study participants. The quantification of protection and risk reduction is usually debatable. In the Tuskegee Syphilis Study, once penicillin was discovered, it is clear that the balance was tipped in the wrong direction.** The Tuskegee Syphilis Study teaches that information reasonably expected to influence a subject's decision regarding continued participation should be revealed. Truly informed consent allows the individual research subject to determine the balance of risks and potential benefits consistent with a subject's understanding of what is in his or her own best interest.

B. The Wichita Jury Study

In 1954, investigators from the University of Chicago conducted a study of the deliberative process by U.S. juries, and this study was named the

Wichita Jury Study (Faden and Beauchamp, 1986). Investigators secretly taped the deliberations of six different juries. The ensuing debate resulted in federal legislation that prohibited the recording of federal grand or petit jury deliberations. The case raised important questions about informed consent. Although the investigators had obtained permission for the study from the relevant courts and opposing counsel, the jurors had no idea that they were being taped or that they were even in a research study. The central issue here was, therefore, not deception in research. The subjects were not deceived about their research participation, but they were totally uninformed.

The criticisms of this study arose from concerns about invasion of privacy. **It is assumed that persons have a right to hold private certain things about themselves; this information can be revealed to others only with their consent. The right not to have one's privacy invaded without consent is consistent with the principle of respect for persons, protecting the dignity and autonomy of each and every individual.** The controversy caused by the Wichita Jury Study evoked much discussion and examination of research practices within the social sciences and solidified notions of informed consent.

C. The Milgram Obedience Studies

From 1960 to 1963, Stanley Milgram conducted studies to investigate the extent to which individuals would demonstrate obedience. These studies are referred to as the Milgram Obedience Studies (Faden and Beauchamp, 1986). Intrigued by the testimony of the Nazi physicians at the Nuremberg trials that they had only been following orders, Milgram wanted to learn why apparently average citizens would inflict harm on a person on the order of another. The central ethical problem posed by these studies was the deceptive manipulation of subjects into presumably uncharacteristic behaviors.

The study involved pairs of individuals who were taken into a laboratory to engage in memory experiments. One member of the pair was a naive subject, and the other was an investigator masquerading as a second subject. A third person was involved, and this person was another investigator who acted as greeter and gave the instructions. The real subject was designated the teacher, and the masquerading subject was the learner. The real subject was told only that the experiment involved the effects of punishment on the learning process. The memory tasks involved word-pair association problems. Punishment for the wrong answer was an electric shock. Although the learner was not really shocked, the teacher was led to believe that he or she was administering a real electric shock. For each wrong answer, the real subject was instructed to give shocks increasing in intensity. Intensity levels were clearly labeled "slight," "moderate," "strong," "very strong," "intense," "extreme intensity," "dangerous," "severe," and finally "XXX," which represented maximally severe. The real subject heard the protests and eventually cries, albeit fake, of the learner. Once the teacher reached the highest possible voltage or refused to go further, the experiment was over. At that point, the subject was debriefed. Approximately 60% of Milgram's subjects were fully obedient, punishing the learner up to the highest shock level.

Just as soon as the work appeared in print, readers condemned the research. Some argued that the deception and the lack of informed consent was a breach of the principle of respect for persons, an autonomy-based argument. Others, believing that the consequences of such an experiment could lead to real harm to subjects, argued that the research breached the principles of nonmaleficence and beneficence. **Here, the heart of the ethical challenge, in addition to concerns about informed consent and deception, was the appropriate balancing of risks to subjects against the potential benefit of the acquired knowledge to society.**

II. CONTEMPORARY CASES IN CLINICAL RESEARCH ETHICS

A. The Jesse Gelsinger Case

Jesse Gelsinger was a young man with ornithine transcarbamylase deficiency (OTC) who died during a gene therapy study at the University of Pennsylvania in 1999 (Smith, 2002). By all accounts, he understood that the experiment would not provide him medical benefit, but he was interested in helping the research field learn more about his disease to help others in the future with the same condition. Within days of receiving the experimental treatment, Gelsinger was dead. All agreed that the cause of death was the experimental gene therapy.

Initially, news reports focused on the sacrifice made by brave persons in the name of scientific progress. As the story unfolded, however, problems in the informed consent process became evident as well as information about the investigator's financial conflicts of interest. These revelations shifted interpretation of the death from a tragedy of a well-informed subject making the ultimate sacrifice for others to one in which a vulnerable subject had been used for commercial interest. It was revealed that although the results of some of Gelsinger's laboratory tests just before injection of the experimental agent did not meet entry criteria, investigators minimized the risks, and considered the differences as not substantive. Information about problems in prior animal studies was not presented during the process of obtaining informed consent. The principal investigator and several other members of the research team had proprietary and/or financial interests in Genovo, Inc., the company that was funding the research. The University of Pennsylvania was also benefiting in several ways from Genovo funding. In time, the Gelsinger case focused the research community on the protection of vulnerable persons from financial interests.

Gelsinger's death resulted in widespread responses in the press, scientific journals, professional association statements, university policies, and proposed government guidelines on conflicts of interest. In this case, however, the flaws in the informed consent process were not as obvious as they were in previous cases of research ethics transgression. The investigators did not include the information from preclinical studies in the process of obtaining informed consent. Such omissions are commonplace. In hindsight, this omission was judged critical. The knowledge, however, has not resulted in any new mechanism or methods for preventing such critical omissions in the future. **Still to be debated is the definition of what preclinical data should be provided to human subjects in the process of obtaining informed consent.**

B. The FIAU Case

In the late 1970s, investigators at Memorial-Sloan Kettering Hospital in New York working with fluoropyrimidine analogs showed that the analogs had robust antiviral effects. Based on this work, NIH researchers hypothesized that a related compound, fialuridine (FIAU), might be useful for persons with HIV infection. A series of studies led to a clinical trial in which 5 of 15 subjects died from liver toxicity and 2 survived only after liver transplantation (Straus, 2002). Among the consequences were a congressional inquiry and full-scale investigations by the NIH, the FDA, and the Institute of Medicine. The FDA concluded that there were flaws in the consent process and flaws in the investigators' interpretation of the data, which resulted in their failure to appreciate the warning signals.

The question remains whether investigators, exonerated in the end by both NIH and the Institute of Medicine, were too close to their own studies to recognize early signs of trouble. In hindsight, the reports of nausea, fatigue, and tingling of extremities from the subjects had been observed in previous clinical trials. In the initial instances, these complaints were attributed to disease progression and/or side effects of medications the subjects were taking or had recently taken. Although perhaps psychologically understandable, an investigator's enthusiasm for success may be a barrier to attributing such side effects to the experimental intervention or to interpreting them as portents of fatal adverse reactions.

This unwitting blind spot, often referred to as **investigator bias,** impairs the conscious appreciation of alarm bells. Investigator bias can lead to attribution of problems to anything but the experimental agent until proven otherwise, rather than the reverse. The FIAU investigators acknowledged this problem and suggested that an unaffiliated scientist should monitor incoming data in real-time. This is an important additional protection that can be expected to become more commonly applied in the future.

C. The Case of Brain Tissue Transplantation in Parkinson's Disease Studies

In the early 1980s, one of the authors of this book (E.D.) was a doctoral student appointed as a research assistant in the Neuropsychiatry Branch of the National Institutes of Mental Health (NIMH). At that time, the branch was receiving much publicity for its groundbreaking work in fetal tissue transplantation for Parkinson's disease. In collaboration with researchers at the Karolinska Institute, Sweden, the NIMH researchers had successfully transplanted fetal rat dopamine-producing cells into the denervated substantia nigra of Parkinson's disease model rats. Although the preclinical results were promising, the U.S. investigators did not think the research was ready for human trials as soon as others did outside the United States. As the U.S. investigators continued this line of research in animals, other researchers began extending this research into human experimentation in other parts of the world (Freed *et al.*, 2001).

Many factors encouraged clinicians and researchers outside the United States to employ this technique to treat Parkinson's disease patients. Videotapes of remarkable patient improvement were shown at professional meetings. Some research studies were conducted. All studies, however, were uncontrolled. Nonetheless, the visibility of these seemingly successful procedures stirred the hope of patient advocates and interest of the media. Ultimately, the need for better treatments for Parkinson's disease, investigator interest, and pressure from patient groups resulted in approval in the United States of a randomized, double-blinded, crossover sham-surgery study for 40 patients, ages 34 to 75 years of age with severe Parkinson's disease. Subjects in the transplantation arm had cultured embryonic mesencephalic tissue implanted bilaterally in the putamen. Sham-surgery subjects had holes drilled into the skull but not into the dura. The primary outcome measure was a subjective global rating of change in severity of disease assessed 1 year after surgery. The design called for those subjects in the sham arm to be crossed over to the transplantation arm if benefit was demonstrated in the transplantation arm subjects.

In the group that included subjects older than 60 years of age, there was no clinically meaningful improvement. There was, however, improvement in the group of younger subjects. Surviving dopamine neurons were present in the putamen in those receiving the transplant. These results were interpreted as a success, but a subset of these younger subjects developed serious problems that halted the crossover portion of the protocol. Of the 33 participants who received transplanted tissue, 5 (15%) developed persistent dystonia and dyskinesia. These adverse reactions continued after reduction or elimination of dopamine-agonist administration.

- Could such an adverse reaction have been anticipated?
- Did the transition from animal to human studies occur too quickly?
- Did the interests of researchers, patient advocates, and the media influence risk/benefit analyses in subtle ways to push the sham-surgery experiment forward too quickly?

In the end, clinical research will always have risks. To bring research risk to zero means no research. Instead, research must proceed with rigorous attempts to reduce risk for subjects to the greatest extent reasonable. Researchers, patient communities, the media, and the public need to try to restrain the hope that must, of course, infuse the research. In doing so, the field will improve the informed consent process, make progress in evaluating the appropriate balance of risks and benefits, and enable important research to go forward while protecting the rights and welfare of human subjects in clinical research.

APPENDIX:
WEB RESOURCES

1. www.ClinicalTrials.gov
   ClinicalTrials.gov provides regularly updated information about federally and privately supported clinical trials involving human research participants. This site provides information about a trial's purpose, who may participate, locations, and phone numbers for more details.

2. http://206.102.88.10/ohsrsite/
   This site takes the reader to the National Institutes of Health (NIH), specifically to the intramural program's Office of Human Subjects Research. This site provides access to Web-based research ethics training and a wealth of research ethics sources.

3. http://www.hhs.gov/ohrp/
   This site is the home page for the U.S. Department of Health and Human Services (DHHS), specifically providing information about the Office for Human Research Protections.

4. http://www.acrpnet.org/
   This is the home page for the Association for Clinical Research Professions (ACRP). This organization offers certification of investigators covering Good Clinical Practices (GCP) and research ethics.

5. The following list contains Web sites with resources, documents, and guidelines on conflicts of interest in research with human participants:
   http://grants1.nih.gov/grants/guide/notice-files/NOT-OD-00-040.html
   http://grants1.nih.gov/grants/guide/notice-files/not95-179.html

http://grants2.nih.gov/grants/policy/coi/
http://www.nih.gov/about/ethics_COI_panelreport.htm
http://grants1.nih.gov/grants/policy/coi/resources.htm
http://www.ohsu.edu/ra/coir/index.shtml
http://www.stanford.edu/dept/DoR/Resources/coi1.html
http://www.irbforum.com/forum/read/2/74/74

6. http://www.pubmed.gov
   Investigators can begin to do their own literature searches by using PubMed, the public access literature database of the NIH Medlars system.

7. http://www.ahrq.gov/research/cbprrole.htm
   This site provides information about participatory, community-based research.

8. http://www.consort-statement.org/
   The CONSORT statement is a research tool endorsed by such publications such as the *Lancet, Annals of Internal Medicine,* and *JAMA* for use in reporting results of randomized trials.

9. http://www.bioethics.net/journal/books.php
   This site provides information about Brown, Robert (2002). Bioethics Online: A Guide to Bioethical Resources on the Internet. New York: Writers Club Press.

10. http://www.hhs.gov/ohrp/humansubjects/guidance/45cfr46.htm
    View this site to see the new guidance clarifying the applicability of the prisoner regulations.

11. http://ohsr.od.nih.gov/guidelines/belmont.html
    The *Belmont Report* is a report of the National Commission for the Protection of Human Subjects of Biomedical and Behavioral Research.

12. http://www.med.umich.edu/irbmed/ethics/Nuremberg/NurembergCode.html
    The Nuremberg Code can be viewed at this Web site.

13. http://www.wma.net/e/policy/b3.htm
    The Declaration of Helsinki can be accessed at this Web site.

14. www.cioms.ch/frame_guidelines_nov_2002.htm
    The International Ethical Guidelines for Biomedical Research Involving Human Subjects were developed by the Council for International Organizations of Medical Sciences (CIOMS).

15. http://www.nihtraining.com/ohsrsite/guidelines/45cfr46.html
See this site for the Common Rule, Title 45 (Public Welfare), and Code of Federal Regulations, Part 46 (Protection of Human Subjects), Subparts A through D.

16. oig.hhs.gov//oei/reports/oei-05-99-00350.pdf
View this site to read the FDA's oversight of clinical investigators.

17. http://www.fda.gov/oc/ohrt/irbs/default.htm
View this site to review the FDA regulations for institutional review boards (21 CFR 56).

18. www.access.gpo.gov/nara/cfr/waisidx_00/21cfr50_00.html
This Web site reviews the FDA's regulations in the document entitled Protection of Human Subjects (21 CFR 50).

19. www.nuffieldbioethics.org/publications/pp_0000000013.asp
This site has published the Ethics of Research Related to Healthcare in Developing Countries.

20. http://grants.nih.gov/grants/funding/women_min/guidelines_amended_10_2001.htm
View this Web site to read Guidelines on the Inclusion of Women and Minorities as Subjects in Clinical Research.

21. http://www.vadscorner.com/internet29.html
This site has published the ICH Harmonized Tripartite Guidelines: Guidelines for Good Clinical Practice (ICH/GCP Guidelines).

22. http://www.apa.org/ethics/
See this site for the American Psychological Association's Ethical Principles of Psychologists and Code of Conduct.

23. http://www.nci.nih.gov/clinicaltrials/understanding/simplification-of-informed-consent-docs
View this site to read the guidelines for writing simplified informed consent forms; these guidelines are from the National Cancer Institute but can be applied to most clinical trials.

24. http://privacyruleandresearch.nih.gov/
This National Institutes of Health site explains HIPAA regulations and information about their implications for clinical research.

25. http://www.hhs.gov/ohrp/assurances/assurances_index.html
This Office for Human Research Protections (OHRP) at the U.S. Department of Health and Human Services provides information on the transition of all existing project assurance documents to the federalwide assurance.

26. http://www.cancer.gov/newscenter/informedcon
    View this site to learn more about assessing decisional capacity in research subjects; these guidelines are from the National Cancer Institute but can be applied to most clinical trials.

27. http://www.hrsa.gov/website.htm
    View this site to learn more about HIPPA, the Health Insurance Portability and Accountability Act of 1996. This is just one of many useful Web sites for information about HIPPA. Typing HIPPA in Google will provide a wealth of HIPPA information. This site, however, provides names, job titles, and contact information for persons within DHHS directly involved with HIPPA administration.

28. http://grants.nih.gov/grants/funding/women_min/guidelines_amended_10_2001.htm
    This Web site provides the up-to-date guidelines on the DHHS policy on the inclusion of women and minorities in clinical research.

29. http://www4.od.nih.gov/orwh/outreach.pdf
    This is the Web site of the Outreach Notebook for the NIH Guidelines on Inclusion of Women and Minorities as Subjects of Clinical Research. As reported in Meinert *et al.* (2003), the Outreach Notebook provides useful information on outreach to these groups.

30. http://www.hhs.gov/ohrp/humansubjects/guidance/prisoner.htm
    View this site for updated DHHS guidance on research involving prisoners. This guidance, updated May 23, 2004, replaces the May 19, 2000 guidance.

REFERENCES

Albin, R. L. (2002). Sham surgery controls: Intracerebral grafting of fetal tissue for Parkinson's disease and proposed criteria for use of sham surgery controls. *J. Med. Ethics* **28(5)**:322–325.

Amatayakul, M. (2003). Another layer of regulation: Research under HIPAA. *J. AHIMA.* **74(1)**:16A–16D.

Anderson, J. A., and Weijer, C. (2002). The research subject as wage earner. *Theor. Med. Bioeth.* **23(4)**:359–376.

Andrews, L. B., Fullarton, J. E., Holtzman, N. A., and Motulsky, A. G. (1994). *Assessing genetic risks: Implications for health and social policy.* Executive Summary: Committee on Assessing Genetic Risks. Institute of Medicine. Washington, DC: National Academies Press.

Annas, G. J. (2005). Family privacy and death—Antigone, war and medical research. *N. Engl. J. Med.* **352(5)**:501–505.

Annas, G. J., and Grodin, M. A. (1992). *The Nazi doctors and the Nuremberg Code: Human rights in human experimentation.* New York: Oxford University.

Appelbaum, P. S., and Grisso, T. (2001). *MacArthur Competence Assessment Tool— Clinical research (MacCAT-CR).* Sarasota, FL: Professional Resource Press.

Arcos-Burgos, M., and Muenke, M. (2002). Genetics of population isolates. *Clin. Genet.* **61(4)**:233–247.

Arean, P. A., Alvidrez, J., Nery, R., Estes, C., and Linkins, K. (2003). Recruitment and retention of older minorities in mental health services research. *Gerontologist* **43(1)**:36–44.

Ashcroft, R. (2001). Responsibilities of sponsors are limited in premature discontinuation of trials. *BMJ* **323(7303)**:53.

Bayoumi, A. M., and Hwang, S. W. (2002). Methodological, practical, and ethical challenges in inner-city health research. *J. Urban Health* **79(4 Suppl)**:S35–S42.

Beecher, H. K. (1966). Ethics and clinical research. *New England J. Med.* **274:**1354–1360.

Beecher, H. K. (1961). Surgery as placebo. *JAMA* **176:**1102–1107.

Bell, J., Whiton, J., and Connelly, S. (1998). *Prepared for the Office of Extramural Research, NIH: Evaluation of NIH implementation of Section 491 of the Public Health Service Act, mandating a program of protection for research subjects.* Alexandria, VA: James Bell and Associates.

Bellin, E., and Dubler, N. N. (2001). The quality improvement/research divide and the need for external oversight. *Am. J. Public Health* **91(9):**1512–1517.

Berg, J. W., Appelbaum, P. S., Lidz, C. W., and Parker, L. S. (2001). *Informed consent: Legal theory and clinical practice.* New York: Oxford University.

Bernard, C. (1865). *An introduction to the study of experimental medicine.* Translated by H. C. Greene. (1927). New York: Dover.

Berry, R. M. (2003). Genetic information and research: Emerging legal issues. *HEC Forum* **15(10):**70–99.

Bersoff, D. N. (1995). *Ethical conflicts in psychology.* Washington, DC: American Psychological Association.

Biesecker, L. G. (2002). Coupling genomics and human genetics to delineate basic mechanisms of development. *Genet. Med.* **4(6 Suppl):**39S–42S.

Bodenheimer, T. (2000). Uneasy alliance—Clinical investigators and the pharmaceutical industry. *N. Engl. J. Med.* **342(20):**1539–1544.

Botkin, J. (2001). Protecting the privacy of family members in survey and pedigree research. *JAMA* **285(2):**207–211.

Carpenter, W. T., Appelbaum, P. S., and Levine, R. J. (2003). The Declaration of Helsinki and clinical trials: A focus on placebo-controlled trials in schizophrenia. *Am. J. Psychiatry* **160(2):**356–362.

Casarett, D., Karlawish, J. H., and Sugarman, J. (2000). Determining when quality improvement initiatives should be considered research: Proposed criteria and potential implications. *JAMA* **283(17):**2275–2280.

Caughlin, S., and Beauchamp, T. L. (1996). *Ethics and epidemiology.* New York: Oxford University.

Chen, D. T., Miller, F. G., and Rosenstein, D. L. (2002). Enrolling decisionally impaired adults in clinical research. *Med. Care* **40(9 Suppl):**V20–V29.

Chen, S. (2001). Negotiating a policy of prudent science and proactive law in the brave new world of genetic information. *Hasting Law J.* **53(1):**243–263.

Cherniack, E. P. (2002). Informed consent for medical research by the elderly. *Exp. Aging Res.* **28(2):**183–198.

Christian, M. J., Goldberg, J. L., Killen, J., Abrams, J. S., McCabe, J. S., Mauer, J. K., and Wittes, R. E. (2002). A central institutional review board for multiinstitutional trials. *N. Engl. J. Med.* **346(19):**1405–1408.

Clark, P. A. (2002). Placebo surgery for Parkinson's disease: Do the benefits outweigh the risks? *J. Law Med. Ethics* **30(1):**58–68.

Cogneau, J., Warck, R., Tichet, J., Royer, B., Cailleau, M., and Balkau, B. (2002). Study of the motivation of physicians participating in public health research. Groupe de Recherche, DESIR. *Sante Publique* **14(20):**191–199.

Committee on Assessing the System for Protecting Human Research Participants. (2003). *Responsible research: A systems approach to protecting research participants.* Washington, DC: Institute of Medicine of the National Academies Press.

Committee on Assessing the System for Protecting Human Research Subjects. (2001). *Preserving public trust: Accreditation and human research participant protection programs.* Washington, DC: Institute of Medicine of the National Academies Press.

CONSORT. (2004). CONSORT: Strength in science, sound ethics. www.consort-statement.org

Cunny, K. A., and Miller, H. W. (1994). Participation in clinical drug studies: Motivations and barriers. *Clin. Ther.* **16(2)**:273–282.

DeRenzo, E. G. Conflicts of interest at the National Institutes of Health: The pendulum swings wildly. *Kennedy Institute of Ethics Journal.* In press.

DeRenzo, E. G. (2003). The rightful goals of a corporation and the obligations of the pharmaceutical industry in a world of bioterrorism. In Moreno, J. D. (Ed.). *In the Wake of Terror: Medicine and Morality in a Time of Crisis.* The MIT Press: NY, pp. 149–166.

DeRenzo, E. G., Biesecker, L. G., and Meltzer, N. (1997). Genetics and the dead: Implications for genetics research with samples from deceased persons. *Amer. J. Med. Genet.* **69**:332–334.

Dickert, N., Emanuel, E., Grady, C. (2002). Paying research subjects: An analysis of current policies. *Ann. Intern. Med.* **136(5)**:368–373.

Dimond, K. (2002). The impact of privacy regulations on clinical research. *J. Biolaw Bus.* **5(3)**:50–53.

Doyal, L., and Tobias, J. S. (2001). *Informed consent in medical research.* London: BMJ Publishing.

Dresser, R. (2002). The ubiquity and utility of the therapeutic misconception. *Soc. Philos. Policy* **19(2)**:271–294.

Durham, M. L. (2002). How research will adapt to HIPAA: A view from within the healthcare delivery system. *Am. J. Law Med.* **28(4)**:491–502.

Eichenwald, K., and Kolata, G. (1999). Drug trials hide conflicts for doctors. *The New York Times.* Sunday, May 16, pp. 1, 28.

Ellenberg, S. S., Fleming, T. R., and DeMets, D. L. (2002). *Data monitoring committees in clinical trials: A practical perspective.* Hoboken, NJ: John Wiley & Sons.

Emanuel, E. J., Crouch, R. A., Arras, J. D., Moreno, J. D., and Grady, C. (Eds). (2003). *Ethical and regulatory aspects of clinical research: Readings and commentary.* Baltimore, MD: Johns Hopkins University.

Emanuel, E. J., Wendler, D., and Grady, C. (2000). What makes clinical research ethical? *JAMA* **283(20)**:2701–2711.

Faden, R., Beauchamp, T. L., and King, N. M. P. (1986). *A history and theory of informed consent.* New York: Oxford University.

Fazzari, M., Heller, G., and Scher, H. I. (2000). The phase II/III transition: Toward the proof of efficacy in cancer clinical trials. *Control Clin. Trials.* **21(4)**:360–368.

Federman, D. D, Hanna, K. E., and Rodriguez, L. L. (2003). *Responsible research: A systems approach to protecting research participants.* Washington, DC: The National Academies Press.

Finkelstein, M. O., Levin, B., and Robbins, H. (1996a). Clinical and prophylactic trials with assured new treatment for those at greatest risk: I. A design proposal. *Amer. J. Pub. Health* **86(5)**:691–695.

Finkelstein, M. O., Levin, B., and Robbins, H. (1996b). Clinical and prophylactic trials with assured new treatment for those at greatest risk: II. Examples. *Amer. J. Pub. Health* **86(5)**:696–702.

Fisher, C. B., and Wallace, S. A. (2000). Through the community looking glass: Reevaluating the ethical and policy implications of research on adolescent risk and sociopathology. *Ethics Behav.* **10(20)**:99–118.

Fleischman, A. R. and Wood, E. B. (2003). Research involving victims of terror—Ethical considerations. In Moreno, J. D. (Ed.). *In the Wake of Terror: Medicine and Morality in a Time of Crisis.* The MIT Press: NY, pp.167–181.

Foster, M. W., Bernsten, D., and Carter, T. H. (1998). A model agreement for genetic research in socially identifiable populations. *Am. J. Hum. Genet.* **63(3)**:696–702.

Foster, M. W., Eisenbraum, A. J., and Carter T. H. (1997). Communal discourse as a supplement to informed consent for genetic research. *Nat. Genet.* **17(3)**:277–279.

Fox, S. J., Wilson, R. H., and Jones, J. W., Jr. (2002). Modified HIPAA privacy rule affects research, marketing, security. *Manag. Care* **11(12)**:46–47.

Freed, C. R., Greene, P. E., Breeze, R. E., Wei-Yann, T., DuMouchel, W., Kao, R., Dillon, S., Winfield, H., Culver, S., Trojanowski, F. C., and Dwyer, R. (2001). For love or money? An exploratory study of why injecting drug users participate in research. *Addiction* **96(9)**:1319–1325.

Fried, E. (2001). The therapeutic misconception, beneficence, and respect. *Account Res.* **8(4)**:331–348.

Gill, D. (2003). Guidelines for informed consent in biomedical research involving pediatric populations as research participants. *Eur. J. Pediatr.* 162(7-8):455–458.

Grisso, T., and Appelbaum, P. S. (1998). *Assessing competence to consent to treatment: A guide for physicians and other health professionals.* New York: Oxford University.

Halpern, S. C., Karlawish, J. H. T., and Berlin, J. A. (2002). The continuing unethical conduct of underpowered clinical trials. *JAMA* **288(3)**:358–362.

Hercberg, S., Hebel, P., Preziosi, P., Briancon, S., Favier, A., Galan, P., Malvy, I., Roussel, A. M., and Schwartz, L. (1995). Motivations of volunteers for participation in an interventional study in the field of nutritional prevention: Results of a pilot study of the SU.VI.MAX project. *Rev. Epidemiol. Sante Publique* **43(2)**:139–146.

Hochhauser, M. (2002). Therapeutic misconception and "recruiting doublespeak" in the informed consent process. *IRB: Ethics Hum. Res.* **24(1)**:11–12.

Horner, J. S. (1998). Research, ethics, and privacy: The limits of knowledge. *Public Health* **112(4)**:217–220.

Horng, S., and Miller, F. G. (2003). Ethical framework for the use of sham procedures in clinical trials. *Crit. Care Med.* **31(3 Suppl)**:S126–S130.

Horrobin, D. F. (2003). Are large clinical trials in rapidly lethal diseases usually unethical? *The Lancet.* **361**:695–697.

Hu, F. F., and Hu, J. H. (2000). Estimation of number of subjects required for comparison of drug versus control in adaptive designs. *Ann. Acad. Med. Singapore* **29(5)**:565–569.

Institute of Medicine. (2001). *Preserving public trust: Accreditation and human research participant protection programs.* Washington, DC: National Academies Press.

Jones, J. (1992). *Bad blood: The Tuskegee syphilis experiment.* New York: Free Press.

Jones, J. W., McCullough, L. B., and Richman, B. W. (2003). The ethics of sham surgery in research. *J. Vasc. Surg.* **37(2)**:482–483.

Jonsen, A. R., Veatch, R. M., and Walters, L. (1998). *Source book in bioethics: A documentary history.* Washington, DC: Georgetown University.

Kagarise, M. J., and Sheldon, G. F. (2000). Translational ethics: A perspective for the new millennium. *Arch. Surg.* **135(1)**:39–45.

Katz, J. (1997). Human sacrifice and human experimentation: Reflections at Nuremberg. *Yale Law School occasional papers, second series. Number 2.* New Haven, CT: Yale University Law School.

Knopman, D., Kahn, J., and Miles, S. (1998). Clinical research designs for emerging treatments for Alzheimer's disease: Moving beyond placebo-controlled trials. *Arch. Neurol.* **55(11)**:1425–1429.

Kolata, G. (2001). Parkinson's research is set back by failure of fetal cell implants. *New York Times.* March 8, Thursday Late Edition final, Page A1.

Korn, E. L., Arbuck, S. G., Pluda, J. M., Simon, R., Kaplan, R. S., and Christian, M. C. (2001). Clinical trial designs for cytostatic agents: Are new approaches needed? *J. Clin. Oncol.* **19(1)**:3154–3155.

Koski, G., and Nightingale, S. L. (2001). Research involving human subjects in developing countries. *N. Engl. J. Med.* **345(2)**:136–138.

Lemmens, T., and Freedman, B. (2000). Ethics review for sale? Conflict of interest and commercial research review boards. *Milbank Q.* **78(4)**:547–584, iii–iv.

Lemmens, T., and Thompson, A. (2001). Noninstitutional commercial review boards in North America: A critical appraisal and comparison with IRBs. *IRB: Ethics Hum. Res.* **25(2)**:1–11.

Levine, R. J., and Gorovitz, S. (2000). *Biomedical research ethics: Updating international guidelines.* Geneva, Switzerland: Council for International Organizations of Medical Sciences.

Levinsky, N. G. (2002). Nonfinancial conflicts of interest. *N. Engl. J. Med.* **347(10)**: 759–761.

Lewis, J. A. (2002). The European regulatory experience. *Stat. Med.* **21(19)**: 2931–2938.

Lewis, J. A., Jonsson, B., Kreutz, G., Sampaio, C., and van Zwieten-Boot, B. (2002). Placebo-controlled trials and the Declaration of Helsinki. *The Lancet* **359(14)**:1337–1340.

Lidz, C. W., and Appelbaum, P. S. (2002). The therapeutic misconception: Problems and solutions. *Med. Care* **40(9)**:V55–V63.

Lievre, M., Menard, J., Bruckert, E., Cogneau, J., Delahaye, F., Giral, P., Leitersdorf, E., Luc, G., Masana, L., Moulin, P., Passa, P., Pouchain, D., and Sjest, G. (2001). Premature discontinuation of clinical trials for reasons not related to efficacy. *BMJ* **322(7286)**:603–605.

Lin, Z. Y., and Zhang, L. X. (2003). Adaptive designs for sequential experiments. *J. Zhejiang Univ. Sci.* **4(2)**:214–220.

Lind, S. E. (1996). Financial issues and incentives related to clinical research and innovative therapies. In Harold Y. Vanderpool (Ed.). *The ethics of research involving human subjects: Facing the 21st century.* Frederick, MD: University Publishing Group.

Livingston, R. B. (1975). Progress report on survey of moral and ethical aspects of clinical investigation: Memorandum to director, NIH, November 4, 1964. In Mark S. Frankel (Ed.). *The development of policy guidelines governing human experimentation in the United States: A case study of public policy making for science and technology. Ethics in Science and Medicine* **2**:43–59.

London, A. J., and Kadane, J. B. (2002). Placebos that harm: Sham surgery controls in clinical trials. *Stat. Methods Med. Res.* **11(5)**:413–427.

Maloney, D. M. (2001). New privacy rule has more tasks for IRBs. *Hum. Res. Rep.* **16(2)**:4.

Marshall, P. A., and Rotimi, C. (2001). Ethical challenges in community-based research. *Am. J. Med. Sci.* **322(5)**:259–263.

Maryland Code: *Health-General*: Title 13. Miscellaneous Health Care Programs: Subtitle 20. Human Subject Research:$13.2003. Institutional Review Board Minutes.

McClure, K. B., DeIorio, N. M., Gunnels, M. D., Ochsner, M. J., Biros, M. H., and Schmidt, T. A. (2003). Attitudes of emergency department patients and visitors regarding emergency exception from informed consent in resuscitation research, community consultation, and public notification. *Acad. Emerg. Med.* **10(4)**:352–359.

Meinert, J. A., Blehar, M. C., Peindl, K. S., Neal-Barnett, A., and Wisner, K. L. (2003). Bridging the gap: Recruitment of African-American women into mental health research studies. *Acad. Psychiatry* **27(1)**:21–28.

Menikoff, J. (2001). Just compensation: Paying research subjects relative to the risk they bear. *Am. J. Bioeth.* **1(2)**:56–58.

Meslin, E. M. (2003). Genetics and bioterrorism: Challenges for science, society, and bioethics. In Moreno, J. D. (Ed.). *In the Wake of Terror: Medicine and Morality in a Time of Crisis.* The MIT Press: NY, pp.199–218.

Miller, F. G., and Rosenstein, D. L. (2003). The therapeutic orientation to clinical trials. *N. Engl. J. Med.* **348(14)**:1383–1386.

Miller, F. G., Rosenstein, D. L., and DeRenzo, E. G. (1998). Professional integrity in clinical research. *JAMA* **280(16)**:1449–1454.

Montgomery, S. A. (1999). Alternatives to placebo-controlled trials in psychiatry: ENCP Consensus Meeting, September 26, 1996, Amsterdam, European College of Neuropsychopharmacology. *Eur. Neuropsychopharmacol.* **9(3)**:265–269.

Moreno, J. D. (2003). *In the wake of terror: Medicine and morality in a time of crisis.* The MIT Press: NY.

Moreno, J. (2001). *Undue risk: Secret state experiments on humans.* Routledge: NY.

Morin, K., Rakatansky, H., Riddick, F. A., Morse, L. J., O'Bannon, J. M., Goldrich, M. S., Ray, P., Weiss, M., Sade, R. M., and Spillman, M. A. (2002). Managing conflicts of interest in the conduct of clinical trials. *JAMA* **287(1)**:78–84.

National Bioethics Advisory Commission. (2001a). *Ethical and policy issues in international research: Clinical trials in developing countries, executive summary.* Bethesda, MD: National Bioethics Advisory Commission.

National Bioethics Advisory Commission. (2001b). *Ethical and policy issues in research involving humans: Summary.* Bethesda, MD: National Bioethics Advisory Commission.

National Bioethics Advisory Commission. (1999). *Research involving human biological materials: Ethical issues and policy guidance. Vol. 1: Report and recommendations.* Bethesda, MD: National Bioethics Advisory Commission.

National Commission for the Protection of Human Subjects of Biomedical and Behavioral Research. (1978). Research involving those institutionalized as mentally infirm: Report and recommendations. DHEW Publication No. (05)78-0006. Washington, DC: U.S. Government Printing Office.

Norton, I. M., and Manson, S. M. (1996). Research in American Indian and Alaska Native communities: Navigating the cultural universe of values and process. *J. Consult. Clin. Psychol.* **64(5):**856–860.

Office of the Inspector General DHHS (1998a). *Institutional review boards: A time for reform.* Washington, DC: DHHS.

Office of the Inspector General DHHS (1998b). *Institutional review boards: Promising approaches.* Washington, DC: DHHS.

Office of the Inspector General DHHS (1998c). *Institutional review boards: The emergence of independent boards.* Washington, DC: DHHS.

Pentz, R. D., Flamm, A. L., Sugarman, J., Cohen, M. Z., Daniel, A. G., Herbst, R. S., and Abbruzzese, J. L. (2002). Study of the media's potential influence on prospective research participants' understanding of and motivations for participation in a high-profile phase I trial. *J. Clin. Oncol.* **20(18):**3785–3791.

Press, E., and Washburn, J. (2000). The kept university. *The Atlantic Monthly* **285(3):** 39–54.

Reverby, S. M. (Ed.). (2000). *Tuskegee's truths.* Chapel Hill, SC: University of South Carolina.

Schooler, N. R., and Baker, R. W. (1999). Providing quality care in the context of clinical research. In Harold A. Pincus, Jeffrey A. Lieberman, and Sandy Ferris (Eds.). *Ethics in psychiatric research: A resource manual for human subjects protection.* Washington, DC: American Psychiatric Association.

Shah, A. N., and Sugarman, J. (2003). Protecting research subjects under the waiver of informed consent for emergency research: Experiences with efforts to inform the community. *Ann. Emerg. Med.* **41(1):**72–78.

Shapiro, H. T., and Meslin, E. M. (2001). Ethical issues in the design and conduct of clinical trials in developing countries. *N. Engl. J. Med.* **345(2):**139–142.

Sharp, R. R., and Foster, M. W. (2002). Community involvement in the ethical review of genetic research: Lessons from American Indian and Alaska Native populations. *Environ. Health Perspect.* **110(2 Suppl):**145–148.

Smith, L., and Byers, J. F. (2002). Gene therapy in the post-Gelsinger era. *JONAS Health Law Ethics Regul.* **4(4):**104–110.

Spilker, B. (2000). *Guide to clinical trials.* Philadelphia, PA: Lippincott Williams & Wilkins.

Stallard, N., and Rosenberger, W. F. (2002). Exact group-sequential designs for clinical trials with randomized play-the-winner allocation. *Stat. Med.* **21(4)**:467–480.

Steinbrook, R. (2004). Financial conflicts of interest at NIH. *N. Engl. J. Med.* **350(4)**:327–330.

Straus, S. E. (2002). Unanticipated risk in clinical research. In John I. Gallin (Ed.). *Principles and practice of clinical research.* San Diego: Academic Press.

Strauss, R. P., Sengupta, S., Quinn, S. C., Goeppinger, J., Spaulding, C., Kegeles, S. M., and Millett, G. (2001). The role of community advisory boards: Involving communities in the informed consent process. *Am. J. Pub. Health* **91(12)**: 1938–1943.

Taylor, A. L., Ziesche, S., Yancy, C., Carson, P., D'Agostino, R., Ferdinand, K., Taylor, M., Adams, K., Sabolinski, M., Worcel, M., and Cohn, J. N.; African-American Heart Failure Trial Investigators. (2004). Combination of isosorbide dinitrate and hydralazine in blacks with heart failure. *N. Eng. J. Med.* **351(11)**:2049–2057.

Temple, R. (2002). Policy developments in regulatory approval. *Stat. Med.* **21(19)**:2939–2948.

Temple, R. J., and Meyer, R. (2003). Continued need for placebo in many cases, even when there is effective therapy. *Arch. Intern. Med.* 162(15):1673–1677.

Thompson, D. F. (1993). Understanding financial conflicts of interest. *N. Engl. J. Med.* **329(8)**:573–576.

van Staden, C. W., and Kruger, C. (2003). Incapacity to give informed consent owing to mental disorder. *J. Med. Ethics* **29(1)**:41–43.

Veatch, R. M. (2002). Indifference of subjects: An alternative to equipoise in randomized clinical trials. *Social Philosophy and Policy.* **19(2)**:295–323.

Warner, T. D., Roberts, L. W., and Nguyen, K. (2003). Do psychiatrists understand research-related experiences, attitudes, and motivations of schizophrenia study participants? *Compr. Psychiatry* **44(3)**:227–233.

Weijer, C. (2002). Placebo trials and tribulations. *CMAJ* 166(5):603–604.

Weijer, C., Goldsand, G., and Emanuel, E. J. (2003). Protecting communities in research: Current guidelines and limits of extrapolation. *Nat. Genet.* **23(3)**:275–280.

Weiss, R. (2005). NIH clears most researchers in conflict-of-interest probe. *The Washington Post.* Febrary 23. p. A1.

White, B. C. (1994). *Competence to consent.* Washington, DC: Georgetown University.

Williams, K. M. (2004). Managing physician financial conflicts of interest in clinical research conducted in the private practice setting. *Food Drug Law J.* **59(1)**:45–77.

Williams, M. A., and Haywood, C., Jr. (2003). Critical care research on patients with advance directives or do-not-resuscitate status: Ethical challenges for clinician/investigators. *Crit. Care Med.* **31(3 Suppl)**:S167–S171.

Yao, Q., and Wei, L. J. (1996). Play the winner for phase II/III clinical trials. *Stat. Med.* **15(21–22)**:2413–2423.

GLOSSARY

Adverse event: Any untoward medical occurrence that may present itself during the study or following treatment or administration of a pharmaceutical product, and which may or may not have a causal relationship with the treatment.

Adverse reaction: An unwanted or harmful side effect experienced following the administration of a drug or combination of drugs and is possibly or suspected to be related to the drug.

Alternatives to study participation: In a protocol, the section that offers alternative standard clinical procedures or treatments potentially advantageous to the subject, including those of no further aggressive intervention and that may include mention of participation in other clinical trials.

Altruism: A person's unselfish regard for the benefit of others, assumed to be the reward of research participants.

Animal research: Research involving whole animals, living or dead, and research on biological materials from animals.

Associate investigator (AI): A collaborating investigator on a clinical trial.

Assurance: A document that institutions must have in place for conducting clinical research with Common Rule agency funding. The document explains how the institution will comply with U.S. federal regulations.

Basic research: Research that involves animals or biological materials from living or dead animals.

Belmont Report: Ethical Principles and Guidelines for the Protection of Human Subjects Research: A U.S. National Commission for the Protection of Human Subjects of Biomedical and Behavioral

Research report issued in 1979 that shaped the way principles of ethics have been codified into legislation and regulations in the United States and that has influenced ethical thinking about clinical research around the world.

Beneficence: The ethical principle that requires that research participants be treated ethically by respecting their decisions, protecting them from harm, and making efforts to secure their well-being.

Benefits section: In a protocol, the section that details if, and if so, what, direct medical benefits a research subject might reasonably expect from study participation and that, at a minimum, knowledge to be gained from the study is anticipated to benefit others in the future through medical progress.

Biologics: Drugs derived from living sources such as viruses, animals, and people.

Certificate of confidentiality: A documented agreement on the part of the DHHS that researchers conducting a particular study will not be required to divulge any personally identifying information about the study's subjects in any administrative or judicial court proceedings other than those already required by law.

Class I device: Devices in this class are governed by the FDA standards that apply to all medical devices prior to the 1976 Amendments. Class I devices are not designed to support or sustain human life or prevent impairment.

Class II device: Device that poses some risk and is subject to controls that continue to evolve.

Class III device: Device that requires premarket approval. Class III devices include those that are life supporting or sustaining, have substantial activity in preventing health impairment, or have the potential to cause injury or illness.

Clinical research: The systematic collection of information from humans and/or from organic material taken from humans to produce generalizable findings; a subset of all scientific research.

Clinical research ethics: The practice of addressing the ethical aspects of research involving human subjects.

Closed futures: The notion that future choices will be limited by being able to predict early in life that one will develop a serious or lethal condition later in life.

Common Rule (45 CFR 46): The regulations governing human subjects research for studies conducted with U.S. federal funding from the Common Rule agencies.

Community-based research: Research that addresses concrete problems and issues of interest to a community that are generated from within the community. Also called participatory research.

Community consent: Consent by the leadership of an identifiable community.

Community consultation: A process of consulting with a whole community, or with a substantially representative group from a whole community, when planning and conducting research.

Compassionate use: A request for the use of a test agent or device for an individual outside the inclusion criteria of an approved protocol or within the inclusion criteria of an as-of-yet-unapproved protocol.

Compliance: In a protocol, the section that describes procedures used to measure subject observance of experimental regimens.

Confidentiality: Protecting the right of privacy by ensuring that information and/or access provided by an individual to a professional, within the context of a trusting (i.e., fiduciary) relationship, will not ordinarily be divulged without permission.

Conflict of commitment: A situation in which professional judgment about the rights and welfare of human subjects may be unduly influenced by a conflicting, nonfinancial interest.

Conflict of interest (financial): A situation in which professional judgment about the rights and welfare of human subjects may be unduly influenced by a conflicting financial interest.

Consent monitor: An individual unaffiliated with the research team who is attached to a study to observe the consent process.

Consequentialist ethical theory: An ethical theory that evaluates an action based on its potential consequences. The most ethically praiseworthy actions, according to this theory, are those that maximize the good for the greatest number.

Council for International Organizations of Medical Sciences (CIOMS) document: A document focused on ethical considerations for performance of research in developing countries and communities.

Data and safety monitoring boards (DSMBs): Oversight committees created to perform unblinded interim reviews of phase III, blinded, randomized, placebo-controlled trials. An increasing number of studies and research in earlier stages of experimental development have incorporated DSMBs into study oversight. DSMBs are also referred to as data monitoring committees (DMCs).

Declaration of Helsinki: An international document to provide ethical guidance for research involving human subjects.

De-identified sample: See **Double-coded sample.**

Deontology: An ethical theory that evaluates an action based on the degree to which the person performing the act meets his or her duties and obligations.

DHHS Office for Human Research Protections (OHRP): The office with which assurance documents are negotiated.

Documentation of informed consent: In the informed consent process, the procedure of obtaining a signature of consent. The signature may be that of a capable adult or of a parent, guardian, or other legally and ethically acceptable person on behalf of a minor or decisionally incapacitated adult.

Double-coded sample: A sample that is labeled with a second coded number that is not related to its original number; also called a de-identified sample. To anonymize the sample, the link between the two codes is destroyed. Also called a de-identified sample.

Double-blinded: When neither the subject nor the investigator knows to which study arm the subject has been assigned.

Drug information: In a protocol, the section that describes the physical properties of experimental agents used in the study, including their formulations, strengths, and other relevant details.

Durable Power of Attorney (DPA) for Research Decisions: A document that assigns an agent to be the responsible decision maker at any time the individual is unable to make his or her own research decisions.

Efficacy endpoints: Study variables evaluated for effectiveness.

Emergency use: When the FDA allows for emergency administration of test agents and/or devices under specified circumstances.

Epidemiological research: Research designed to study processes, characteristics, or other facets of particular populations or phenomenon.

Equipoise: The ethical justification for randomization; the notion that one arm has the potential to be as beneficial as any other study arm.

Evidenced-based research: See **Outcomes research.**

Exclusion criteria: In a protocol, the section that identifies the characteristics that would disqualify potential subjects and/or necessitate removal of a subject if the characteristics happen to appear during the study.

Federal Food, Drug, and Cosmetic Act of 1938 (FDC): Sweeping legislation that extended the FDA's control so that it could also regulate cosmetics, pharmaceutical drugs, and therapeutic devices.

Federalwide project assurance: The name of the assurance document that a research organization negotiates with the federal government covering the conduct of studies funded by a Common Rule agency.

Follow-up: Procedures or contact by the researcher after completion of a study's primary procedures.

Food and Drug Act of 1906: Act that prohibited interstate commerce in misbranded and adulterated foods, drinks, and drugs.

Healthy subject: A volunteer with no diagnosed and/or apparent physical or mental disease or condition.

Hypothesis-generating research: Research intended to investigate previously unexplored or under-explored areas to begin the data accumulation process needed to develop hypotheses.

Hypothesis-testing research: Research designed to produce statistical support or refutation of a formally articulated research hypothesis.

Inclusion criteria: In a protocol, the section in which medical, demographic, and psychosocial conditions or characteristics of subjects should be specified in precise detail.

Independent ethics committees (IECs): The international counterparts of IRBs in the United States. Also called research ethics committees (RECs) or simply ethics committees (ECs).

Independent IRBs: Institutional review boards set up largely by for-profit companies to provide IRB reviews for a fee.

Index subject: The primary subject of a study involving persons related, in some way, to the primary subject.

Informed consent: Explicit agreement to participate in a research study given by a decisionally capable adult.

Institutional review boards (IRBs): The review bodies required by law and by international guidance documents to approve and monitor the conduct of human subjects research.

Introduction: In a protocol, the section that explains the purpose of the study and its scientific importance.

Investigator bias: Unconscious inclination to observe hoped-for scientific outcomes and/or to interpret scientific data in a way that is consistent with hoped-for scientific outcomes; this bias is created by an investigator's enthusiasm for supporting anticipated scientific outcomes.

Justice: The ethical principle that requires a fair distribution of benefits and burdens.

Justification: In a protocol, the section that includes a description of specific characteristics of study design, such as proposed subjects, blinding and randomization strategies, and why these study components are optimal for the proposed study.

Literature review: In a protocol, the section that presents information from the existing scientific literature to explain and justify the proposed study.

Maximally tolerated dose (MTD): The dose just below that which produces unacceptable toxicities.

Minimal risk: Risk that is inherent in the daily lives of healthy individuals.

Modeling: A computer strategy that can be used to justify the involvement of humans in research.

New drug or device application: Application necessary for most pharmaceutical research involving untested drugs or devices. Either an investigational new drug (IND) or an investigational device exemption (IDE) number is required prior to initiation.

Nuremberg Code: Ethical code resulting from the atrocities committed by Nazi physician/investigators during World War II. The core notion set forth by the code is that the voluntary consent of a research participant is essential.

Objectives section: In a protocol, the section that presents in clear and concise scientific language the question to be asked or hypothesis to be tested.

On-study subject: Subject already enrolled in the protocol.

Open-label: All participants and investigators know what agent the subject is taking or device the subject is testing.

Open-label extension: A study added on at the end of a randomized trial to provide an experimental drug in an unblinded fashion for an extended period of time.

Outcomes research: Research in which approved drugs/devices or existing standards of practice are tested against each other and/or against placebo controls. In outcomes research, or evidence-based research, studies are conducted to evaluate established but unvalidated treatment practices.

Participatory research: See **Community-based research.**

Permission: Explicit agreement to study participation of the child or decisionally impaired adult given by a parent on behalf of a child or by a research surrogate on behalf of a decisionally impaired adult.

Pharmacodynamics: The study of how medications affect the body (i.e., the biological and clinical effects of an administered drug).

Pharmacogenomics: A growing field intended to identify differences in gene sequences that can predict differences in responsiveness or sensitivity to specific drug molecules.

Pharmacokinetics: The study of the absorption, distribution, metabolism, and elimination of a drug.

Phase I trials: The phase of drug or device development studies in which a drug or device is tested in humans for the first time. These trials usually have a small number of subjects who may be healthy volunteers.

Phase II trials: Trials designed to begin to accrue efficacy data and continue to identify safety problems. The primary goal of a phase II drug trial is often to define a maximally tolerated dose (MTD). Phase II trials usually also have small numbers of subjects, but have more subjects than phase I trials.

Phase III trials: Trials that are often multicenter and/or multinational, with efficacy as a primary end point. Phase III trials are the final phase for a drug or device to be submitted to the FDA for approval. Phase III trials involve large numbers of subjects, including subgroups representing an ever-widening range of potential patients for whom the drug or device is ultimately intended.

Phase IV trials: Trials conducted after an agent or device has been approved for clinical use.

Pilot: A study of only a few subjects in which the design, materials, and/or procedures anticipated for a larger trial are tested for feasibility.

Placebo arm: An arm of a trial in which the administered study agent is an inert substance.

Précis: In a protocol, a brief summary of what the study is about.

Principal investigator (PI): The primary and ultimately responsible investigator of a human research protocol.

Privacy: As a positive right, privacy means that a person has the right to control access to and distribution of personal information, property, and/or knowledge of behaviors. As a negative right, privacy ensures absence of interference or the right to be left alone.

Proband: The index subject in a genetic study involving multiple members of the same family.

Proprietary IRBs: Institutional review boards set up by for-profit research sponsors to review specific sponsor's research studies. Little is known about the membership, functions, and processes of proprietary IRBs.

Quality assurance (QA) research: Research conducted in hospitals and other health care delivery organizations to ensure that the quality of care provided is adequate.

Quality improvement (QI) research: Research intended to evaluate and continually upgrade standards in health care organizations.

Quality-of-life (QOL) information: A wide spectrum of data related to subject well-being.

Quality-of-life study: A common add-on study that often employs survey questionnaires to be completed by a subject to indicate how his or her quality of life has been or is being affected by the disease process and/or the study participation.

Radiation safety committees (RSCs): Institutional bodies that are responsible for implementing the regulations of the U.S. Nuclear Regulatory Commission (NRC).

Randomization: A process of selecting groups for comparison of safety and/or efficacy of one intervention over another.

Randomized clinical trial (RCT): A trial in which subjects are allocated to the various arms via a random selection process.

Recruitment section: In a protocol, the section that presents a description of the subjects to be recruited and a description of recruitment procedures.

Relinking: Determining the original coding on a sample based on a link between the second coding and the original.

Research coordinator: A person who is responsible for overseeing and conducting a wide range of research activities.

Research ethics committees (RECs): See **Independent ethics committees (IECs)**.

Research subject: A living person.

Respect for persons: The ethical principle that requires respect for each individual's values, perspectives, and capacities that obligates researchers to assist individuals to exercise self-determination, and the provision of appropriate protections for individuals who have limitations on autonomous behavior.

Risk, burden, and discomfort section: In a protocol, the section that details the potential risks, discomforts, and/or inconveniences a subject can be expected to encounter during study participation. These include medical and nonmedical risks.

Scientific research: The systematic collection of information to produce generalizable findings.

Sham surgery: The placebo arm in a surgical trial.

Short form: A less detailed consent form, which is sufficient if all the required elements for ethically and legally valid informed consent have been presented orally to the subject or the subject's rightful surrogate.

Single-blinded: When the subjects, but not the investigator, are blinded to the study intervention.

Special populations: Any subject group or community with qualities or characteristics that requires specific consideration of additional protections beyond those needed to protect the rights and welfare of a fully autonomous healthy adult.

Standard consent form: A form that includes all required elements of consent and any additional elements required by the needs of subjects in a particular study.

Statistics and data collection, data management, and record keeping: In a protocol, the section that describes how the data will be collected, recorded, and maintained.

Study design: The processes involved in organizing data collection and analysis to answer a research question or to test a scientific hypothesis, including selection of the optimal population for study, data points for analysis, and analysis strategies.

Study monitors: Individuals or organizations that provide sponsors with a range of services to ensure that the study is conducted properly and in accordance with the approved protocol.

Study procedures and methodology: In a protocol, the section that describes the manipulations that will be carried out, in what sequence, and by whom.

Study report forms: Forms devised on a per-study basis to record necessary study data. Also called case report forms.

Subject selection: In a protocol, the section that includes justification for the proposed subject population as well as the inclusion and exclusion criteria.

Substantive ethics section: In a protocol, the section that delineates the specific ethical issues raised by the particular study, presents the reasoning for how the ethical issues raised are being addressed, and states the ethical justification(s) for the approach(es) taken.

Summary report of the subject's personal participation: A lay rewriting of any medical information that is provided to the subject and that may be given to his or her community physician or that goes directly, with the participant's permission, to the subject's community treating clinician.

Surrogate: Someone who makes decisions for an individual's clinical care and/or research participation after the research subject or the potential subject has been judged incapable of decision making or someone who makes a research study decision for a minor child.

Therapeutic misconception: The belief on the part of a research subject that research participation, even in a randomized trial, is going to provide the subject with direct medical benefit.

Translational research: Research designed to move basic research findings into therapeutics and to accelerate the flow of insights from the bench to the marketplace.

Underpowering: When a study lacks the statistical power to have a reasonable expectation of answering the study question or adequately testing the study hypothesis.

Virtue ethics: The ethical theory that evaluates an action based on the character and virtuous intent of the person performing the action.

Vulnerable subject: A subject who, for whatever reason, has, or may have, constraints on his or her ability to act as a fully autonomous individual.

Washout period: The period prior to a study during which participants are taken off specific, or possibly any, medications they have been taking.

INDEX

A

ACRP. *See* Association of Clinical
   Research Professionals
Adult patient volunteers. *See also*
   Patient provisions; Research
   participants; Vulnerable subjects
   community consent for, 17,
      150–151
   confidentiality of, 161–163
   consent of, 32, 71–72, 100
   data analysis of, 71
   direct-benefit research for, 51–52
   DPA for, 90–92, 180
   healthy, 68–71
   with interest conflicts, 13–14,
      115–116, 240
   IRB review of, 68–69
   with language barriers, 66, 69–70,
      74–75
   pregnant women, 70–71, 191–192,
      250–251
   protection of, 17, 21, 24–25, 67–68,
      76, 80, 88, 161–162
   psychiatric impairment in, 73–74
   with questionable capacity, 76
   recruitment of, 73
   refractory populations for, 70–72
   regulations for, 4, 64, 68
   with socioeconomic disadvantages,
      75–76
Adverse reactions/events
   to medications, 203
   reporting of, 204–205
Altruism, 102, 116
Applied research, 46–47
Assessments. *See also* Capacity
      assessment
   of adverse reactions/events,
      203–205
   of consent capacity, 66, 76, 84–88,
      142–143, 199
   of laboratory studies, 199
   of observational methods, 199–201
   of physical/patient history, 197–199
   of quality-of-life measurements,
      201–202
   of sexual maturity, 199
   of video/audio taping, 201

Associate investigator, 13, 124
Association of Clinical Research
    Professionals, 30

B

Basic research, 46–47
The Belmont Report, 17, 28, 68, 245
Beneficence, 18
Benefits. *See* Direct-benefit research;
    Research Benefits
Biologics, 257
Bioterrorism, 258–259
Blinding, 53, 57, 164–165, 186–187

C

Capacity assessment
    analysis of, 86–87
    criteria for, 84–88
    diagnostic labels in, 76
    difficulties of, 87–88
    for psychiatric research, 246–247
    for valid consent, 66, 84–88,
        142–143, 199, 246–247
Case histories
    classical, 262–265
    contemporary, 263–264
Classical case histories
    Milgram Obedience Studies,
        264–265
    Tuskegee Syphilis Study, 262–263
    Wichita Jury Study, 263–264
Clinical investigator. *See* Principal
    investigator
Clinical trials, 57–59
Clinical volunteers. *See* Research par-
    ticipants
Closure, study. *See* Study closure
Common Rule, 27–28, 32, 35–36,
    250–251
Communities research, special. *See*
    Special communities research
Community consent, 17, 150–151
Community input, 94–95
Community-based research, 252–253
Comparator arms, 55–56
Compensation/Payment, therapeutic
    misconception of, 115–116
Completion, study. *See* Study comple-
    tion
Confidentiality. *See also* Disclosure
    certificate of, 173, 192

in consent documents, 154–156, 174
    management of, 160–163
    of minors, 162–163
    for multiple family participants, 161
    protection of, 161–162
    provisions of, 163–168, 171–174
    regulation of, 160
    in subject counseling, 167
    of tissue use, 229–230
    tradition of, 159–160
    withholding information for,
        168–171
    writing about, 173–175
Conflict of interest
    financial, 14, 35, 38–39, 103
    in genetic research, 240
    personal/institutional, 13–14, 38–39,
        115–116, 124, 218–219
Consent capacity, assessment of, 66,
    76, 84–88, 142–143, 199
Consent documentation. *See also*
    Disclosure
    for alterations/waivers, 136–137,
        150, 155–156
    assent/surrogacy format for,
        148–149, 152–155
    confidentiality in, 154–156, 174
    for direct-benefit research, 154–155
    electronic, 132
    for family members, 148
    forms for, 107, 174
    for health services research,
        156–157
    language of, 132
    for minors/unable adults, 77–78,
        143–145
    for patient provisions, 164–165
    for prospective subjects, 146
    for quality improvement projects,
        156–157
    risks in, 153–154
    short form, 157
    for surrogate permission, 89–90,
        146, 148–150
    timing of, 158
    translations of, 158
Consent, informed. *See also*
    Confidentiality; Disclosure;
    Special population protection
    of adult patient volunteers, 32,
        71–72, 100

of community, 17, 150–151
confidentiality in, 154–156, 174
for direct-benefit research,
    154–155
disclosure of, 134–138, 155–156
for follow-up information, 141,
    202–203
for medically indicated procedures,
    138–142
of minors, 77–78, 143–146
process of, 129–134
for psychiatric research, 246–247
recruiting subjects with, 119
regulations for, 93, 101, 133–134,
    136–137, 143–144
risks in, 105–106, 135–137, 153–154
in special populations, 83
for substudies, 139–142
for tissue use, 230
tradition/purpose of, 127–128
valid consent, 66, 141–146, 199
of vulnerable subjects, 101,
    105–106, 143–146
writing protocol for, 146–151
Consent monitors, 93, 180
Consent process
electronic media in, 131–132
phases of, 129–131
risk in, 100, 105–106, 135–137,
    153–154
timing of, 132
Consent, valid
assessing capacity for, 66, 84–88,
    142–143, 199, 246–247
of minors, 143–146
substantive ethics of, 180–181
Consequentialist ethical theory,
    20–22
Contemporary case histories
Case of the Brain Tissue
    Transplantation, 267–268
FIAU case, 266–277
Jesse Gelsinger Case, 265–266
Contract research organizations,
    217–218

D

Data collection, 215–216
Data management
academic/pharmaceutical collabo-
    rations, 218–219

data analysis, 71
data collection, instructions for,
    215–216
data entry, 216–217
record keeping, 219–220
research coordinators, 217–219
Data Monitoring Committee. *See* Data
    Safety Monitoring Board
Data Safety Monitoring Board, 37–38,
    53
Debriefing. *See* Disclosure
The Declaration of Helsinki
origin of, 4, 15–17
physician conflict in, 13, 124
placebo regulation in, 55–56
subject selection regulation, 25, 64
Deontology, 22–23
Department of Health and Human
    Services
adult's regulations by, 71
The Common Rule, 27–28, 32,
    35–36, 250–251
Department of Education, 28
federal agencies in, 27–28
minors' regulations by, 77
prisoners' regulations by, 257–258
project assurances for, 35–36
tissue regulations by, 230–231
Device testing, 196–197
DHHS. *See* Department of Health and
    Human Services
Direct-benefit research
consent for, 154–155
evaluation of, 103–104
expected, 50–52, 102–105,
    114–115
for fetal research, 80–81
guidelines for, 52
IRB review of, 51
for minors, 78–79, 145–146
no-, 50–52, 114–115
personal, 50–51
for research participants, 51–52,
    78–79
risk in, 100–102, 104–105
sponsor's obligations for, 112
writing about, 117–118
Disclosure
of conflict information, 38–39
consent waivers for, 136–137, 150,
    155–156

Disclosure (*continued*)
  deception/risks in, 135–137
  for IRB review, 13–14, 35, 38–39
  of medically indicated procedures,
    138–142
  of research information, 134–138,
    171–173
Document. *See* Consent documenta-
    tion; Landmark Documents
Double-blinding, 53, 186–187
DPA. *See* Durable Power of Attorney
Drugs
  accountability for, 189–190
  biologics development, 257
  compliance with, 191–192
  concomitant therapies, 192
  dosing/administration of, 189–191
  open-label extensions with,
    192–194
  regulations of, 188, 189
  testing of, 187–189
  undesirable responses to, 204–205
DSMB. *See* Data Safety Monitoring
    Board
Durable Power of Attorney
  protection of, 90, 180
  sample forms, 91–92
Duty-based ethics. *See* Deontology

E

Emergency medicine research, 251–252
Epidemiological research, 255–256
Ethical analysis. *See also* Ethics, sub-
    stantive
  consequentialist ethical theory,
    20–22
  evolution of, 6
  guidelines for, 14–17
  principles of, 18–20, 178–181
  of study design, 19–20, 43–45, 50, 103
Ethical conduct, of physician/princi-
    pal investigator, 13, 21, 23–25, 102
Ethical judgment, 18–19, 50, 103
Ethical review boards, 31–34. *See
    also* Institutional Review Board
Ethical tension
  from scientific goals, 11–12
  in socioeconomic trials, 75–76
Ethics, substantive
  compliance with, 175–177
  existing model for, 177–178

guidelines for, 178–179
  language of, 179–180
  risk in, 180–181
Evidence-based research, 50
Evolving research areas
  biologics, 257
  bioterrorism research, 258–259
  community-based research,
    252–253
  emergency medicine research,
    251–252
  epidemiological research, 255–256
  genetic research, 237–245
  pregnant women/fetal research,
    250–251
  prisoner research, 257–258
  psychiatric research, 245–249
  quality improvement/quality assur-
    ance research, 253–254
  surgical research, 256
  translational research, 254–255
  women/minority population
    research, 249–250
Exclusion criteria, 30, 96, 106–107
Experimental agents, 58

F

FDA. *See* Federal Drug
    Administration
Federal Drug Administration. *See also*
    Drugs
  development of, 28–29
  IDE/IND review by, 48–49
  minors' regulations by, 77–78
  placebo regulation by, 55–56
  toxicity regulations of, 28–30
Federalwide Assurance, 36
Fetal research
  direct-benefit for, 80–81
  regulations for, 80–81
  risk in, 80, 250–251
Financial conflicts, 14, 35, 38–39, 103
Follow-up, 141, 202–203
Funding. *See* Sponsors, Clinical
    Research
FWA. *See* Federalwide Assurance

G

Genetics research. *See also* Tissue use
  community risks of, 240–241
  independent studies, 241–242

minors' participation in, 244
regulations for, 244–245
review of, 237–239
subject conflict in, 240
subject's risk in, 238–241
use/storage of samples, 243–244

H
Health services research, 156–157
Healthy adult volunteers, 68–71
Human biological material. *See also*
    Tissue use
categorizing samples of, 223–225
writing about, 232–235
Human subject, 148
Hypothesis
ethical analysis of, 44–45
guideline questions for, 45
sources for, 43–44
writing of, 61

I
IDE. *See* Investigational Device
    Exemption
Inclusion criteria, 67–68, 96, 106–107
IND. *See* Investigational New Drugs
Independent Ethics Committee,
    31–34
Independent human research review,
    31–34
Informed consent. *See* Consent,
    informed
Injuries, research related, 113
Institutional Review Board
accreditation of, 33–34
adult volunteer review by, 68–69
direct-benefit review by, 51
DSMB reports for, 37–38
emergency medicine research
    review by, 252
for-profit independent, 34–35
FWA for, 36
IDE/IND review by, 48–49
information disclosure to, 13–14,
    35, 38–39
institutional not-for-profit, 34–35
minors' review by, 78
phase IV trial review by, 59
of prisoners' research, 257–258
process of, 5, 31–33, 36
project assurance for, 36

proprietary, 34–35
protocol review by, 34–35
study design review by, 34
vulnerable subject's review by, 67
The International Guidelines, 16–17
Investigational Device Exemption
emergency use of, 50
IRB review of, 48–49
for pharmaceutical industry, 47–49
Investigational New Drugs
emergency use of, 50
IRB review of, 48–49
for pharmaceutical industry, 47–48
Investigator. *See* Principal
    investigator
IRB. *See* Institutional Review Board

J
Justice, 18, 69

L
Laboratory studies, 199
Landmark documents
The Belmont Report, 17, 28, 68, 245
The Declaration of Helsinki, 4, 13,
    15–17, 25, 55–56, 64, 124
importance of, 14–17
*The International Ethical
    Guidelines*, 16–17
The Nuremberg Code, 4, 15, 25,
    105, 143–144
Language barriers
adult patient volunteers with, 66,
    69–70, 74–75
interpreters for, 93–94, 158
Literature review, 60–61

M
Marketing studies, 59
Maximally tolerated dose, 58
Medically indicated procedures,
    138–142
Methods. *See* Procedures
Minority populations, 81–83,
    249–250
Minors' research
confidentiality for, 162–163
consent for, 77–78, 143–146
direct-benefit of, 78–79, 145–146
genetic research, 244
psychiatric research, 248–249

Minors' research (*continued*)
 regulations for, 64, 77–78
 risk in, 66, 78–79, 238–240
 sexual maturity in, 199
 surrogate permission for, 89–90,
  146, 148–150
 toddlers/infants as, 80
Monitoring criteria, 107–108
Multiple studies, 123–125

N

National Institute of Health
 ethical policy of, 177–178
 funding by, 29–30
 independent review policies of,
  31–32
 radiation regulations by, 30
 surrogate permission policy of, 150
NIH. *See* National Institute of Health
The Nuremberg Code, 4, 15, 25, 105,
  143–144

O

Observational methods, 200–201
Open-label design, 57
Outcomes research, 50

P

Participants, research. *See* Research
  participants; Subjects, recruiting;
  Subjects, selecting
Patient provisions
 to counseling, 167
 to destructive information, 170–171
 to personal information, 168
 for randomizing, 164–165
 at study conclusion, 164–167,
  171–172
 during study participation, 163–164
 to uninterpretable data, 168–170
Pediatrics. *See* Minors' research
Peer review, 31–32
Pharmaceutical industry
 academic collaborations with,
  218–219
 funding by, 30, 75
 IDE/IND for, 47–48
 outcomes research by, 50
Pharmacogenomics, 140
Pharmacokinetics/pharmacodynam-
  ics, 211–212

Phase I trials, 57
Phase II trials, 58, 210–211
Phase III trials, 58, 210–211
Phase IV trials, 58–59
Phases of clinical trial
 I–IV, 57–59
 term-of-art, 57
Physician. *See also* Principal
  investigator
 conflicts of, 13, 124
 ethical conduct of, 13, 21, 23–25,
  100, 102
 non-research affiliated, 88, 180
 recruiting subjects by, 120–124
Placebo controls
 in psychiatric research, 247–248
 regulation of, 55–56, 212–214
 sham surgery as, 196
 statistical analysis of, 212–214
 in study design, 54
Population characterization, 96
Population justification, 96
Population protection. *See* Special
  population protection
Précis, 59–60
Pregnant women volunteers, 70–71,
  191–192, 250–251
Principal investigator
 capacity assessment criteria for,
  84–88
 ethical conduct of, 13, 21, 23–25,
  100, 102
 financial conflicts of, 14, 35, 38–39,
  103
 NIH review of, 31
 non-research physicians, 88, 180
 personal conflicts of, 13–14, 38–39,
  103
 project assurance by, 35–36
 recruiting subjects by, 120–124
 regulations certification for, 29–30
 reporting adverse events by,
  204–205
Prisoners' research, 257–258
Privacy. *See* Confidentiality
Procedures. *See also* Assessments;
  Data management; Drugs; Human
  biological material; Risk, minimization of; Statistics
 for adverse reactions/events,
  203–205

assessment of, 197
device testing, 196–197
drug testing, 187–189
follow-up, 141, 202–203
for laboratory studies, 199
medically indicated, 138–142
observational methods, 200–201
for obtaining valid consent, 199
for physical/patient history,
    197–199
for quality-of-life measurements,
    201–202
for record keeping, 219–220
reducing bias in, 186
for surgical trials, 193–197
for video/audio taping, 201
Professional research subject, 123
Project assurance, 35–36
Protection. *See* Special population
    protection
Protocol. *See also* Ethics, substantive;
    Human biological material;
    Procedures; Study design; Writing
    approval regulations for, 18, 36–37
    blinding in, 53, 57, 164–165,
        186–187
    continuing review of, 36–37
    ethical analysis of, 18–20, 50
    ethical compliance of, 175–177
    introduction of, 60
    IRB review of, 34–35
    justification of, 19–20, 60–61,
        179–180
    literature review for, 60–61
    précis of, 59–60
    randomizing for, 53, 56, 164–165, 186
    rescue end points for, 106–107
    rescue intervention for, 108–109
    risk minimization of, 105–106,
        116–118, 180
    RSC review of, 30
    subject confidentiality in, 173–174
    subject withdrawal in, 107–109
    for surgical trials, 193–196
    template for, 6–10
    writing of, 59–61
Provisions. *See* Patient provisions
Psychiatric research
    consent capacity in, 246–247
    minors' participation in, 248–249
    placebo controls for, 247–248

regulations for, 245–246
surrogate consent in, 246–247

Q

Quality assurance, 157–158, 253–254
Quality improvement projects,
    157–158, 253–254
Quality improvement/quality assur-
    ance research, 253–254
Quality-of-life measurements,
    201–202

R

Radiation Safety Committee
    review by, 30
    U.S. Nuclear Regulatory
        Commission, 30
Randomization
    with comparator arms, 56
    double-blinding for, 53, 186–187
    DSMB review of, 53
    patient provisions for, 164–165
    procedures for, 186
Record keeping, 219–220
Regulations. *See also* Department of
    Health and Human Services;
    Ethics, substantive; Institutional
    Review Board; Landmark
    documents
    for adverse reactions/events,
        204–205
    for community consent, 151
    for comparator arms, 55–56
    for confidentiality, 160
    for conflict, 13–14, 35, 38–39
    for consent, 93, 101, 133–134,
        136–137, 143–144
    for continuing review, 36–37
    of drug testing, 188–189
    of ethical compliance, 175–177
    of ethics committees, 31–34
    of FDA, 28–30, 48–49, 55–56, 77–78
    for fetal research, 80–81
    for genetic research, 244–245
    guidance with, 5
    for international research, 29
    for investigator certification, 29–30
    for minors, 64, 77–78
    for placebo controls, 55–56,
        212–214
    for prisoners' research, 257–258

Regulations (*continued*)
  for project assurance, 35–36
  for protocol approval, 18, 36–37
  for psychiatric research, 245–246
  for radiation safety, 30
  for recruiting subjects, 120–121
  for rescue intervention, 109
  for research participants, 4, 64, 68
  for risk, 98–99, 105–106
  for special communities, 81–83,
      249–250
  for surrogate permission, 89, 146,
      148–150
  for tissue use, 230–231
  for toxicity, 28–30
  of U.S. government, 5, 27–30
  for vulnerable subjects, 68
Rescue end points, 106–107
Rescue interventions, 106–109
Research benefits. *See also* Direct-
    benefit research; Societal benefits
  analysis of, 114–115
  balancing risks and, 97–99, 102–105
  maximization of, 113–116, 209
  societal risk from, 98–102
  of tissue use, 228–229
  of using compensation, 115–116
  writing about, 117–118
Research Ethics Committee, 31
Research participants. *See also* Adult
    patient volunteers;
    Confidentiality; Consent,
    informed; Minors' research;
    Patient provisions; Subjects,
    recruiting; Subjects, selecting;
    Vulnerable subjects
  adult regulations for, 4, 64, 68
  blinding of, 53, 57, 164–165, 186–187
  conflicts for, 13–14, 115–116, 240
  consent of
    community, 17, 150–151
    informed, 32, 71–72, 100
  counseling for, 167
  in direct-benefit research, 51–52,
      78–79
  DPA for, 90–92, 180
  inclusion/exclusion of, 30, 67–68,
      96, 106–107
  information provisions of, 163–168
  with language barriers, 66, 69–70,
      74–75

minors as, 64, 77–80, 143–146
need for, 23–24
patient subjects as, 64–65
prisoners as, 257–258
professional, 125
protection of, 17, 21, 24–25, 67–68,
    76, 80, 88, 161–162
randomization of, 53, 56, 164–165,
    186
rights of, 4, 12–13, 16, 19–20
risk for, 11, 18–19, 24, 32, 49, 67–68,
    238–240
teens as, 79
toddlers/infants as, 80
with valid consent, 66, 142–146, 199
vulnerable subjects as, 66–68
withdrawal of, 107–109
women as, 70–71, 191–192
Risk
  of altruistic behavior, 102, 116
  assessment of, 97–102
  balancing benefits and, 97–99,
      102–105
  in consent process, 100, 105–106,
      135–137, 153–154
  in direct-benefit research, 100–102,
      104–105
  in disclosure process, 135–137
  excessive/unreasonable risk, 98
  in genetic research, 238–241
  minimization of
    compensation/payments for,
        115–116
    for completing study, 111–112
    for fetal research, 80, 151–152
    inclusion/exclusion criteria for,
        30, 67–68, 96, 106–107
    informed consent for, 105–106
    maximizing benefits for, 113–116
    for pregnant women, 250–251
    in research related injuries, 113
    with statistics, 209
    for study closure, 110–111
    with substantive ethics, 178–181
  in minors' research, 66, 78–79
  of participant withdrawal, 107–109
  in protocol, 105–106, 116–118, 180
  in psychiatric research, 247–248
  regulations for, 98–99, 105–106
  for research participants, 11, 18–19,
      24, 32, 49, 67–68, 238–240

for society, 98–102
in special communities research,
82–83
in study design, 11, 18–19, 24, 32,
102–105
of tissue use, 228–229
writing about, 105–106, 116–118
RSC. *See* Radiation Safety Committee

S

Safety parameter criteria, 107–108
Scientific considerations
in clinical trials, 4
for efficiency, 24–25
in study design, 18–20, 50
Scientific goals, 11–12
Scientific judgments, 18–20, 50
Sexual maturity, 199
Sham surgery, 196
Societal benefits
balancing risk with, 98–102
expectations of, 100
Special communities research, 81–83,
249–250, 252–253
Special population protection. *See
also* Minors' research; Vulnerable
subjects
capacity assessment for, 84–88
consent in, 83
consent monitors for, 93, 180
DPA for, 90–92, 180
in genetic research, 238–240
non-research physicians for, 88, 180
surrogate permission for, 89–90,
146, 148–150
Sponsors, clinical research
Common Rule agencies, 27–28, 32,
35–36, 250–251
NIH, 29–30
obligations of, 111–112
pharmaceutical industry, 30, 75
study closure by, 110
for translational research, 254–255
Statistics. *See also* Data management;
Procedures
analysis of, 207–208
for computer modeling, 214
data collection, 215
for pharmacokinetics/pharmacody-
namics, 211–212
for placebo controls, 212–214

qualitative/quantitative data,
208–209
risk/benefits from, 209
sample size/power calculations,
209–210
variables/end points, 210–211
Study closure, 110–111, 164–165
Study completion, 111–112, 141,
164–167, 171–173, 202–203
Study design. *See also* Consent,
informed; Direct-benefit research;
Ethics, substantive; Human biological material; Procedures;
Protocol; Statistics; Writing
applied research, 46–47
basic research, 46–47
community input for, 94–95
comparator arms in, 55–56
double-blinding for, 53, 186–187
ethical analysis of, 19–20, 43–45,
50, 103
ethical principles of, 18–20, 178–181
of genetics research, 241–242
hypothesis, research for, 43–45
IDE/IND in, 47–48
IRB review of, 34
justification for, 19–20, 45–46
open-label, 57
outcomes research for, 50
patient provisions in, 163–168
placebo controls in, 54
predicting consequences of, 21–22
of psychiatric research, 246–249
randomizing for, 53, 164–165, 186
recruiting subjects in, 119–124
risk in, 11, 18–19, 24, 32, 102–105
subject counseling in, 167
of surgical trials, 193–198
of trial phases, 57–59
Sub-group analysis, 58
Subject withdrawal, 107–109, 228
Subjects, recruiting
community consent for, 17, 150–151
distancing tactics for, 123
gatekeeping in, 121–122
informed consent process for,
119–121
of minority populations, 249–250
for multiple studies, 123–125
patient, 64–65, 73
process of, 122–123

Subjects, recruiting (*continued*)
  recruiter responsibilities in,
    120–122
  regulations for, 120–121
  women, 249–250
  writing about, 125
Subjects, selecting
  adult regulations for, 13, 21, 64–65,
    68–71
  community consent for, 17, 150–151
  in direct-benefit research, 51–52,
    63–68, 78–79
  ethical order for, 63–64
  inclusion/exclusion criteria for,
    67–68, 96
  patient subjects, 64–65
  pediatric regulations for, 64
  population characterization for, 96
  population justification for, 96
  in special communities, 81–83
  teens, 79
  toddlers and infants, 80
  women, 70–71, 191–193
  writing about, 95–96
Substantive ethics. *See* Ethics, substantive
Surgical Research, 256
Surgical trials
  justification for, 195–196
  risk assessment in, 193–196
Surrogate permission, 89–90, 146,
  148–150, 246–247

T
Timing, of informed consent, 132, 159
Tissue use
  from deceased patients, 230–231
  for genetic research, 243–244
  review of, 224–227, 232–233
  risks in, 228–229
  sharing samples for, 229–230
  storage procedures for, 227–229,
    233–235
Toxicity, 28–30, 51–52, 58
Translational research, 254–255

U
Uninterpretable data, 168–170

V
Valid consent. *See* Consent, valid
Video/audio taping, 201
Virtue ethics, 23–24
Volunteers. *See* Research participants
Vulnerable subjects. *See also* Special
  population protection
  adults as, 67
  coercion of, 66
  consent for, 101, 105–106, 143–146
  genetic research risk for, 238–240
  IRB review of, 67
  minors as, 67, 77–79
  recruiting of, 122
  regulations for, 68

W
Washout period, 108–109
Withdrawal. *See* Subject withdrawal
Women volunteers, 70–71, 191–192,
  249–251
Writing
  about benefits, 117–118
  about confidentiality, 173–174
  about consent/assent/surrogacy,
    146–151
  of consent/assent/surrogacy docu-
    ments, 151–158, 174
  about human biological material,
    234–237
  of hypothesis, 61
  literary review of, 60–61
  of protocol, 59–61
  about rescue interventions, 106–109
  about risk assessment, 97–102,
    106–107
  about risk/burden/discomfort,
    116–118
  about subject recruitment, 125
  about subject selection, 95–96
  about substantive ethics, 178–181